W9-ATY-613

Disease Management
SOURCEBOOK

Second Edition

Health Reference Series

Second Edition

Disease Management
SOURCEBOOK

*Basic Consumer Health Information about Coping with
Chronic and Serious Illnesses, Navigating the Healthcare
System, Communicating with Healthcare Providers,
Assessing Healthcare Quality, and Making Informed
Healthcare Decisions, Including Facts about Second
Opinions, Hospitalization, Surgery, and Medications*

*Along with a Section about Children with Chronic
Conditions, Information about Legal, Financial, and
Insurance Issues, a Glossary of Related Terms, and
Directories of Additional Resources*

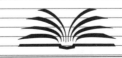

OMNIGRAPHICS

615 Griswold, Ste. 901, Detroit, MI 48226

Bibliographic Note
Because this page cannot legibly accommodate all the copyright notices, the Bibliographic
Note portion of the Preface constitutes an extension of the copyright notice.

* * *

Health Reference Series
Keith Jones, *Managing Editor*
***

OMNIGRAPHICS
A PART OF RELEVANT INFORMATION
***

Copyright © 2017 Omnigraphics
ISBN 978-0-7808-1545-2
E-ISBN 978-0-7808-1546-9

Library of Congress Cataloging-in-Publication Data

Names: Omnigraphics, Inc.

Title: Disease management sourcebook: basic consumer health information about
coping with chronic and serious illnesses, navigating the health care system,
communicating with health care providers, assessing health care quality, and
making informed health care decisions, including facts about second opinions,
hospitalization, surgery, and medications; along with a section about children
with chronic conditions, information about legal, financial, and insurance issues, a
glossary of related terms, and directories of additional resources.

Description: Second edition. | Detroit, MI: Omnigraphics, [2017] | Series: Health
reference series | Includes bibliographical references and index.

Identifiers: LCCN 2016059261 (print) | LCCN 2017003760 (ebook) | ISBN
9780780815452 (hardcover: alk. paper) | ISBN 9780780815469 (ebook) | ISBN
9780780815469 (eBook)

Subjects: LCSH: Chronic diseases--Treatment. | Consumer education.

Classification: LCC RC108 .D58 2017 (print) | LCC RC108 (ebook) | DDC
616/.044--dc23

LC record available at https://lccn.loc.gov/2016059261

Table of Contents

Part III: Health Literacy and Making Informed Health Decisions

Part IV: Prescription (Rx) and Over-the-Counter (OTC) Medications

Part VI: Children and Chronic Disease

Part VII: Legal, Financial, and Insurance Issues That Impact Disease Management

Part VIII: Additional Help and Information

Preface

About This Book

Making informed healthcare decisions is vital to everyone. It is particularly important to the estimated 117 million Americans who are living with chronic illnesses, such as cardiovascular disease, diabetes, and cancer. Health literacy is the degree to which individuals have the capacity to obtain, process, and understand basic health information and services needed to make appropriate health decisions. It is estimated that only 12 percent of adults have proficient health literacy. In other words, nearly nine out of ten adults may lack the skills needed to manage their health and prevent disease. These adults were more likely to report their health as poor and are more likely to lack health insurance than adults with proficient health literacy. Low literacy has been linked to poor health outcomes such as higher rates of hospitalization and less frequent use of preventive services. Both of these outcomes are associated with higher healthcare costs.

Disease Management Sourcebook, Second Edition, addresses these concerns by providing facts about navigating the healthcare system, communicating with healthcare providers, and finding and evaluating health information. It discusses patient rights and responsibilities, privacy, medical errors, and healthcare fraud. It explains assistive technologies available to help people who have chronic illnesses and provides tips for dealing with legal, financial, and health insurance matters. Facts about medications—including prescription, generic, over-the-counter, and counterfeit drugs—are included. The book's end section features a glossary and directories of resources for patients and their families and caregivers.

How to Use This Book

This book is divided into parts and chapters. Parts focus on broad areas of interest. Chapters are devoted to single topics within a part.

Part I: Facts about Serious and Chronic Illnesses presents an overview of disease management in the United States. It includes information about risk factors for chronic disease and symptoms that may indicate serious health conditions or medical emergencies. It describes common screening and diagnostic tests and offers tips for finding support after receiving a diagnosis.

Part II: Working with Healthcare Providers and the Healthcare System provides information about effective communication in a doctor's office or hospital setting. Topics include making decisions in consultation with the doctor, second opinions, understanding medical specialties and alternative medicine, clinical trials, and laboratory services. Basic information is also provided about choosing a hospital and undergoing surgery, and issues related to healthcare quality are addressed.

Part III: Health Literacy and Making Informed Health Decisions discusses the skills that are essential for making knowledgeable healthcare choices. This includes finding the most reliable and up-to-date health information. The rapidly changing world of health information technology is discussed. Information on mobile health applications and evaluating online health information is provided, along with information on personal and electronic health records. Patient privacy rights, informed consent, medical errors, and healthcare fraud are also discussed.

Part IV: Prescription (Rx) and Over-the-Counter (OTC) Medications provides information about what medications do and how to use them safely. It discusses purchasing and using prescription, generic, and over-the-counter drugs. Details on common drug interactions, adverse drug reactions, drug name confusion, purchasing prescription drugs online, counterfeit and misused drugs, and imported drugs and safety concerns are also provided.

Part V: Managing Chronic Disease offers guidelines for self-management practices, including tips for dealing with pain, stress, and depression. Infection prevention, assistive technology, home modifications, and transitional and palliative care options are explained. A chapter offering tips for caregivers of individuals with chronic disease is also included.

Part VI: Children and Chronic Disease presents facts for parents and caregivers about serious illness in children, home healthcare, and the pediatric intensive care unit. It offers guidelines to help families and schools provide medical support for students with asthma, diabetes, and other chronic conditions, and it provides information about finding camps for children with special health needs.

Part VII: Legal, Financial, and Insurance Issues That Impact Disease Management includes information about healthcare benefit laws, the Affordable Care Act, the Americans with Disabilities Act, and the Family and Medical Leave Act. It describes advance directives and discusses hospital bills and access to free or reduced-cost healthcare. It also includes information on the health insurance Marketplace, and provides guidelines for purchasing health insurance. In addition it discusses topics such as health savings accounts, medical discount plans and cards, the insurance needs of people with known medical risk factors, and the insurance claim process.

Part VIII: Additional Help and Information includes a glossary of related terms and directories of resources for information about disease management, health insurance, and financial assistance for medical treatments.

Bibliographic Note

This volume contains documents and excerpts from publications issued by the following U.S. government agencies: Centers for Disease Control and Prevention (CDC); Centers for Medicare and Medicaid Services (CMS); Federal Bureau of Prisons (BOP); National Cancer Institute (NCI); National Center for Complementary and Integrative Health (NCCIH); National Criminal Justice Reference Service (NCJRS); National Human Genome Research Institute (NHGRI); National Institute of Arthritis and Musculoskeletal and Skin Diseases (NIAMS); National Institute of Mental Health (NIMH); National Institute of Neurological Disorders and Stroke (NINDS); National Institute on Aging (NIA); National Institute on Drug Abuse (NIDA); National Institutes of Health (NIH); *NIH News in Health*; Office of Disease Prevention and Health Promotion (ODPHP); Office of Minority Health (OMH); Office on Women's Health (OWH); Substance Abuse and Mental Health Services

Administration (SAMHSA); U.S. Department of Health and Human Services (HHS); U.S. Department of Veterans Affairs (VA); and U.S. Food and Drug Administration (FDA).

In addition, this volume contains copyrighted documents from the following organization: The Nemours Foundation

It may also contain original material produced by Omnigraphics and reviewed by medical consultants.

About the Health Reference Series

The *Health Reference Series* is designed to provide basic medical information for patients, families, caregivers, and the general public. Each volume takes a particular topic and provides comprehensive coverage. This is especially important for people who may be dealing with a newly diagnosed disease or a chronic disorder in themselves or in a family member. People looking for preventive guidance, information about disease warning signs, medical statistics, and risk factors for health problems will also find answers to their questions in the *Health Reference Series*. The *Series*, however, is not intended to serve as a tool for diagnosing illness, in prescribing treatments, or as a substitute for the physician/patient relationship. All people concerned about medical symptoms or the possibility of disease are encouraged to seek professional care from an appropriate health care provider.

A Note about Spelling and Style

Health Reference Series editors use *Stedman's Medical Dictionary* as an authority for questions related to the spelling of medical terms and the *Chicago Manual of Style* for questions related to grammatical structures, punctuation, and other editorial concerns. Consistent adherence is not always possible, however, because the individual volumes within the *Series* include many documents from a wide variety of different producers, and the editor's primary goal is to present material from each source as accurately as is possible. This sometimes means that information in different chapters or sections may follow other guidelines and alternate spelling authorities.

Medical Review

Omnigraphics contracts with a team of qualified, senior medical professionals who serve as medical consultants for the *Health Reference*

Series. As necessary, medical consultants review reprinted and originally written material for currency and accuracy. Citations including the phrase, "Reviewed (month, year)" indicate material reviewed by this team. Medical consultation services are provided to the *Health Reference Series* editors by:

Dr. Senthil Selvan, MBBS, DCH, MD
Dr. K. Sivanandham, MBBS, DCH, MS (Research), PhD

Our Advisory Board

We would like to thank the following board members for providing initial guidance on the development of this series:

- Dr. Lynda Baker, Associate Professor of Library and Information Science, Wayne State University, Detroit, MI

- Nancy Bulgarelli, William Beaumont Hospital Library, Royal Oak, MI

- Karen Imarisio, Bloomfield Township Public Library, Bloomfield Township, MI

- Karen Morgan, Mardigian Library, University of Michigan-Dearborn, Dearborn, MI

- Rosemary Orlando, St. Clair Shores Public Library, St. Clair Shores, MI

Health Reference Series *Update Policy*

The inaugural book in the *Health Reference Series* was the first edition of *Cancer Sourcebook* published in 1989. Since then, the *Series* has been enthusiastically received by librarians and in the medical community. In order to maintain the standard of providing high-quality health information for the layperson the editorial staff at Omnigraphics felt it was necessary to implement a policy of updating volumes when warranted.

Medical researchers have been making tremendous strides, and it is the purpose of the *Health Reference Series* to stay current with the most recent advances. Each decision to update a volume is made on an individual basis. Some of the considerations include how much new information is available and the feedback we receive from people who use the books. If there is a topic you would like to see added to the update list, or an area of medical concern you feel has not been adequately addressed, please write to:

Managing Editor
Health Reference Series
Omnigraphics
615 Griswold, Ste. 901
Detroit, MI 48226

Part One

Facts about Serious and Chronic Illnesses

Chapter 1

Chronic Disease in the United States

Chronic Diseases: The Leading Cause of Death and Disability in the United States[1]

Chronic diseases and conditions—such as heart disease, stroke, cancer, type 2 diabetes, obesity, and arthritis—are among the most common, costly, and preventable of all health problems.

- As of 2012, about half of all adults—117 million people—had one or more chronic health conditions. One of four adults had two or more chronic health conditions.

- Seven of the top 10 causes of death in 2010 were chronic diseases. Two of these chronic diseases—heart disease and cancer—together accounted for nearly 48 percent of all deaths.

This chapter includes text excerpted from documents published by three public domain sources. Text under headings marked 1 are excerpted from "Chronic Disease Overview," Centers for Disease Control and Prevention (CDC), August 26, 2015; Text under headings marked 2 are excerpted from "Preventing Chronic Disease: Eliminating the Leading Preventable Causes of Premature Death and Disability in the United States," Centers for Disease Control and Prevention (CDC), July 22, 2015; Text under headings marked 3 are excerpted from "Chronic Disease Prevention and Health Promotion," Centers for Disease Control and Prevention (CDC), November 29, 2016.

3

- Obesity is a serious health concern. During 2009-2010, more than one-third of adults, or about 78 million people, were obese (defined as body mass index [BMI] ≥30 kg/m²). Nearly one of five youths aged 2–19 years was obese (BMI ≥95th percentile).

- Arthritis is the most common cause of disability. Of the 53 million adults with a doctor diagnosis of arthritis, more than 22 million say they have trouble with their usual activities because of arthritis.

- Diabetes is the leading cause of kidney failure, lower-limb amputations other than those caused by injury, and new cases of blindness among adults.

Health Risk Behaviors That Cause Chronic Diseases[1]

Health risk behaviors are unhealthy behaviors you can change. Four of these health risk behaviors—lack of exercise or physical activity, poor nutrition, tobacco use, and drinking too much alcohol—cause much of the illness, suffering, and early death related to chronic diseases and conditions.

- In 2011, more than half (52 percent) of adults aged 18 years or older did not meet recommendations for aerobic exercise or physical activity. In addition, 76 percent did not meet recommendations for muscle-strengthening physical activity.

- About half of U.S. adults (47 percent) have at least one of the following major risk factors for heart disease or stroke: uncontrolled high blood pressure, uncontrolled high low-density lipoprotein (LDL) cholesterol, or are current smokers. Ninety percent of Americans consume too much sodium, increasing their risk of high blood pressure.

- In 2011, more than one-third (36 percent) of adolescents and 38 percent of adults said they ate fruit less than once a day, while 38 percent of adolescents and 23 percent of adults said they ate vegetables less than once a day.

- More than 42 million adults—close to 1 of every 5—said they currently smoked cigarettes in 2012. Cigarette smoking accounts for more than 480,000 deaths each year. Each day, more than 3,200 youth younger than 18 years smoke their first cigarette, and another 2,100 youth and young adults who smoke every now and then become daily smokers.

- Drinking too much alcohol is responsible for 88,000 deaths each year, more than half of which are due to binge drinking. About 38 million U.S. adults report binge drinking an average of 4 times a month, and have an average of 8 drinks per binge, yet most binge drinkers are not alcohol dependent.

The Cost of Chronic Diseases and Health Risk Behaviors[1]

In the United States, chronic diseases and conditions and the health risk behaviors that cause them account for most healthcare costs.

- Eighty-six percent of all healthcare spending in 2010 was for people with one or more chronic medical conditions.

- The total costs of heart disease and stroke in 2010 were estimated to be $315.4 billion. Of this amount, $193.4 billion was for direct medical costs, not including costs of nursing home care.

- Cancer care cost $157 billion in 2010 dollars.

- The total estimated cost of diagnosed diabetes in 2012 was $245 billion, including $176 billion in direct medical costs and $69 billion in decreased productivity. Decreased productivity includes costs associated with people being absent from work, being less productive while at work, or not being able to work at all because of diabetes.

- The total cost of arthritis and related conditions was about $128 billion in 2003. Of this amount, nearly $81 billion was for direct medical costs and $47 billion was for indirect costs associated with lost earnings.

- Medical costs linked to obesity were estimated to be $147 billion in 2008. Annual medical costs for people who are obese were $1,429 higher than those for people of normal weight in 2006.

- For the years 2009–2012, economic cost due to smoking is estimated to be more than $289 billion a year. This cost includes at least $133 billion in direct medical care for adults and more than $156 billion for lost productivity from premature death estimated from 2005 through 2009.

- The economic costs of drinking too much alcohol were estimated to be $223.5 billion, or $1.90 a drink, in 2006. Most of these costs were due to binge drinking and resulted from losses in workplace productivity, healthcare expenses, and crimes related to excessive drinking.

Chronic Disease: Burden and Implications[2]

When compared with 16 other high-income "peer" countries, the United States is less healthy in key areas, including obesity, diabetes, heart disease, chronic lung disease, and disability.

Diabetes is the leading cause of:

- Kidney failure.

- Lower-limb amputations other than those caused by injury.

- New cases of blindness among adults.

  Chronic diseases are the leading causes of death and disability:

- Arthritis is the most common cause of disability.

- Of the 53 million adults with a doctor's diagnosis of arthritis, more than 22 million say arthritis causes them to have trouble with their usual activities.

Minority Population and Chronic Conditions[3]

Heart disease, cancer, diabetes, and stroke are among the most common causes of illness, disability, and death in the United States. These chronic conditions—and the factors that lead to them—can be more common or severe for minority groups (specifically, non-Hispanic blacks, Hispanics, American Indians, Alaska Natives, Asians, Native Hawaiians, and Pacific Islanders). For example,

- Non-Hispanic blacks are 40 percent more likely to have high blood pressure than are non-Hispanic whites, and they are less likely to manage this condition.

- The rate of diagnosed diabetes is 77 percent higher among non-Hispanic blacks, 66 percent higher among Hispanics, and 18 percent higher among Asians than among non-Hispanic whites.

- American Indians and Alaska Natives are 60 percent more likely to be obese than non-Hispanic whites.

- Life expectancy for non-Hispanic blacks is 75.1 years, compared to 78.9 years for non-Hispanic whites.

Racial and ethnic minority populations often receive poorer quality of care and face more barriers in seeking care, including preventive care and chronic disease management, than do non-Hispanic whites. These disparities can lead to poor health outcomes and higher healthcare costs.

Statistics on a Few Chronic Diseases[3]

Alzheimer Disease

- Alzheimer disease (AD) affects mainly older adults, and the growth in the number of older adults is unprecedented.

- In 2014, 46 million adults living in the United States—15 percent of the population—were 65 or older.

- In 2016, total payments for healthcare, long-term care, and hospice for people with AD and other dementias are estimated to be $236 billion.

Arthritis

- In the United States, 23 percent of all adults, or about 53 million people, have arthritis. It is a leading cause of disability.

- About half of U.S. adults with heart disease or diabetes and one-third of people who are obese also have arthritis.

- Eight million working-age adults report that their ability to work is limited because of their arthritis.

Diabetes

- Diabetes was the seventh leading cause of death in the United States in 2013 (and may be underreported).

- Diabetes is the leading cause of kidney failure, lower-limb amputations, and adult-onset blindness.

- More than 20 percent of healthcare spending is for people with diagnosed diabetes.

Cancer[1]

- In 2016, an estimated 1,685,210 new cases of cancer will be diagnosed in the United States and 595,690 people will die from the disease.

- The most common cancers in 2016 are projected to be breast cancer, lung and bronchus cancer, prostate cancer, colon and rectum cancer, bladder cancer, melanoma of the skin, non-Hodgkin lymphoma, thyroid cancer, kidney and renal pelvis cancer, leukemia, endometrial cancer, and pancreatic cancer.

- The number of new cases of cancer (cancer incidence) is 454.8 per 100,000 men and women per year (based on 2008–2012 cases).

- The number of cancer deaths (cancer mortality) is 171.2 per 100,000 men and women per year (based on 2008–2012 deaths).

- Cancer mortality is higher among men than women (207.9 per 100,000 men and 145.4 per 100,000 women). It is highest in African American men (261.5 per 100,000) and lowest in Asian/Pacific Islander women (91.2 per 100,000). (Based on 2008–2012 deaths.)

- The number of people living beyond a cancer diagnosis reached nearly 14.5 million in 2014 and is expected to rise to almost 19 million by 2024.

- Approximately 39.6 percent of men and women will be diagnosed with cancer at some point during their lifetimes (based on 2010–2012 data).

- In 2014, an estimated 15,780 children and adolescents ages 0 to 19 were diagnosed with cancer and 1,960 died of the disease.

Heart Disease[2]

- About 610,000 people die of heart disease in the United States every year–that's 1 in every 4 deaths.

- Heart disease is the leading cause of death for both men and women. More than half of the deaths due to heart disease in 2009 were in men.

- Coronary heart disease (CHD) is the most common type of heart disease, killing over 370,000 people annually.

- Every year about 735,000 Americans have a heart attack. Of these, 525,000 are a first heart attack and 210,000 happen in people who have already had a heart attack.

1. Text under the heading "Heart Disease" is excerpted from "Heart Disease Facts," Centers for Disease Control and Prevention (CDC), August 10, 2015.
2. Text under the heading "Cancer" is excerpted from "Cancer Statistics," National Cancer Institute (NCI), March 14, 2016.

Chronic Diseases Are a Major Cause of Disability and Lost Productivity[2]

- 12.6 percent of the population have a disability, including 43.8 percent of those aged 75 or older.

- Lost productivity resulting from chronic conditions and risk factors is associated with enormous costs for those remaining in the workforce and for those who leave the workforce prematurely because of disability.

Chapter 2

Family Health History Is Important to Your Health

A Family Tree for Health

A family health history is a written record of a family's health. The history contains information about a family's medical conditions, lifestyle habits (for example, whether anyone in the family has smoked), and where and how family members grew up. It's like a family tree for health.

What a Family Health History May Reveal

You can use a family health history to see if you, your children, or your grandchildren might face an increased risk of developing serious health problems. These health problems might be common ones, such as heart disease, cancer, or diabetes. They could also be less common diseases that are passed from one generation to the next, such as hemophilia or sickle cell anemia.

People can't change the genes they inherit from their parents, but they can change things like diet, physical activity, and medical care to try to prevent diseases that run in the family. This is good news

---

This chapter includes text excerpted from "Creating a Family Health History: Why Create a Family Health History?" NIHSeniorHealth, National Institute on Aging (NIA), May 2015.

because many diseases result from a combination of a person's genes, lifestyle, and environment.

Actions That May Reduce Disease Risk

A healthcare professional can use a family health history to help assess a person's risk of certain diseases. The professional might recommend actions to lower the chance of getting those diseases.

Actions to reduce the risk of disease may involve:

- lifestyle changes, such as eating healthier foods or exercising more
- getting certain medical tests
- taking medicines that are more effective based on your specific genes

For example, a son with a family history of diabetes might be told to lose weight and exercise more. A daughter who is considering having a baby might get tested to see if she carries a gene for a rare condition that runs in the family.

How You and Your Family May Benefit

For older adults, a family health history might help explain why you have developed certain health conditions. But it is important to know that simply getting older increases the risk of many diseases, too.

Creating and sharing your family health history with your healthcare professional can help you be healthier. But perhaps the biggest benefit is providing information that may help your children and grandchildren live longer, healthier lives.

Family History and Disease Risk

Many things influence your overall health and likelihood of developing a disease. Sometimes, it's not clear what causes a disease. Many diseases are thought to be caused by a combination of genetic, lifestyle, and environmental factors. The importance of any particular factor varies from person to person.

If you have a disease, does that mean your children and grandchildren will get it, too? Not necessarily. They may have a greater chance of developing the disease than someone without a similar family history. But they are not certain to get the disease.

Health Problems That May Run in Families

Common health problems that can run in a family include:

- Alzheimer disease/dementia
- arthritis
- asthma
- blood clots
- cancer
- depression
- diabetes
- heart disease
- high cholesterol
- high blood pressure
- pregnancy losses and birth defects
- stroke

Heritable Diseases

Some diseases are clearly heritable. This means the disease comes from a mutation, or harmful change, in a gene inherited from one or both parents. Genes are small structures in your body's cells that determine how you look and tell your body how to work. Examples of heritable diseases are Huntington disease, cystic fibrosis, and muscular dystrophy.

Role of Lifestyle and Environment

Genes are not the only things that cause disease. Lifestyle habits and environment also play a major part in developing disease. Diet, weight, physical activity, tobacco and alcohol use, occupation, and where you live can each increase or decrease disease risk. For example, smoking increases the chance of developing heart disease and cancer. For common diseases like heart disease and cancer, habits like smoking or drinking too much alcohol may be more important in causing disease than genes.

Sun exposure is the major known environmental factor associated with the development of skin cancer of all types. However, other environmental and genetic factors can also increase a person's risk. The best defense against skin cancer is to encourage sun-protective behaviors, regular skin examinations, and skin self-awareness in an effort to decrease high-risk behaviors and optimize early detection of problems.

Clues to Your Disease Risk

Creating a family health history helps you know about diseases and disease risks. It can also show the way a disease occurs in a family. For example, you may find that a family member had a certain disease at an earlier age than usual (10 to 20 years before most people get it). That can increase other family members' risk.

Risk also goes up if a relative has a disease that usually does not affect a certain gender, for example, breast cancer in a man. Certain combinations of diseases within a family—such as breast and ovarian cancer, or heart disease and diabetes—also increase the chance of developing those diseases.

Some Risk Factors Are Not Apparent

Even if they appear healthy, people could be at risk for developing a serious disease that runs in the family. They could have risk factors that they cannot feel, such as high blood pressure. They might not even know the disease runs in their family because they've lost touch with family members with the disease or because other family members with the disease have kept the information private. Another possibility is that family members who might have developed the disease died young in accidents or by other means. They might also be adopted and not share genes with members of their adoptive family.

Getting Professional Advice

Family members who think they might be at risk for a disease based on their family health history can ask their healthcare professionals for advice. The professional may order a test to see if the person has the disease or a risk factor for the disease. For instance, a mammogram can detect possible breast cancer, and a colonoscopy can find colon cancer. Many diseases are more treatable if they are caught early.

The first step toward better understanding of your family's health is to learn more about the health of close relatives such as parents, brothers and sisters, and children. Creating a family health history is one way to do that.

Chapter 3

When to See a Doctor: Symptoms of Serious Health Conditions

The following symptoms could be signs of serious health conditions and should be checked by a doctor or nurse. It is important to note that you might feel symptoms in one part of your body that could actually mean a problem in another part. Even if the symptoms don't seem related, they could be. Keep track of your symptoms. If you have any of these symptoms, make an appointment to see your doctor. Listen to what your body is telling you, and be sure to describe every symptom in detail to your doctor.

Signs of a Heart Attack

The most common sign of a heart attack is mild or strong pain or discomfort in the center of the chest. It can last more than a few minutes, or it can go away and come back.

Other common signs of a heart attack include:

- Pain or discomfort in one or both arms, back, neck, jaw, or stomach

This chapter includes text excerpted from "Symptoms of Serious Health Conditions," National Women's Health Information Center (NWHIC), Office on Women's Health (OWH), September 10, 2008. Reviewed January 2017.

- Shortness of breath (feeling like you can't get enough air)
- Nausea or vomiting
- Feeling faint or woozy
- Breaking out in a cold sweat

Some women may feel very tired, sometimes for days or weeks before a heart attack occurs. Women may also have heartburn, a cough, or heart flutters or lose their appetite.

Signs of a Stroke

A stroke happens fast. The most common signs of a stroke are sudden:

- Numbness or weakness of the face, arm, or leg, especially on one side of the body
- Trouble seeing in one or both eyes
- Trouble walking, dizziness, or loss of balance or coordination
- Confusion or trouble speaking or understanding
- Severe headache with no known cause

If you have any of these symptoms or see anyone with these symptoms, call 911 right away. Every minute counts!

Symptoms of Reproductive Health Problems

- Bleeding or spotting between periods
- Itching, burning, or irritation (including bumps, blisters, or sores) of the vagina or genital area
- Pain or discomfort during sex
- Severe or painful bleeding with periods
- Moderate to severe pelvic or abdominal pain
- Unusual (for you) vaginal discharge of any type or color or with strong odor
- Pain or other problems while urinating or moving bowels

Symptoms of Breast Problems

- Hard lump or knot in or near the breast or in your underarm
- Dimpling, puckering, or ridges of the skin on the breast
- Change in the size or shape of your breast
- Clear or bloody fluid that leaks out of nipple
- Itchy or scaly sore or rash on the nipple
- Unusual swelling, warmth, or redness

Symptoms of Lung Problems

- Coughing up blood or mucus
- Shortness of breath
- Wheezing
- A cough that won't go away
- Uncomfortable or painful breathing
- A feeling of tightness in the chest

Symptoms of Stomach or Digestive Problems

- Bleeding from the rectum
- Blood or mucus in the stool (including diarrhea) or black or clay-colored stools
- Change in bowel habits or not being able to control bowels
- Constipation, diarrhea, or both
- Heartburn or acid reflux (feels like burning in throat or mouth)
- Stomach pain or discomfort, such as bloating
- Nausea and vomiting
- Unexplained weight loss or weight gain

Symptoms of Bladder Problems

- Difficult or painful urination
- Frequent urination, intense urges to urinate, or loss of bladder control

- Urine that is bloody, cloudy, dark, or strong smelling
- Long-term pain in the back or sides

Symptoms of Skin Problems

- Changes in the skin, such as changes in existing moles or new growths
- Moles that are no longer round or have irregular borders
- Moles that change colors or change in size (usually get bigger)
- Frequent flushing (a sudden feeling of heat)
- Jaundice (when the skin and whites of the eyes turn yellow)
- Painful, crusting, scaling, or oozing sores that don't heal
- Sensitivity to sun

Symptoms of Muscle or Joint Problems

- Muscle pains and body aches that are persistent, or that come and go often
- Numbness, tingling (pins and needles sensation), or discomfort in hands, feet, or limbs
- Pain, stiffness, swelling, or redness in or around joints

Symptoms of Mental Health Problems

These symptoms can have a physical cause and are usually treatable:

- Anxiety and constant worry
- Depression: feeling empty, sad all the time, or worthless
- Extreme fatigue, even when rested
- Extreme tension that can't be explained
- Flashbacks and nightmares about traumatic events
- No interest in getting out of bed or doing regular activities, including eating or sex
- Thoughts about suicide and death

- Seeing or hearing things that aren't there (hallucinations)
- Seeing things differently from what they are (delusions)
- "Baby Blues" that haven't gone away two weeks after giving birth and seem to get worse over time
- Thoughts about harming yourself or your baby after giving birth
- Desire to starve or vomit on purpose
- Desire to binge on food excessively

Chapter 4

Is It a Medical Emergency?

Patients with chronic medical conditions often become so accustomed to managing their own treatment, from pills and injections to pain control, that they often wait too long to call their doctor when the condition worsens. As a result, studies show that the majority of frequent visitors to emergency rooms are patients with chronic illnesses. And since emergency care can cost two-to-three times as much as an office visit, clearly it's better to make an appointment with the regular doctor than wait until an ER trip becomes necessary. But how can a patient and his or her family tell when the situation worsens to the point that there is no alternative?

When to Go to the Emergency Room

In some instances, such as with injuries that result in copious bleeding, it's fairly obvious when emergency treatment is necessary. But when people deal with the symptoms of chronic illnesses on a daily basis, it can be more difficult to determine the point at which home care is no longer an option. The best way for the patient and caregivers to gain this knowledge is to have a conversation with the doctor and ask for a detailed description of the types of signs associated with the particular condition that could indicate an emergency. By becoming intimately familiar with the day-to-day symptoms and management of the condition, patients and their families will be better prepared to determine steps to be taken if the illness worsens.

"Is It a Medical Emergency?" © 2017 Omnigraphics. Reviewed January 2017.

In general, some signs that a visit to an emergency room or a call to 911 may be necessary include:

- stopped breathing, or extreme difficulty breathing
- loss of consciousness
- uncontrollable bleeding
- pain that is significantly beyond that normally experienced as a result of the condition
- severe pain in the chest or jaw
- changes in vision
- high fever, especially with a stiff neck
- sudden headache
- seizures
- uncontrollable vomiting
- changes in mental state, such as confusion
- sudden paralysis, weakness, or dizziness
- unusual abdominal pain
- severe allergic reaction, such as in response to a new medication
- coughing or vomiting blood
- the patient's sense that something about the condition has changed

Note that when the patient is a child who is too young to describe symptoms or changes in a medical condition, it falls to the parent or guardian to be vigilant for signs that might constitute an emergency. All of the above indicators are applicable to infants and toddlers, as well, but other signs can include:

- turning blue
- continuing loose stools
- hard to wake up
- fast heartbeat for an extended period of time
- dry mouth

- dry diapers for more than 18 hours

- a body part that is cold or pale

What to Do in an Emergency Situation

The advice given most often about emergencies is to remain calm. And as trite as that might sound, a panic-stricken relative or caregiver won't be able to respond appropriately or describe the situation to a first-responder or medical professional in such a way as to ensure the fastest and best treatment for the patient. And if the patient is alone when the emergency occurs, his or her physical response to panic (rapid heartbeat, increased breathing rate, sweating, dizziness) can exacerbate the condition itself. In addition to maintaining composure, other steps to be taken include the following:

- **Call 911 if necessary.** Certain situations leave no room for doubt that an immediate trained response is required. For example, if the patient has stopped breathing, is bleeding pro- fusely, or has lost consciousness, he or she needs qualified EMTs and ambulance.

- **Assess the need for first aid.** In extreme, life-threatening cases, such as when breathing has stopped or there is no pulse, CPR or other first aid needs to be administered immediately. Caregivers for patients with some chronic conditions should undergo training in order to learn proper first-aid techniques.

- **Resist the urge to transport the patient.** Although it may seem faster than waiting for an ambulance, transport- ing a patient in extreme distress, such as lost consciousness or stopped breathing, can delay treatment and make matters worse. Better to call 911 and follow the operator's instructions.

- **Prepare for the ER visit.** If it's determined that the patient may be transported safely, advanced preparation can save time at the hospital. Bring a list of the patient's medications, aller- gies, and immunizations, as well as the name and contact infor- mation of his or her regular doctor.

- **If unsure what to do, call a professional.** If the situation is not immediately life-threatening, and you're not sure an ER visit is necessary, call the patient's doctor or other medical pro- fessional familiar with his or her condition. In addition, many health systems and insurance companies offer 24-hour consultation lines, which can help make an assessment.

Urgent Care Facilities

Urgent-care facilities are available for patients whose doctors are unavailable or when illness occurs outside of the physician's normal office hours, and they can serve as a viable alternative to the emergency room in certain cases.. Although many of their services are designed to treat such medical situations as flu, sprains and fractures, fever, and minor lacerations, they are quite well-equipped to handle many of the problems associated with chronic illnesses. For example, if the condition results in dehydration, an urgent-care center can provide IV fluids while monitoring the patient's vital signs, or if pain intensifies beyond the control of the patient's normal medication, the clinic can respond with appropriate treatment.

Being Prepared

Obviously, it's not possible to prevent all medical emergencies, especially in the case of patients with chronic conditions. But advanced preparation can lessen the severity and allay some anxiety if an emergency does occur. Some ways to prepare for an emergency include:

- Keep contact information handy for doctors, hospitals, urgent-care clinics, professional caregivers, and emergency advice lines.

- Have a list of medications (including dosages), allergies, and immunizations ready in advance.

- Ask the doctor for a written medical history for the patient to keep ready for EMTs or emergency-room personnel.

- Keep an appropriately equipped first-aid kit on hand.

- Be sure the patient is seeing his or her doctor for regularly scheduled appointments and is following the doctor's instructions carefully.

- Learn first-aid basics, including CPR.

Depending on the particular condition, there may be other, more specific ways to prepare for a crisis situation. The best thing to do is to discuss this with the physician supervising the case and ask about additional steps you can take to be prepared.

References

1. Kaneshiro, Neil K., MD, MHA. "When to Use the Emergency Room–Child," MedlinePlus.com, November 20, 2014.

2. Martin, Laura J., MD, MPH, ABIM. "When to Use the Emergency Room–Adult," MedlinePlus.com, October 27, 2014.

3. "Medical Emergency," Tufts University Office of Emergency Management, n.d.

4. English, Taunya. "Chronic Conditions: When Do You Call the Doctor?" Center for Advancing Health, n.d.

5. "What to Do in an Emergency," American College of Emergency Physicians, n.d.

6. "When should I go to the Emergency Department?" Progressive Emergency Physicians, n.d.

Chapter 5

Common Screening and Diagnostic Tests

Chapter Contents

Section 5.1

Laboratory and Diagnostic Tests

This section contains text excerpted from the following sources:
Text under the heading "Lab Tests for Screening" is excerpted from
"Laboratory Tests," U.S. Food and Drug Administration (FDA),
June 5, 2014; Text under the heading "Common Screening and
Diagnostic Tests" is excerpted from "Common Screening and
Diagnostic Tests," Office on Women's Health (OWH),
U.S. Department of Health and Human Services (HHS),
September 10, 2008. Reviewed January 2017.

Lab Tests for Screening

This section provides information about lab tests your doctor may
use to screen for certain diseases or conditions.

What Are Lab Tests?

Laboratory tests are medical procedures that involve testing sam-
ples of blood, urine, or other tissues or substances in the body.

Why Does Your Doctor Use Lab Tests?

Your doctor uses laboratory tests to help:

- identify changes in your health condition before any symptoms
  occur

- diagnose a disease or condition before you have symptoms

- plan your treatment for a disease or condition

- evaluate your response to a treatment, or

- monitor the course of a disease over time

How Are Lab Tests Analyzed?

After your doctor collects a sample from your body, it is sent to a
laboratory. Laboratories perform tests on the sample to see if it reacts

to different substances. Depending on the test, a reaction may mean you do have a particular condition or it may mean that you do not have the particular condition. Sometimes laboratories compare your results to results obtained from previous tests, to see if there has been a change in your condition.

What Do Lab Tests Show?

Lab tests show whether or not your results fall within normal ranges. Normal test values are usually given as a range, rather than as a specific number, because normal values vary from person to person. What is normal for one person may not be normal for another person.

Some laboratory tests are precise, reliable indicators of specific health problems, while others provide more general information that gives doctors clues to your possible health problems. Information obtained from laboratory tests may help doctors decide whether other tests or procedures are needed to make a diagnosis or to develop or revise a previous treatment plan. All laboratory test results must be interpreted within the context of your overall health and should be used along with other exams or tests.

What Factors Affect Your Lab Test Results?

Many factors can affect test results, including:

- sex
- age
- race
- medical history
- general health
- specific foods
- drugs you are taking
- how closely your follow preparatory instructions
- variations in laboratory techniques
- variation from one laboratory to another

Common Screening and Diagnostic Tests

Table 5.1. Few Screening Tests

Name of Test	Definition
Angiography	Exam of your blood vessels using X-rays. The doctor inserts a small tube into the blood vessel and injects dye to see the vessels on the X-ray.
Barium enema	A lubricated enema tube is gently inserted into your rectum. Barium flows into your colon. An X-ray is taken of the large intestine.
Biopsy	A test that removes cells or tissues for examination by a pathologist to diagnose for disease. The tissue is examined under a microscope for cancer or other diseases.
Blood test	Blood is taken from a vein in the inside elbow or back of the hand to test for a health problem.
Bone mineral density (BMD) test	Special X-rays of your bones are used to test if you have osteoporosis, or a weakening of the bones.
Clinical breast exam (CBE)	A doctor, nurse, or other health professional uses his or her hands to examine your breasts and underarm areas to find lumps or other problems.
Chest X-ray	An X-ray of the chest, lungs, heart, large arteries, ribs, and diaphragm.
Colonoscopy	An examination of the inside of the colon using a colonoscope, inserted into the rectum. A colonoscope is a thin, tube-like instrument with a light and lens for viewing. It may also have a tool to remove tissue to be checked under a microscope for disease.
Computed tomography (CT or CAT) scan	The patient lies on a table and X-rays of the body are taken from different angles. Sometimes, a fluid is used to highlight parts of the body in the scan.
Echocardiography	An instrument (that looks like a microphone) is placed on the chest. It uses sound waves to create a moving picture of the heart. A picture appears on a TV monitor, and the heart can be seen in different ways.
Electrocardiography (EKG or ECG)	A test that records the electrical activity of the heart, using electrodes placed on the arms, legs, and chest.
Electroencephalography (EEG)	A test that measures the electrical activity of the brain, using electrodes that are put on the patient's scalp. Sometimes patients sleep during the test.

Table 5.1. Continued

Name of Test	Definition
Exercise stress test	Electrodes are placed on the chest, arms, and legs to record the heart's activity. A blood pressure cuff is placed around the arm and is inflated every few minutes. Heart rate and blood pressure are taken before exercise starts. The patient walks on a treadmill or pedals a stationary bicycle. The pace of the treadmill is increased. The response of the heart is monitored. The test continues until target heart rate is reached. Monitoring continues after exercise for 10 to 15 minutes or until the heart rate returns to normal.
Fecal occult blood test (FOBT)	Detects hidden blood in a bowel movement. There are two types: the smear test and flushable reagent pads.
Laparoscopy	A small tube with a camera is inserted into the abdomen through a small cut in or just below the belly button to see inside the abdomen and pelvis. Other instruments can be inserted in the small cut as well. It is used for both diagnosing and treating problems inside the abdomen.
Magnetic resonance imaging (MRI)	A test that uses powerful magnets and radio waves to create a picture of the inside of your body without surgery. The patient lies on a table that slides onto a large tunnel-like tube, which is surrounded by a scanner. Small coils may be placed around your head, arm, leg, or other areas.
Mammogram	X-rays of the breast taken by resting one breast at a time on a flat surface that contains an X-ray plate. A device presses firmly against the breast. An X-ray is taken to show a picture of the breast. Mammography is used to screen healthy women for signs of breast cancer. It can also be used to evaluate a woman who has symptoms of disease. It can, in some cases, detect breast cancers before you can feel them with your fingers.
Medical history	The doctor or nurse talks to the patient about current and past illnesses, surgeries, pregnancies, medications, allergies, use of alternative therapies, vitamins and supplements, diet, alcohol and drug use, physical activity, and family history of diseases
Pap test	The nurse or doctor uses a small brush to take cells from the cervix (opening of the uterus) to look at under a microscope in a lab.

Table 5.1. Continued

Name of Test	Definition
Pelvic exam	A doctor or nurse asks about the patient's health and looks at the vaginal area. The doctor or nurse checks the fallopian tubes, ovaries, and uterus by putting two gloved fingers inside the vagina. With the other hand, the doctor or nurse will feel from the outside for any lumps or tenderness.
Physical exam	The doctor or nurse will test for diseases, assess your risk of future medical problems, encourage a healthy lifestyle, and update your vaccinations.
Positron emission tomography (PET) scan	The patient is injected with a radioactive substance, such as glucose. A scanner detects any cancerous areas in the body. Cancerous tissue absorbs more of the substance and looks brighter in images than normal tissue.
Sigmoidoscopy	The sigmoidoscope is a small camera attached to a flexible tube. This tube, about 20 inches long, is gently inserted into the colon. As the tube is slowly removed, the lining of the bowel is examined.
Spirometry	The patient breathes into a mouthpiece that is connected to an instrument called a spirometer. The spirometer records the amount and the rate of air that is breathed in and out over a specified time. It measures how well the lungs exhale.
Ultrasound	A clear gel is put onto the skin over the area being examined. An instrument is then moved over that area. The machine sends out sound waves, which reflect off the body. A computer receives these waves and uses them to create pictures of the body.

Section 5.2

Screening Tests for Women

This section includes text excerpted from "Women: Stay Healthy at Any Age," Agency for Healthcare Research and Quality (AHRQ), U.S. Department of Health and Human Services (HHS), May 2014.

Screenings are tests that look for diseases before you have symptoms. Blood pressure checks and mammograms are examples of screenings.

You can get some screenings, such as blood pressure readings, in your doctor's office. Others, such as mammograms, need special equipment, so you may need to go to a different office.

After a screening test, ask when you will see the results and who to talk to about them.

Breast Cancer: Talk with your healthcare team about whether you need a mammogram.

***BRCA 1* and *2* Genes:** If you have a family member with breast, ovarian, or peritoneal cancer, talk with your doctor or nurse about your family history. Women with a strong family history of certain cancers may benefit from genetic counseling and *BRCA* genetic testing.

Cervical Cancer: Starting at age 21, get a Pap smear every 3 years until you are 65 years old. Women 30 years of age or older can choose to switch to a combination Pap smear and human papillomavirus (HPV) test every 5 years until the age of 65. If you are older than 65 or have had a hysterectomy, talk with your doctor or nurse about whether you still need to be screened.

Colon Cancer: Between the ages of 50 and 75, get a screening test for colorectal cancer. Several tests—for example, a stool test or a colonoscopy—can detect this cancer. Your healthcare team can help you decide which is best for you. If you are between the ages of 76 and 85, talk with your doctor or nurse about whether you should continue to be screened.

Depression: Your emotional health is as important as your physical health. Talk to your healthcare team about being screened for depression, especially if during the last 2 weeks:

- You have felt down, sad, or hopeless.
- You have felt little interest or pleasure in doing things.

Diabetes: Get screened for diabetes (high blood sugar) if you have high blood pressure or if you take medication for high blood pressure.

Diabetes can cause problems with your heart, brain, eyes, feet, kidneys, nerves, and other body parts.

Hepatitis C Virus (HCV): Get screened one time for HCV infection if:

- You were born between 1945 and 1965.
- You have ever injected drugs.
- You received a blood transfusion before 1992.

If you currently are an injection drug user, you should be screened regularly.

High Blood Cholesterol: Have your blood cholesterol checked regularly with a blood test if:

- You use tobacco.
- You are overweight or obese.
- You have a personal history of heart disease or blocked arteries.
- A male relative in your family had a heart attack before age 50 or a female relative, before age 60.

High Blood Pressure: Have your blood pressure checked at least every 2 years. High blood pressure can cause strokes, heart attacks, kidney and eye problems, and heart failure.

Human Immunodeficiency Virus (HIV): If you are 65 or younger, get screened for HIV. If you are older than 65, talk to your doctor or nurse about whether you should be screened.

Lung Cancer: Talk to your doctor or nurse about getting screened for lung cancer if you are between the ages of 55 and 80, have a 30 pack-year smoking history, and smoke now or have quit within the past 15 years. (Your pack-year history is the number of packs of cigarettes smoked per day times the number of years you have smoked.) Know that quitting smoking is the best thing you can do for your health.

Overweight and Obesity: The best way to learn if you are overweight or obese is to find your body mass index (BMI). You can find your BMI by entering your height and weight into a BMI calculator, such as the one available at: www.nhlbi.nih.gov/guidelines/obesity/BMI/bmicalc.htm.

A BMI between 18.5 and 25 indicates a normal weight. Persons with a BMI of 30 or higher may be obese. If you are obese, talk to your doctor or nurse about getting intensive counseling and help with changing your behaviors to lose weight. Overweight and obesity can lead to diabetes and cardiovascular disease.

Osteoporosis (Bone Thinning): Have a screening test at age 65 to make sure your bones are strong. The most common test is a dual energy X-ray absorptiometry (DEXA) scan—a low-dose X-ray of the spine and hip. If you are younger than 65 and at high risk for bone fractures, you should also be screened. Talk with your healthcare team about your risk for bone fractures.

Sexually Transmitted Infections (STIs): Sexually transmitted infections can make it hard to get pregnant, may affect your baby, and can cause other health problems.

- Get screened for chlamydia and gonorrhea infections if you are 24 years or younger and sexually active. If you are older than 24 years, talk to your doctor or nurse about whether you should be screened.

- Ask your doctor or nurse whether you should be screened for other sexually transmitted infection.

You know your body better than anyone else. Always tell your healthcare team about any changes in your health, including your vision and hearing. Ask them about being checked for any condition you are concerned about, not just the ones here. If you are wondering about diseases such as Alzheimer disease or skin cancer, for example, ask about them.

Get Preventive Medicines If You Need Them

Aspirin: If you are 55 or older, ask your healthcare team if you should take aspirin to prevent strokes. Your healthcare team can help you decide whether taking aspirin to prevent stroke is right for you.

Breast Cancer Drugs: Talk to your doctor about your risks for breast cancer and whether you should take medicines that may reduce those risks. Medications to reduce breast cancer have some potentially serious harms, so think through both the potential benefits and harms.

Folic Acid: If you of an age at which you can get pregnant, you should take a daily supplement containing 0.4 to 0.8 mg of folic acid.

Vitamin D to Avoid Falls: If you are 65 or older and have a history of falls, mobility problems, or other risks for falling, ask your doctor about taking a vitamin D supplement to help reduce your chances of falling. Exercise and physical therapy may also help.

Immunizations:

- Get a flu shot every year.

- Get shots for tetanus, diphtheria, and whooping cough. Get tetanus booster if it has been more than 10 years since your last shot.

- If you are 60 or older, get a shot to prevent shingles.

- If you are 65 or older, get a pneumonia shot.

- Talk with your healthcare team about whether you need other vaccinations. You can also find which ones you need by going to: www.cdc.gov/vaccines.

Take Steps to Good Health

- Be physically active and make healthy food choices.

- Get to a healthy weight and stay there. Balance the calories you take in from food and drink with the calories you burn off by your activities.

- Be tobacco free. For tips on how to quit, go to www.smokefree. gov. To talk to someone about how to quit, call the National Quitline: 1-800-QUITNOW (784-8669).

- If you drink alcohol, have no more than one drink per day. A standard drink is one 12-ounce bottle of beer or wine cooler, one 5-ounce glass of wine, or 1.5 ounces of 80-proof distilled spirits.

Section 5.3

Screening Tests for Men

This section includes text excerpted from "Men: Stay Healthy at Any Age," Agency for Healthcare Research and Quality (AHRQ), U.S. Department of Health and Human Services (HHS), March 2014.

Screenings are tests that look for diseases before you have symptoms. Blood pressure checks and tests for high blood cholesterol are examples of screenings.

You can get some screenings, such as blood pressure readings, in your doctor's office. Others, such as colonoscopy, a test for colon cancer, need special equipment, so you may need to go to a different office.

After a screening test, ask when you will see the results and who you should talk to about them.

Abdominal Aortic Aneurysm (AAA): If you are between the ages of 65 and 75 and have ever been a smoker, (smoked 100 or more cigarettes in your lifetime) get screened once for abdominal aortic aneurysm (AAA). AAA is a bulging in your abdominal aorta, your largest artery. An AAA may burst, which can cause dangerous bleeding and death.

An ultrasound, a painless procedure in which you lie on a table while a technician slides a medical device over your abdomen, will show whether an aneurysm is present.

Colon Cancer: Have a screening test for colorectal cancer starting at age 50. If you have a family history of colorectal cancer, you may need to be screened earlier. Several different tests can detect this cancer. Your doctor can help you decide which is best for you.

Depression: Your emotional health is as important as your physical health. Talk to your doctor or nurse about being screened for depression, especially if during the last 2 weeks:

- You have felt down, sad, or hopeless.

- You have felt little interest or pleasure in doing things.

Diabetes: Get screened for diabetes (high blood sugar) if you have high blood pressure or if you take medication for high blood pressure.

Diabetes can cause problems with your heart, brain, eyes, feet, kidneys, nerves, and other body parts.

Hepatitis C virus (HCV): Get screened one time for HCV infection if:

- You were born between 1945 and 1965.

- You have ever injected drugs.

- You received a blood transfusion before 1992.

If you currently are an injection drug user, you should be screened regularly.

High Blood Cholesterol: If you are 35 or older, have your blood cholesterol checked regularly with a blood test. High cholesterol increases your chance of heart disease, stroke, and poor circulation. Talk to your doctor or nurse about having your cholesterol checked starting at age 20 if:

- You use tobacco.

- You are overweight or obese.

- You have diabetes or high blood pressure.

- You have a history of heart disease or blocked arteries.

- A man in your family had a heart attack before age 50 or a woman, before age 60.

High Blood Pressure: Have your blood pressure checked at least every 2 years. High blood pressure can cause strokes, heart attacks, kidney and eye problems, and heart failure.

Human Immunodeficiency Virus (HIV): If you are 65 or younger, get screened for HIV. If you are older than 65, ask your doctor or nurse whether you should be screened.

Lung Cancer: Talk to your doctor or nurse about getting screened for lung cancer if you are between the ages of 55 and 80, have a 30 pack-year smoking history, and smoke now or have quit within the past 15 years. (Your pack-year history is the number of packs of cigarettes smoked per day times the number of years you have smoked.) Know that quitting smoking is the best thing you can do for your health.

Overweight and Obesity: The best way to learn if you are overweight or obese is to find your body mass index (BMI). You can find your BMI by entering your height and weight into a BMI calculator, such as the one available at: www.nhlbi.nih.gov/guidelines/obesity/BMI/bmicalc.htm.

A BMI between 18.5 and 25 indicates a normal weight. Persons with a BMI of 30 or higher may be obese. If you are obese, talk to your doctor or nurse about getting intensive counseling and help with changing your behaviors to lose weight. Overweight and obesity can lead to diabetes and cardiovascular disease.

You know your body better than anyone else. Always tell your doctor or nurse about any changes in your health, including your vision and hearing. Ask them about being checked for any condition you are concerned about, not just the ones here. If you are wondering about diseases such as Alzheimer disease or skin cancer, for example, ask about them.

Get Preventive Medicines If You Need Them

Aspirin: If you are 45 or older, your doctor or nurse can help you decide whether taking aspirin to prevent a heart attack is right for you.

Vitamin D to Avoid Falls: If you are 65 or older and have a history of falls, mobility problems, or other risks for falling, ask your doctor about taking a vitamin D supplement to help reduce your chances of falling. Exercise and physical therapy may also help.

Immunizations:

- Get a flu shot every year.

- If you are 60 or older, get a shot to prevent shingles.

- If you are 65 or older, get a pneumonia shot.

- Get a shot for tetanus, diphtheria, and whooping cough. Get a tetanus booster if it has been more than 10 years since your last shot.

- Talk with your healthcare team about whether you need other vaccinations. You can also find which ones you need by going to: www.cdc.gov/vaccines.

Take Steps to Good Health

- Be physically active and make healthy food choices.

- Get to a healthy weight and stay there. Balance the calories you take in from food and drink with the calories you burn off by your activities.

- Be tobacco free. For tips on how to quit, go to www.smokefree. gov. To talk to someone about how to quit, call the National Quitline: 1-800-QUITNOW (1-800-784-8669).

- If you drink alcohol, have no more than one drink per day. A standard drink is one 12-ounce bottle of beer or wine cooler, one 5-ounce glass of wine, or 1.5 ounces of 80-proof distilled spirits.

Chapter 6

After Your Diagnosis: Finding Information and Support

Your doctor gave you a diagnosis that could change your life. This chapter can help you take the next steps. Every person is different, of course, and every person's disease or condition will affect them differently. But research shows that after getting a diagnosis, many people have some of the same reactions and needs.

Five Basic Steps

This chapter describes five basic steps to help you cope with your diagnosis, make decisions, and get on with your life.

Step one: Take the time you need: Do not rush important decisions about your health. In most cases, you will have time to carefully examine your options and decide what is best for you.

Step two: Get the support you need: Look for support from family and friends, people who are going through the same thing you are, and those who have "been there." They can help you cope with your situation and make informed decisions.

Step three: Talk with your doctor: Good communication with your doctor can help you feel more satisfied with the care you receive.

This chapter includes text excerpted from "Next Steps after Your Diagnosis," Agency for Healthcare Research and Quality (AHRQ), U.S. Department of Health and Human Services (HHS), June 2016.

Research shows it can even have a positive effect on things such as symptoms and pain. Getting a "second opinion" may help you feel more confident about your care.

Step four: Seek out information: When learning about your health problem and its treatment, look for information that is based on a careful review of the latest scientific findings published in medical journals.

Step five: Decide on a treatment plan: Work with your doctor to decide on a treatment plan that best meets your needs.

As you take each step, remember this: Research shows that patients who are more involved in their healthcare tend to get better results and be more satisfied.

Step One: Take the Time You Need

A Diagnosis Can Change Your Life in an Instant

Like so many other people in your situation, you might be feeling one or more of the following emotions after getting your diagnosis:

- afraid
- alone
- angry
- anxious
- ashamed
- confused
- depressed
- helpless
- in denial
- numb
- overwhelmed
- panicky
- powerless
- relieved (that you finally know what's wrong)
- sad
- shocked
- stressed

It is perfectly normal to have these feelings. It is also normal, and very common, to have trouble taking in and understanding information after you receive the news—especially if the diagnosis was a surprise. And it can be even harder to make decisions about treating or managing your disease or condition.

Take Time to Make Your Decisions

No matter how the news of your diagnosis has affected you, do not rush into a decision. In most cases, you do not need to take action right away. Ask your doctor how much time you can safely take.

Taking the time you need to make decisions can help you:

- feel less anxious and stressed

- avoid depression

- cope with your condition

- feel more in control of your situation

- play a key role in decisions about your treatment

Step Two: Get the Support You Need

You Do Not Have to Go through It Alone

Sometimes the emotional side of illness can be just as hard to deal with as the physical side. You may have fears or concerns. You may feel overwhelmed. No matter what your situation, having other people to turn to will help you know you are not alone.

Here are the kinds of support you might want to seek:

Family and friends. Talking to family and friends you feel close to can help you cope with your illness or condition. Just knowing that someone is there can be a comfort.

Sometimes it is hard to ask for help. And sometimes your family and friends want to help, but they do not want to intrude, or they do not know how to ask or what to offer. Think about specific ways people can help you. One idea is to ask someone to come with you to a doctor's appointment to help ask questions, take notes, and talk with you afterward.

If you do not have family or friends who can provide support, other people or groups can.

Support or self-help groups. Support groups are made up of people with the same disease or condition who get together to share information and concerns and to help one another.

Support groups may or may not be led by experts. Self-help groups are similar to support groups but usually are led by the participants. The names "support group" and "self-help group" sometimes are used to refer to either kind.

Research on support groups shows that participants feel less anxious, experience less depression, have a better quality of life, and have more success coping with their disease or condition. Similar findings have been reported for self-help groups.

Online support or self-help groups. The internet has support or self-help groups for people whose concerns and situations may be similar to yours. You can also find "message boards," where you can post questions and get answers. These online communities can help you connect with people who can give you support and provide information.

But be careful. Not every idea or treatment you come across in these groups will be scientifically proven to be safe and effective. If you read about something interesting and new, check it out with your doctor.

Counselor or therapist. A good counselor or therapist can help you cope with sadness, depression, and feelings of being overwhelmed. If you think this kind of help might be right for you, ask your doctor or other healthcare professional to recommend someone in your area.

People like you. You might want to meet and talk with someone in your own situation. Someone who has "been there" can talk about the real-life outcomes of their treatment choices as well as how they have learned to live with their disease or condition. Some advocacy or support groups can help you make this kind of contact.

Step Three: Talk with Your Doctor

Your Doctor Is Your Partner in Healthcare

You probably have many questions about your disease or condition. The first person to ask is your doctor.

It is fine to seek more information from other sources; in fact, it is important to do so. But consider your doctor your partner in healthcare—someone who can discuss your situation with you, explain your options, and help you make decisions that are right for you.

It is not always easy to feel comfortable around doctors. But research has shown that good communication with your doctor can actually be good for your health. It can help you to:

- Feel more satisfied with the care you receive.

- Have better outcomes (end results), such as reduced pain and better recovery from symptoms.

Being an active member of your healthcare team also helps to reduce your chances of medical mistakes, and it helps you get high-quality care.

Of course, good communication is a two-way street. Here are some ways to help make the most of the time you spend with your doctor:

Prepare for Your Visit

- Think about what you want to get out of your appointment. Write down all your questions and concerns.

- Prepare and bring to your doctor visit a list of all the medicines you take.

- Consider bringing along a trusted relative or friend. This person can help ask questions, take notes, and help you remember and understand everything once you leave the doctor's office.

Give Information to Your Doctor

- Do not wait to be asked.

- Tell your doctor everything he or she needs to know about your health—even the things that might make you feel embarrassed or uncomfortable.

- Tell your doctor how you are feeling—both physically and emotionally.

- Tell your doctor if you are feeling depressed or overwhelmed.

Get Information from Your Doctor

- Ask questions about anything that concerns you. Keep asking until you understand the answers. If you do not, your doctor may think you understand everything that is said.

- Ask your doctor to draw pictures if that will help you understand something.

- Take notes.

- Tape record your doctor visit, if that will be helpful to you. But first ask your doctor if this is okay.

- Ask your doctor to recommend resources such as websites, booklets, or tapes with more information about your disease or condition.

Do Not Hesitate to Seek a Second Opinion

A second opinion is when another doctor examines your medical records and gives his or her views about your condition and how it should be treated.

You might want a second opinion to:

- Be clear about what you have.

- Know all of your treatment choices.

- Have another doctor look at your choices with you.

It is not pushy or rude to want a second opinion. Most doctors will understand that you need more information before making important decisions about your health.

Check to see whether your health plan covers a second opinion. In some cases, health plans require second opinions.

Here are some ways to find a doctor for a second opinion:

- Ask your doctor. Request someone who does not work in the same office, because doctors who work together tend to share similar views.

- Contact your health plan or your local hospital, medical society, or medical school.

Get Information about Next Steps

- Get the results of any tests or procedures. Discuss the meaning of these results with your doctor.

- Make sure you understand what will happen if you need surgery.

- Talk with your doctor about which hospital is best for your healthcare needs.

Finally, if you are not satisfied with your doctor, you can do two things:

- Talk with your doctor and try to work things out.

- Switch doctors, if you are able to.

It is very important to feel confident about your care.

Ten Important Questions to Ask Your Doctor after a Diagnosis

These ten basic questions can help you understand your disease or condition, how it might be treated, and what you need to know and do before making treatment decisions.

1. What is the technical name of my disease or condition, and what does it mean in plain English?

2. What is my prognosis (outlook for the future)?

3. How soon do I need to make a decision about treatment?

4. Will I need any additional tests, and if so what kind and when?

5. What are my treatment options?

6. What are the pros and cons of my treatment options?

7. Is there a clinical trial (research study) that is right for me?

8. Now that I have this diagnosis, what changes will I need to make in my daily life?

9. What organizations do you recommend for support and information?

10. What resources (booklets, websites, audiotapes, videos, digital video disks (DVDs), etc.) do you recommend for further information?

Step Four: Seek Out Information

Now that you know your treatment options, you can learn which ones are backed up by the best scientific evidence. "Evidence-based" information—that is, information that is based on a careful review of the latest scientific findings in medical journals—can help you make decisions about the best possible treatments for you.

Evidence-Based Information Comes from Research on People Like You

Evidence-based information about treatments generally comes from two major types of scientific studies:

- **Clinical trials** are research studies on human volunteers to test new drugs or other treatments. Participants are randomly assigned to different treatment groups. Some get the research treatment, and others get a standard treatment or may be given a placebo (a medicine that has no effect), or no treatment. The results are compared to learn whether the new treatment is safe and effective.

- **Outcomes research** looks at the impact of treatments and other healthcare on health outcomes (end results) for patients and populations. End results include effects that people care about, such as changes in their quality of life.

Take advantage of the evidence-based information that is available. Health information is everywhere—in books, newspapers, and magazines, and on the internet, television, and radio. However, not all information is good information. Your best bets for sources of evidence-based information include the Federal Government, national nonprofit organizations, medical specialty groups, medical schools, and university medical centers.

Steer Clear of Deceptive Advertisements and Information

While searching for information either on or off the internet, beware of "miracle" treatments and cures. They can cost you money and your health, especially if you delay or refuse proper treatment. Here are some tip-offs that a product truly is too good to be true:

- Phrases such as "scientific breakthrough," "miraculous cure," "exclusive product," "secret formula," or "ancient ingredient."

- Claims that the product treats a wide range of ailments.

- Use of impressive-sounding medical terms. These often cover up a lack of good science behind the product.

- Case histories from consumers claiming "amazing" results.

- Claims that the product is available from only one source, and for a limited time only.

- Claims of a "money-back guarantee."

- Claims that others are trying to keep the product off the market.

- Ads that fail to list the company's name, address, or other contact information.

Step Five: Decide on a Treatment Plan

At this point, you have learned about your disease or condition and how it can be treated or managed. Your information may have come from the following sources:

- Your doctor.

- Second opinions from one or more other doctors.

- Other people who are or were in the same situation as you.

- Information sources such as websites, health or medical libraries, and nonprofit groups.

Work with Your Doctor to Make Decisions

When you are ready to make treatment decisions, you and your doctor can discuss:

- The treatments that have been found to work well, or not work well, for your particular condition.

- The pros and cons of each treatment option.

Make sure that your doctor knows your preferences and feelings about the different treatments—for example, whether you prefer medicine over surgery.

Once you and your doctor decide on one or more treatments that are right for you, you can work together to develop a treatment plan. This plan will include everything that will be done to treat or manage your disease or condition—including what you need to do to make the plan work. Remember, being an active member of your healthcare team helps to reduce your chances of medical mistakes, and it helps you get high-quality care.

Take Another Deep Breath

You have taken important steps to cope with your diagnosis, make decisions, and get on with your life. Remember two things:

- Call on others for support as you need it.

- Make use of evidence-based information for any future health decisions.

Part Two

Working with Healthcare Providers and the Healthcare System

Chapter 7

Talking with Your Healthcare Provider

How well you and your doctor talk to each other is one of the most important parts of getting good healthcare. Unfortunately, talking with your doctor isn't always easy. In the past, the doctor typically took the lead and the patient followed. Today, a good patient-doctor relationship is a partnership. You and your doctor can work as a team.

Creating a basic plan before you go to the doctor can help you make the most of your visit. The tips in this chapter will make it easier for you and your doctor to cover everything you need to talk about.

Make a List of Your Symptoms

Talking about your health means sharing information about how you feel. Sometimes it can be hard to remember everything that is bothering you during your doctor visit. Making a list of your symptoms before your visit will help you not forget to tell the doctor anything.

Symptoms can be physical, such as pain, fever, a lump or bump, unexplained weight gain or loss, change in energy level, or having a hard time sleeping. Symptoms can also involve your thoughts and your feelings. For example, you would want to tell your doctor if you are often confused, or if you feel sad a lot.

This chapter includes text excerpted from "Talking with Your Doctor," NIHSeniorHealth, National Institute on Aging (NIA), June 2015.

What to Include

When you list your symptoms, be specific. Your list should include:

- what the symptom is
- when it started
- what time of day it happens and how long it lasts
- how often it happens
- anything that makes it worse or better
- anything it prevents you from doing

List Your Medications

Your doctor needs to know about ALL the medications you take. Medications include:

- prescription drugs
- over-the-counter (non-prescription) drugs
- vitamins, herbal remedies or supplements
- laxatives
- eye drops

Sometimes doctors may ask you to bring all your medications in a bag to your visit. Other doctors suggest making a list of all your medications to bring to your visit.

Note Dosages, Frequency, Side Effects

If you do make a list of the medications you take, do not forget to write down how much you take and how often you take it. Make sure to tell the doctor if a dose has changed or if you are taking a new medicine since your last visit.

Write down or bring all your medications even if you think that one or some of them are not important. The doctor needs to know everything you take because sometimes medicines cause problems when taken together. Also, sometimes a medicine you take for one health problem, like a headache, can cause another health problem to get worse. Write down any medication allergies you have and any bad side effects you have had with the medicines you take. Also, write down which medications work best for you.

To provide the best care, your doctor must understand you as a person and know what your life is like.

Do You Use Assistive Devices?

Be sure to let your doctor know if you use any assistive devices to help you in your daily activities. Assistive devices can help you see, hear, stand, reach, balance, grasp items, go up or down stairs, and move around. Devices used by older adults may include canes, walkers, scooters, hearing aids, reachers, grab bars, and stair lifts.

What Are Your Everyday Habits?

Be prepared to tell your doctor about where you live, if you drive or how you get around, what you eat, how you sleep, what you do each day, what activities you enjoy, what your sex life is like, and if you smoke or drink alcohol.

Be open and honest. It will help your doctor to better understand your medical conditions and figure out the best treatment choices for you.

Any Life Changes?

Sometimes things happen in life that are sad or stressful. Your doctor needs to know about any life changes that have occurred since your last visit because they can affect your health. Examples of life changes are divorce, death of a loved one, or changing where you live.

Your list should include all your life changes but does not need to go into detail. It can be short like "had to sell home and move in with daughter."

Any Other Medical Encounters?

Also, write down and tell your doctor if you had to go to the emergency room, stay in the hospital or see a different doctor, such as a specialist, since your last visit. It may be helpful to bring that doctor's contact information.

What Else to Bring

Bring your insurance cards, names and phone numbers of your other doctors, and the phone number of the pharmacy you use. Also, bring your medical records if your doctor does not have them.

Chapter 8

Making Decisions with Your Doctor

Giving and getting information are two important steps in talking with your doctor. The third big step is making decisions about your care.

Find Out about Different Treatments

You will benefit most from a treatment when you know what is happening and are involved in making decisions. Make sure you understand what your treatment involves and what it will or will not do. Have the doctor give you directions in writing and feel free to ask questions. For example: "What are the pros and cons of having surgery at this stage?" or "Do I have any other choices?"

If your doctor suggests a treatment that makes you uncomfortable, ask if there are other treatments that might work. If cost is a concern, ask the doctor if less expensive choices are available. The doctor can work with you to develop a treatment plan that meets your needs.

Here are some things to remember when deciding on a treatment:

- **Discuss choices.** There are different ways to manage many health conditions, especially chronic conditions like high blood pressure and cholesterol. Ask what your options are.

This chapter includes text excerpted from "Talking with Your Doctor: A Guide for Older People," National Institute on Aging (NIA), National Institutes of Health (NIH), July 29, 2016.

- **Discuss risks and benefits.** Once you know your options, ask about the pros and cons of each one. Find out what side effects might occur, how long the treatment would continue, and how likely it is that the treatment will work for you.

- **Consider your own values and circumstances.** When thinking about the pros and cons of a treatment, don't forget to consider its impact on your overall life. For instance, will one of the side effects interfere with a regular activity that means a lot to you? Is one treatment choice expensive and not covered by your insurance? Doctors need to know about these practical matters and can work with you to develop a treatment plan that meets your needs.

Questions to ask about treatment:

- Are there any risks associated with the treatment?

- How soon should treatment start? How long will it last?

- Are there other treatments available?

- How much will the treatment cost? Will my insurance cover it?

Learn about Prevention

Doctors and other health professionals may suggest you change your diet, activity level, or other aspects of your life to help you deal with medical conditions. Research has shown that these changes, particularly an increase in exercise, have positive effects on overall health.

Until recently, preventing disease in older people received little attention. But things are changing. We now know that it's never too late to stop smoking, improve your diet, or start exercising. Getting regular checkups and seeing other health professionals such as dentists and eye specialists helps promote good health. Even people who have chronic diseases, like arthritis or diabetes, can prevent further disability and, in some cases, control the progress of the disease.

If a certain disease or health condition runs in your family, ask your doctor if there are steps you can take to help prevent it. If you have a chronic condition, ask how you can manage it and if there are things you can do to prevent it from getting worse. If you want to discuss health and disease prevention with your doctor, say so when you make your next appointment. This lets the doctor plan to spend more time with you.

It is just as important to talk with your doctor about lifestyle changes as it is to talk about treatment. For example: "I know that you've told me to eat more dairy products, but they really disagree with me. Is there something else I could eat instead?" or "Maybe an exercise class would help, but I have no way to get to the senior center. Is there something else you could suggest?"

As with treatments, consider all the alternatives, look at pros and cons, and remember to take into account your own point of view. Tell your doctor if you feel his or her suggestions won't work for you and explain why. Keep talking with your doctor to come up with a plan that works.

Questions to ask about prevention:

- Is there any way to prevent a condition that runs in my family—before it affects me?

- Are there ways to keep my condition from getting worse?

- How will making a change in my habits help me?

- Are there any risks in making this change?

- Are there support groups or community services that might help me?

Evaluating Health Information Online

Many people search online to find information about medical problems and health issues. However, not all health information on the web is of equal quality. How do you find websites that are accurate and reliable? The following questions may be useful to consider when you look at a health-related website.

- Who is responsible for the content? Is it a government agency (.gov), national nonprofit organization, or professional association? An individual? A commercial organization?

- If you are reading an article or blog, what are the author's credentials? Is the author affiliated with any major medical institutions?

- Who reviews the material? Is there a medical or scientific advisory board that reads the medical content before it is made available to the public?

- Are sources cited for the statistical information? For example, it's easy enough to say "4 out of 5 doctors agree..." but where did that statistic come from?

- Is the purpose and goal of the sponsoring organization clearly stated?

- Is there a way to contact the sponsor for more information or to verify information presented?

- Is the site supported by public funds or donations? If it includes advertisements, are they separate from content?

- Because health information gets outdated so quickly, does the website post the source and date for the information?

- If you have to register, is it clear how your personal information will be used? Does the site have a clear privacy policy?

- Is the website trying to sell you something?

Don't forget to talk with your doctor about what you've learned online.

Chapter 9

Getting a Second Opinion

What's a Second Opinion?

A second opinion is when a doctor other than your regular doctor gives his or her view about your health problem and how it should be treated. Getting a second opinion can help you make a more informed decision about your care.

Medicare Part B (Medical Insurance) helps pay for a second opinion before surgery. When your doctor says you have a health problem that needs surgery, you have the right to:

- Know and understand your treatment choices.

- Have another doctor look at those choices with you (second opinion).

- Participate in treatment decisions by making your wishes known.

This chapter contains text excerpted from the following sources: Text beginning with the heading "What's a Second Opinion?" is excerpted from "Getting a Second Opinion before Surgery," Centers for Medicare and Medicaid Services (CMS), July 2016; Text beginning with the heading "Importance of Getting a Second Opinion" is excerpted from "How to Get a Second Opinion," Office on Women's Health (OWH), U.S. Department of Health and Human Services (HHS), September 10, 2008. Reviewed January 2017.

When Should I Get a Second Opinion?

If your doctor says you need surgery to diagnose or treat a health problem that isn't an emergency, you should consider getting a second opinion. It's up to you to decide when and if you'll have surgery. You might also want a second opinion if your doctor tells you that you should have certain kinds of major non-surgical procedures.

Medicare doesn't pay for surgeries or procedures that aren't medically necessary, like cosmetic surgery. This means that Medicare won't pay for second opinions for surgeries or procedures that aren't medically necessary.

Don't wait for a second opinion if you need emergency surgery.

Some types of emergencies may require surgery right away, like:

- Acute appendicitis

- Blood clot or aneurysm

- Accidental injuries

How Do I Find a Doctor for a Second Opinion?

Make sure the doctor giving the second opinion accepts Medicare. To find a doctor for a second opinion, you can:

- Visit Medicare.gov/physiciancompare to find doctors who accept Medicare.

- Call 1-800-MEDICARE (1-800-633-4227). TTY users should call 1-877-486-2048. Ask for information about doctors who accept Medicare.

- Ask your doctor for the name of another doctor to see for a second opinion. Don't hesitate to ask—most doctors want you to get a second opinion. You can also ask another doctor you trust to recommend a doctor.

What Should I Do before Getting a Second Opinion?

Before you visit the second doctor, you should:

- Ask the first doctor to send your medical records to the doctor giving the second opinion. That way, you may not have to repeat the tests you already had.

- Call the second doctor's office and make sure they have your records.

- Write down a list of questions to take with you to the appointment.

- Ask a family member or friend to go to the appointment with you.

During the visit with the second doctor, you should:

- Tell the doctor what surgery you're thinking about having.

- Tell the doctor what tests you already had.

- Ask the questions you have on your list and encourage your friend or loved one to ask any questions that he or she may have.

The second doctor may ask you to have additional tests performed as a result of the visit. Medicare will help pay for these tests just as it helps pay for other services that are medically necessary.

What If the First and Second Opinions Are Different?

If the second doctor doesn't agree with the first, you may feel confused about what to do. In that case, you may want to:

- Talk more about your condition with your first doctor.

- Talk to a third doctor. Medicare helps pay for a third opinion.

Getting a second or third opinion doesn't mean you have to change doctors. You decide which doctor you want to do your surgery.

How Much Does Medicare Pay for a Second Opinion?

Medicare Part B helps pay for a second (or third) opinion and related tests just as it helps pay for other services that are medically necessary. If you have Part B and are in Original Medicare:

- Medicare pays 80 percent of the Medicare-approved amount.

- Your share is usually 20 percent of the Medicare-approved amount after you pay your yearly Part B deductible.

Do Medicare Advantage Plans Cover Second Opinions?

If you're in a Medicare Advantage Plan (like a Health Maintenance Organization (HMO) or preferred provider organization (PPO), you have the right to get a second opinion. If the first two opinions are different, your plan will help pay for a third opinion.

Even though you have the right to get a second opinion, you should keep these things in mind:

- Some plans will only help pay for a second opinion if you have a referral (a written OK) from your primary care doctor.

- Some plans will only help pay for a second opinion from a doctor who's in your plan's provider network.

- If you're in a Medicare Advantage Plan, call your plan for more information

If you have Medicaid, it might also pay for second surgical opinions. To find out, call your Medicaid office. You can get the phone number by:

- Visiting Medicare.gov/contacts.

- Calling 1-800-MEDICARE (1-800-633-4227). TTY users should call 1-877-486-2048.

Importance of Getting a Second Opinion

Even though doctors may get similar medical training, they can have their own opinions and thoughts about how to practice medicine. They can have different ideas about how to diagnose and treat conditions or diseases. Some doctors take a more conservative, or traditional, approach to treating their patients. Other doctors are more aggressive and use the newest tests and therapies. It seems like we learn about new advances in medicine almost every day.

Many doctors specialize in one area of medicine, such as cardiology or obstetrics or psychiatry. Not every doctor can be skilled in using all the latest technology. Getting a second opinion from a different doctor might give you a fresh perspective and new information. It could provide you with new options for treating your condition. Then you can make more informed choices. If you get similar opinions from two doctors, you can also talk with a third doctor.

Tips: What to Do

- **Ask your doctor for a recommendation.** Ask for the name of another doctor or specialist, so you can get a second opinion.

Don't worry about hurting your doctor's feelings. Most doctors welcome a second opinion, especially when surgery or long-term treatment is involved.

- **Ask someone you trust for a recommendation.** If you don't feel comfortable asking your doctor for a referral, then call another doctor you trust. You can also call university teaching hospitals and medical societies in your area for the names of doctors. Some of this information is also available on the Internet.

- **Check with your health insurance provider.** Call your insurance company before you get a second opinion. Ask if they will pay for this office visit. Many health insurance providers do. Ask if there are any special procedures you or your primary care doctor needs to follow.

- **Ask to have medical records sent to the second doctor.** Ask your primary care doctor to send your medical records to the new doctor. You need to give written permission to your current doctor to send any records or test results to a new doctor. You can also ask for a copy of your own medical records for your files. Your new doctor can then examine these records before your office visit.

- **Learn as much as you can.** Ask your doctor for information you can read. Go to a local library. Find a teaching hospital or university that has medical libraries open to the public. The information you find can be hard to understand, or just confusing. Make a list of your questions, and bring it with you when you see your new doctor.

- **Do not rely on the Internet or a telephone conversation.** When you get a second opinion, you need to be seen by a doctor. That doctor will perform a physical examination and perhaps other tests. The doctor will also thoroughly review your medical records, ask you questions, and address your concerns.

Chapter 10

Medical Specialties: Definitions

Below are definitions of medical specialties for physicians followed by a list of specialties for other healthcare professionals.

Addiction medicine: Specialists in addiction medicine treat substance abuse and addiction.

Allergy / Immunology: Specialists in allergy and immunology treat conditions that involve the immune system. Examples include allergies, immune deficiency diseases, and autoimmune diseases.

Anesthesiology: Anesthesiologists provide anesthesia for patients who are having surgery or other procedures. They also treat pain and care for patients with critical illnesses or severe injuries.

Cardiac electrophysiology: Cardiac electrophysiologists use technical procedures to evaluate heart rhythms.

Cardiac surgery / Thoracic surgery: Thoracic surgeons treat problems in the chest, including problems affecting the heart, lungs, or windpipe.

Cardiovascular disease (Cardiology): Cardiologists treat diseases of the heart and blood vessels.

This chapter includes text excerpted from "Specialty Definitions," Centers for Medicare and Medicaid Services (CMS), June 27, 2013. Reviewed January 2017.

Chiropractic: Chiropractors manipulate specific parts of the body (often the spine) to prevent and treat diseases.

Colorectal surgery (Proctology): Colorectal surgeons treat diseases of the lower digestive tract.

Critical care (Intensivist): Intensivist treat critically ill or injured patients.

Dermatology: Dermatologists treat skin conditions.

Diagnostic radiology: Diagnostic radiologists use imaging, such as X-rays or ultrasound, to diagnose diseases.

Emergency medicine: Emergency medicine specialists take care of patients with critical illnesses or injuries.

Endocrinology: Endocrinologists treat diseases that involve the internal (endocrine) glands. Examples include diabetes and diseases of the thyroid, pituitary, or adrenal glands.

Family practice: Family practitioners provide primary care for people of all ages. They treat illnesses, provide preventive care, and coordinate the care provided by other health professionals.

Gastroenterology: Gastroenterologists treat diseases of the digestive organs, including the stomach, bowels, liver, and gallbladder.

General practice: General practitioners provide primary care. They treat illnesses, provide preventive care, and coordinate the care provided by other health professionals.

General surgery: General surgeons take care of patients who may need surgery.

Geriatric medicine: Geriatricians provide primary care for elderly patients.

Gynecological oncology: Gynecological oncologists treat cancers of the female reproductive organs.

Hand surgery: Hand surgeons perform surgery for patients with problems that affect the hand, wrist, or forearm.

Hematology: Hematologists treat diseases of the blood, spleen, and lymph. Examples include anemia, sickle cell disease, hemophilia, and leukemia.

Hospice and palliative care: Physicians manage pain and other distressing symptoms of serious illnesses. "Hospice care" is palliative care for patients who are expected to have six months or less to live.

Infectious disease: Infectious disease physicians treat patients with all types of infectious diseases.

Internal medicine: Internists treat diseases of the internal organs that don't require surgery. They also provide primary care for teenagers, adults, and elderly people.

Interventional cardiology: Interventional cardiologists are heart and circulatory system specialists who use minimally invasive catheterization techniques to diagnose and treat coronary arteries, the peripheral vascular system, heart valves, and congenital heart defects.

Interventional pain management: Interventional pain management specialists use special procedures to treat and manage pain. For example, they may use cryoablation (a procedure involving extreme cold) to stop a nerve from working for a long period of time.

Interventional radiology: Interventional radiologists perform procedures guided by various types of imaging. For example, they may use imaging to find a clogged spot in an artery and to guide a procedure to unclog it.

Maxillofacial surgery: Maxillofacial surgeons perform surgery on the teeth, jaws, and surrounding tissues.

Medical oncology: Medical oncologists treat cancer with chemotherapy, hormonal therapy, biological therapy, and targeted therapy. They may also coordinate cancer care given by other specialists.

Nephrology: Nephrologists treat disorders of the kidneys.

Neurology: Neurologists treat diseases of the brain, spinal cord, and nerves.

Neuropsychiatry: Neuropsychiatrist treat patients with behavioral disturbances related to nervous system problems.

Neurosurgery: Neurosurgeons perform surgery to treat problems in the brain, spine, and nerves.

Nuclear medicine: Nuclear medicine specialists use radioactive materials to diagnose and treat diseases.

Obstetrics / Gynecology: Obstetricians and gynecologists take care of women during pregnancy and childbirth (called obstetrics). They also treat disorders of the female reproductive system (called gynecology).

Ophthalmology: Ophthalmologists are physicians who specialize in the care of the eyes. They prescribe glasses and contact lenses, diagnose and treat eye conditions, and perform eye surgery.

Optometry: Optometrists are eye care professionals who perform eye examinations, prescribe corrective lenses, and treat some eye diseases that don't require surgery.

Oral surgery (Dentist only): Oral surgeons are dentists who use surgery to treat problems in the mouth and nearby areas.

Orthopedic surgery: Orthopedic surgeons treat diseases, injuries, and deformities of the bones and muscles.

Osteopathic manipulative medicine: Osteopathic physicians often use a treatment method called osteopathic manipulative treatment. This is a hands-on approach to make sure that the body is moving freely.

Otolaryngology: Otolaryngologists treat conditions of the ears, nose, and throat (ENT) and related areas of the head and neck.

Pain management: Pain management specialists take care of patients with pain.

Pathology: Pathologists examine body tissues and interpret laboratory test results.

Pediatric medicine: Pediatricians provide primary care for infants, children, and teenagers.

Peripheral vascular disease: Peripheral vascular disease physicians treat diseases of the circulatory system other than those of the brain and heart.

Physical medicine and rehabilitation: Physical medicine and rehabilitation specialists are physicians who treat patients with short-term or long-term disabilities.

Plastic and reconstructive surgery: Plastic and reconstructive surgeons perform procedures to improve the appearance or function of parts of the body.

Podiatry: Podiatrists specialize in caring for the foot and treating foot diseases.

Preventive medicine: Preventive medicine specialists work to promote the health and well-being of individuals or groups of people.

Primary care: Primary care physicians treat illnesses, provide preventive care, and coordinate the care provided by other health professionals. Physicians in family practice, general practice, geriatric medicine, and internal medicine provide primary care.

Psychiatry: Psychiatrists treat mental, addictive, and emotional disorders.

Psychiatry (Geriatric): Geriatric psychiatrists treat mental and emotional disorders in elderly people.

Pulmonary disease: Pulmonologists treat diseases of the lungs and airways.

Radiation oncology: Radiation oncologists use radiation to treat cancer.

Rheumatology: Rheumatologists treat problems involving the joints, muscles, bones, and tendons.

Sleep medicine: Sleep medicine physicians treat problems related to sleep or the sleep-wake cycle.

Sports medicine: Sports medicine specialists treat problems related to participation in sports or exercise.

Surgical oncology: Surgical oncologists specialize in the surgical diagnosis and treatment of cancer.

Thoracic surgery: Thoracic surgeons treat problems in the chest, including problems affecting the heart, lungs, or windpipe.

Urology: Urologists treat problems in the male and female urinary tract and the male reproductive system.

Vascular surgery: Vascular surgeons treat diseases of the circulatory system, other than the brain and heart.

Other Healthcare Professional Specialties

Anesthesiologist assistant. Anesthesiologist assistants work under the direction of an anesthesiologist as a part of the anesthesia care team.

Audiology. Audiologists have advanced training and evaluate hearing or balance problems. They provide hearing aids and counsel people about how to cope with hearing loss.

Certified nurse midwife (CNM). Certified nurse midwives are registered nurses who have earned a master's degree in nursing and met other requirements. They practice in hospitals and medical clinics. They may also deliver babies in birthing centers and attend home births.

Certified registered nurse anesthetist (CRNA). Certified registered nurse anesthetists are registered nurses who have earned a master's degree in nursing and met other requirements. They provide anesthesia, working with other healthcare professionals.

Clinical nurse specialist (CNS). Clinical nurse specialists are registered nurses who have earned a master's degree in nursing and met other requirements. They handle a range of physical and mental health problems.

Clinical psychologist. Clinical psychologists have a doctorate in psychology and have advanced training in promoting mental health and helping people cope with problems.

Clinical social worker (CSW). Clinical social workers have earned a master's degree, and help people deal with life changes and challenges, including mental disorders.

Nurse practitioner (NP). Nurse practitioners are registered nurses who have earned a master's degree in nursing and met other requirements. They provide primary and preventive care, prescribe medicines, and treat common minor illnesses and injuries.

Occupational therapy (OT). Occupational therapists help people who are recovering from injuries to regain skills. They also support people who are going through changes related to aging. They provide home assessments, teach people to use adaptive equipment (such as devices to help with bathing, dressing, or eating), and work with family members and caregivers. OTs are state-licensed and nationally certified to practice

Physical therapy (PT). Physical therapists provide rehabilitation to help people move, reduce pain, restore function, and prevent disability. PTs are state-licensed and nationally certified to practice.

Physician assistant (PA). Physician assistants are graduates of accredited PA educational programs. They're licensed to practice medicine with a physician's supervision. They examine patients, diagnose and treat illnesses, order lab tests, prescribe medicines, perform procedures, assist in surgery, and counsel patients.

Registered dietitian (RD) / Nutrition professional. Registered dietitians and other nutrition professionals are food and nutrition experts. They teach patients about nutrition. They also provide medical nutrition therapy.

Speech-language pathology (SLP). Speech-language pathologists, sometimes called speech therapists, treat communication and swallowing disorders. They're state-licensed and nationally certified in speech-language pathology.

Chapter 11

Selecting a Complementary and Alternative Medicine (CAM) Practitioner

Complementary Health Approach

Millions of Americans use complementary health approaches. Like any decision concerning your health, decisions about whether to use complementary approaches are important. This chapter will assist you in your decision making about complementary health products and practices.

What Do "Complementary," Alternative," and "Integrative" Mean?

"Complementary and alternative medicine," "complementary medicine," "alternative medicine," "integrative medicine"—you may have

This chapter contains text excerpted from the following sources: Text beginning with the heading "Complementary Health Approach" is excerpted from "Are You Considering a Complementary Health Approach?" National Center for Complementary and Integrative Health (NCCIH), September 6, 2016; Text under the heading "Things to Know When Selecting a Complementary Health Practitioner" is excerpted from "6 Things to Know When Selecting a Complementary Health Practitioner," National Center for Complementary and Integrative Health (NCCIH), October 11, 2016.

seen these terms on the Internet and in marketing, but what do they really mean? While the terms are often used to mean the array of healthcare approaches with a history of use or origins outside of mainstream medicine, they are actually hard to define and may mean different things to different people.

The terms complementary and integrative refer to the use of non-mainstream approaches together with conventional medical approaches.

Alternative health approaches refer to the use of non-mainstream products or practices in place of conventional medicine. National Center for Complementary and Integrative Health (NCCIH) advises against using any product or practice that has not been proven safe and effective as a substitute for conventional medical treatment or as a reason to postpone seeing your healthcare provider about any health problem. In some instances, stopping—or not starting—conventional treatment can have serious consequences. Before making a decision not to use a proven conventional treatment, talk to your healthcare providers.

How Can I Get Reliable Information about a Complementary Health Approach?

It's important to learn what scientific studies have discovered about the complementary health approach you're considering. Evidence from research studies is stronger and more reliable than something you've seen in an advertisement or on a website, or something someone told you about that worked for them.

Understanding a products' or practice's potential benefits, risks, and scientific evidence is critical to your health and safety. Scientific research on many complementary health approaches is relatively new, so this kind of information may not be available for each one. However, many studies are underway, including those that NCCIH supports, and knowledge and understanding of complementary approaches are increasing all the time. Here are some ways to find reliable information:

- **Talk with your healthcare providers.** Tell them about the complementary health approach you're considering and ask any questions you may have about safety, effectiveness, or interactions with medications (prescription or nonprescription) or dietary supplements.

- **Visit the NCCIH** website **(nccih.nih.gov).** The "Health Information" page has an A–Z list of complementary health products and practices, which describes what the science says about them, and links to other objective sources of online information. The website also has contact information for the NCCIH Clearinghouse, where information specialists are available to assist you in searching the scientific literature and to suggest useful NCCIH publications.

- **Visit your local library or a medical library.** Ask the reference librarian to help you find scientific journals and trustworthy books with information on the product or practice that interests you.

Are Complementary Health Approaches Safe?

As with any medical product or treatment, there can be risks with complementary approaches. These risks depend on the specific product or practice. Each needs to be considered on its own. However, if you're considering a specific product or practice, the following general suggestions can help you think about safety and minimize risks.

- Be aware that individuals respond differently to health products and practices, whether conventional or complementary. How you might respond to one depends on many things, including your state of health, how you use it, or your belief in it.

- Keep in mind that "natural" does not necessarily mean "safe." (Think of mushrooms that grow in the wild: some are safe to eat, while others are not.)

- Learn about factors that affect safety. For a practice that is administered by a practitioner, such as chiropractic, these factors include the training, skill, and experience of the practitioner. For a product such as a dietary supplement, the specific ingredients and the quality of the manufacturing process are important factors.

- If you decide to use a practice provided by a complementary health practitioner, choose the practitioner as carefully as you would your primary healthcare provider.

- If you decide to use a dietary supplement, such as an herbal product, be aware that some products may interact in harmful ways with medications (prescription or over-the-counter) or other dietary supplements, and some may have side effects on their own.

- Tell all your healthcare providers about any complementary or integrative health approaches you use. Give them a full picture of what you do to manage your health. This will help ensure coordinated and safe care.

How Can I Determine Whether Statements Made about the Effectiveness of a Complementary Health Approach Are True?

Before you begin using a complementary health approach, it's a good idea to ask the following questions:

- Is there scientific evidence (not just personal stories) to back up the statements?

- What is the source? Statements that manufacturers or other promoters of some complementary health approaches may make about effectiveness and benefits can sound reasonable and promising. However, the statements may be based on a biased view of the available scientific evidence.

- Does the Federal Government have anything to report about the product or practice?

- Visit the NCCIH website or contact the NCCIH Clearinghouse to see if NCCIH has information about the product or practice.

- Visit the U.S. Food and Drug Administration (FDA) online at www.fda.gov to see if there is any information available about the product or practice.

- Information specifically about dietary supplements can be found on the FDA's website at www.fda.gov/Food/DietarySupplements and on the website of the National Institutes of Health (NIH) Office of Dietary Supplements (ODS) at ods.od.nih.gov.

- Visit the FDA's webpage on recalls and safety alerts at www.fda. gov/Safety/Recalls. The FDA has a rapid public notification system to provide information about tainted dietary supplements.

- Check with the Federal Trade Commission (FTC) at www.ftc.gov to see if there are any enforcement actions for deceptive advertising regarding the therapy. Also, visit the site's Consumer Information section at www.consumer.ftc.gov.

- How does the provider or manufacturer describe the approach?

- Beware of terms like "scientific breakthrough," "miracle cure," "secret ingredient," or "ancient remedy."

- If you encounter claims of a "quick fix" that depart from previous research, keep in mind that science usually advances over time by small steps, slowly building an evidence base.

- Remember: if it sounds too good to be true—for example, claims that a product or practice can cure a disease or works for a variety of ailments—it usually is.

Is That Health Website Trustworthy?

If you're visiting a health website for the first time, these five quick questions can help you decide whether the site is a helpful resource.

- **Who?** Who runs the website? Can you trust them?

- **What?** What does the site say? Do its claims seem too good to be true?

- **When?** When was the information posted or reviewed? Is it up-to-date?

- **Where?** Where did the information come from? Is it based on scientific research?

- **Why?** Why does the site exist? Is it selling something?

Are Complementary Health Approaches Tested to See If They Work?

While scientific evidence now exists regarding the effectiveness and safety of some complementary health approaches, there remain many yet-to-be-answered questions about whether others are safe, whether they work for the diseases or medical conditions for which they are promoted, and how those approaches with health benefits may work.

I'm Interested in an Approach That Involves Seeing a Complementary Health Practitioner. How Do I Go about Selecting a Practitioner?

Your primary healthcare provider or local hospital may be able to recommend a complementary health practitioner.

The professional organization for the type of practitioner you're seeking may have helpful information, such as licensing and training requirements. Many states have regulatory agencies or licensing boards for certain types of complementary health practitioners; they may be able to help you locate practitioners in your area.

Make sure any practitioner you're considering is willing to work in collaboration with your other healthcare providers.

Things to Know When Selecting a Complementary Health Practitioner

If you're looking for a complementary health practitioner to help treat a medical problem, it is important to be as careful and thorough in your search as you are when looking for conventional care.

Here are some tips to help you in your search:

1. **If you need names of practitioners in your area, first check with your doctor or other healthcare provider.** A nearby hospital or medical school, professional organizations, state regulatory agencies or licensing boards, or even your health insurance provider may be helpful. Unfortunately, the NCCIH cannot refer you to practitioners.

2. **Find out as much as you can about any potential practitioner, including education, training, licensing, and certifications.** The credentials required for complementary health practitioners vary tremendously from state to state and from discipline to discipline.

Once you have found a possible practitioner, here are some tips about deciding whether he or she is right for you:

1. **Find out whether the practitioner is willing to work together with your conventional healthcare providers.** For safe, coordinated care, it's important for all of the professionals involved in your health to communicate and cooperate.

2. **Explain all of your health conditions to the practitioner, and find out about the practitioner's training and experience in working with people who have your conditions.** Choose a practitioner who understands how to work with people with your specific needs, even if general well-being is your goal. And, remember that health conditions can affect the safety of complementary approaches; for

example, if you have glaucoma, some yoga poses may not be safe for you.

3. **Don't assume that your health insurance will cover the practitioner's services.** Contact your health insurance provider and ask. Insurance plans differ greatly in what complementary health approaches they cover, and even if they cover a particular approach, restrictions may apply.

4. **Tell all your healthcare providers about the complementary approaches you use and about all practitioners who are treating you.** Keeping your healthcare providers fully informed helps you to stay in control and effectively manage your health.

Chapter 12

An Introduction to Clinical Studies

What Is a Clinical Study?

A clinical study involves research using human volunteers (also called participants) that is intended to add to medical knowledge. There are two main types of clinical studies: clinical trials (also called interventional studies) and observational studies. ClinicalTrials.gov includes both interventional and observational studies.

In a clinical trial, participants receive specific interventions according to the research plan or protocol created by the investigators. These interventions may be medical products, such as drugs or devices; procedures; or changes to participants' behavior, such as diet. Clinical trials may compare a new medical approach to a standard one that is already available, to a placebo that contains no active ingredients, or to no intervention. Some clinical trials compare interventions that are already available to each other. When a new product or approach is being studied, it is not usually known whether it will be helpful, harmful, or no different than available alternatives (including no intervention). The investigators try to determine the safety and efficacy of the intervention by measuring certain outcomes in the participants. For example, investigators may give a drug or treatment to participants who have high blood pressure to see whether their blood pressure decreases.

This chapter includes text excerpted from "Learn about Clinical Studies," ClinicalTrials.gov, National Institutes of Health (NIH), December 2015.

Clinical trials used in drug development are sometimes described by phase. These phases are defined by the U.S. Food and Drug Administration (FDA).

Some people who are not eligible to participate in a clinical trial may be able to get experimental drugs or devices outside of a clinical trial through an Expanded Access Program (EAP).

Observational Studies

In an observational study, investigators assess health outcomes in groups of participants according to a research plan or protocol. Participants may receive interventions (which can include medical products such as drugs or devices) or procedures as part of their routine medical care, but participants are not assigned to specific interventions by the investigator (as in a clinical trial). For example, investigators may observe a group of older adults to learn more about the effects of different lifestyles on cardiac health.

Who Conducts Clinical Studies?

Every clinical study is led by a principal investigator, who is often a medical doctor. Clinical studies also have a research team that may include doctors, nurses, social workers, and other healthcare professionals.

Clinical studies can be sponsored, or funded, by pharmaceutical companies, academic medical centers, voluntary groups, and other organizations, in addition to Federal agencies such as the National Institutes of Health (NIH), the U.S. Department of Defense (DoD), and the U.S. Department of Veterans Affairs (VA). Doctors, other healthcare providers, and other individuals can also sponsor clinical research.

Where Are Clinical Studies Conducted?

Clinical studies can take place in many locations, including hospitals, universities, doctors' offices, and community clinics. The location depends on who is conducting the study.

How Long Do Clinical Studies Last?

The length of a clinical study varies, depending on what is being studied. Participants are told how long the study will last before they enroll.

Reasons for Conducting Clinical Studies

In general, clinical studies are designed to add to medical knowledge related to the treatment, diagnosis, and prevention of diseases or conditions. Some common reasons for conducting clinical studies include:

- Evaluating one or more interventions (for example, drugs, medical devices, approaches to surgery or radiation therapy) for treating a disease, syndrome, or condition

- Finding ways to prevent the initial development or recurrence of a disease or condition. These can include medicines, vaccines, or lifestyle changes, among other approaches

- Evaluating one or more interventions aimed at identifying or diagnosing a particular disease or condition

- Examining methods for identifying a condition or the risk factors for that condition

- Exploring and measuring ways to improve the comfort and quality of life through supportive care for people with a chronic illness

Participating in Clinical Studies

A clinical study is conducted according to a research plan known as the protocol. The protocol is designed to answer specific research questions and safeguard the health of participants. It contains the following information:

- The reason for conducting the study

- Who may participate in the study (the eligibility criteria)

- The number of participants needed

- The schedule of tests, procedures, or drugs and their dosages

- The length of the study

- What information will be gathered about the participants

Who Can Participate in a Clinical Study?

Clinical studies have standards outlining who can participate. These standards are called eligibility criteria and are listed in the protocol. Some research studies seek participants who have the illnesses or conditions that will be studied, other studies are looking for healthy participants, and some studies are limited to a predetermined group of people who are asked by researchers to enroll.

Eligibility. The factors that allow someone to participate in a clinical study are called inclusion criteria, and the factors that disqualify someone from participating are called exclusion criteria. They are based on characteristics such as age, gender, the type and stage of a disease, previous treatment history, and other medical conditions.

How Are Participants Protected?

Informed consent is a process used by researchers to provide potential and enrolled participants with information about a clinical study. This information helps people decide whether they want to enroll or continue to participate in the study. The informed consent process is intended to protect participants and should provide enough information for a person to understand the risks of, potential benefits of, and alternatives to the study. In addition to the informed consent document, the process may involve recruitment materials, verbal instructions, question-and-answer sessions, and activities to measure participant understanding. In general, a person must sign an informed consent document before joining a study to show that he or she was given information on the risks, potential benefits, and alternatives and that he or she understands it. Signing the document and providing consent is not a contract. Participants may withdraw from a study at any time, even if the study is not over.

Institutional review boards. Each federally supported or conducted clinical study and each study of a drug, biological product, or medical device regulated by FDA must be reviewed, approved, and monitored by an institutional review board (IRB). An IRB is made up of doctors, researchers, and members of the community. Its role is to make sure that the study is ethical and that the rights and welfare of participants are protected. This includes making sure that research risks are minimized and are reasonable in relation to any potential benefits, among other responsibilities. The IRB also reviews the informed consent document.

In addition to being monitored by an IRB, some clinical studies are also monitored by data monitoring committees (also called data safety and monitoring boards).

Various Federal agencies, including the Office of Human Subjects Research Protection (OHRP) and FDA, have the authority to determine whether sponsors of certain clinical studies are adequately protecting research participants.

Relationship to Usual Healthcare

Typically, participants continue to see their usual healthcare providers while enrolled in a clinical study. While most clinical studies provide participants with medical products or interventions related to the illness or condition being studied, they do not provide extended or complete healthcare. By having his or her usual healthcare provider work with the research team, a participant can make sure that the study protocol will not conflict with other medications or treatments that he or she receives.

Considerations for Participation

Participating in a clinical study contributes to medical knowledge. The results of these studies can make a difference in the care of future patients by providing information about the benefits and risks of therapeutic, preventative, or diagnostic products or interventions.

Clinical trials provide the basis for the development and marketing of new drugs, biological products, and medical devices. Sometimes, the safety and the effectiveness of the experimental approach or use may not be fully known at the time of the trial. Some trials may provide participants with the prospect of receiving direct medical benefits, while others do not. Most trials involve some risk of harm or injury to the participant, although it may not be greater than the risks related to routine medical care or disease progression. (For trials approved by IRBs, the IRB has decided that the risks of participation have been minimized and are reasonable in relation to anticipated benefits.) Many trials require participants to undergo additional procedures, tests, and assessments based on the study protocol. These requirements will be described in the informed consent document. A potential participant should also discuss these issues with members of the research team and with his or her usual healthcare provider.

Questions to Ask

Anyone interested in participating in a clinical study should know as much as possible about the study and feel comfortable asking the research team questions about the study, the related procedures, and any expenses. The following questions may be helpful during such a discussion. Answers to some of these questions are provided in the informed consent document. Many of the questions are specific to clinical trials, but some also apply to observational studies.

- What is being studied?

- Why do researchers believe the intervention being tested might be effective? Why might it not be effective? Has it been tested before?

- What are the possible interventions that I might receive during the trial?

- How will it be determined which interventions I receive (for example, by chance)?

- Who will know which intervention I receive during the trial? Will I know? Will members of the research team know?

- How do the possible risks, side effects, and benefits of this trial compare with those of my current treatment?

- What will I have to do?

- What tests and procedures are involved?

- How often will I have to visit the hospital or clinic?

- Will hospitalization be required?

- How long will the study last?

- Who will pay for my participation?

- Will I be reimbursed for other expenses?

- What type of long-term follow-up care is part of this trial?

- If I benefit from the intervention, will I be allowed to continue receiving it after the trial ends?

- Will results of the study be provided to me?

- Who will oversee my medical care while I am participating in the trial?

- What are my options if I am injured during the study?

Chapter 13

Clinical Trials: An Overview

What Are Clinical Trials and Why Do People Participate?

Clinical trials are part of clinical research and at the heart of all medical advances. Clinical trials look at new ways to prevent, detect, or treat disease. Treatments might be new drugs or new combinations of drugs, new surgical procedures or devices, or new ways to use existing treatments. The goal of clinical trials is to determine if a new test or treatment works and is safe. Clinical trials can also look at other aspects of care, such as improving the quality of life for people with chronic illnesses.

People participate in clinical trials for a variety of reasons. Healthy volunteers say they participate to help others and to contribute to moving science forward. Participants with an illness or disease also participate to help others, but also to possibly receive the newest treatment and to have the additional care and attention from the clinical trial staff. Clinical trials offer hope for many people and an opportunity to help researchers find better treatments for others in the future.

Types of Clinical Trials

There are different types of clinical trials.

- **Natural history studies** provide valuable information about how disease and health progress.

This chapter includes text excerpted from "NIH Clinical Research Trials and You," National Institutes of Health (NIH), April 29, 2016.

- **Prevention trials** look for better ways to prevent a disease in people who have never had the disease or to prevent the disease from returning. Better approaches may include medicines, vaccines, or lifestyle changes, among other things.

- **Screening trials** test the best way to detect certain diseases or health conditions.

- **Diagnostic trials** determine better tests or procedures for diagnosing a particular disease or condition.

- **Treatment trials** test new treatments, new combinations of drugs, or new approaches to surgery or radiation therapy.

- **Quality of life trials** (or supportive care trials) explore and measure ways to improve the comfort and quality of life of people with a chronic illness.

Phases of Clinical Trials

Clinical trials are conducted in "phases." Each phase has a different purpose and helps researchers answer different questions.

- **Phase I trials:** Researchers test an experimental drug or treatment in a small group of people (20–80) for the first time. The purpose is to evaluate its safety and identify side effects.

- **Phase II trials:** The experimental drug or treatment is administered to a larger group of people (100–300) to determine its effectiveness and to further evaluate its safety.

- **Phase III trials:** The experimental drug or treatment is administered to large groups of people (1,000–3,000) to confirm its effectiveness, monitor side effects, compare it with standard or equivalent treatments, and collect information that will allow the experimental drug or treatment to be used safely.

- **Phase IV trials:** After a drug is approved by the U.S. Food and Drug Administration (FDA) and made available to the public, researchers track its safety, seeking more information about a drug or treatment's risks, benefits, and optimal use.

Some Concepts to Understand

Typically, clinical trials compare a new product or therapy with another that already exists to determine if the new one is as successful as, or better than, the existing one. In some studies, participants may be assigned to receive a placebo (an inactive product that resembles the test product, but without its treatment value).

Comparing a new product with a placebo can be the fastest and most reliable way to demonstrate the new product's therapeutic effectiveness. However, placebos are not used if a patient would be put at risk—particularly in the study of treatments for serious illnesses—by not having effective therapy. Most of these studies compare new products with an approved therapy. Potential participants are told if placebos will be used in the study before they enter a trial.

Randomization is the process by which two or more alternative treatments are assigned to volunteers by chance rather than by choice. This is done to avoid any bias with investigators assigning volunteers to one group or another. The results of each treatment are compared at specific points during a trial, which may last for years. When one treatment is found superior, the trial is stopped so that the fewest volunteers receive the less beneficial treatment.

In single-or double-blind studies, also called single-or double-masked studies, the participants do not know which medicine is being used, so they can describe what happens without bias. "Blind" (or "masked") studies are designed to prevent members of the research team or study participants from influencing the results. This allows scientifically accurate conclusions. In single-blind ("single-masked") studies, only the patient is not told what is being administered. In a double-blind study, only the pharmacist knows; members of the research team are not told which patients are getting which medication, so that their observations will not be biased. If medically necessary, however, it is always possible to find out what the patient is taking.

What Do I Need to Know If I Am Thinking about Participating?

Risks and Benefits

Clinical trials involve risks, just as routine medical care and the activities of daily living. When weighing the risks of research, you can consider two important factors:

the degree of harm that could result from participating in the study, and the chance of any harm occurring

Most clinical studies pose the risk of minor discomfort, which lasts only a short time. However, some study participants experience complications that require medical attention. In rare cases, participants have been seriously injured or have died of complications resulting from their participation in trials of experimental therapies. The specific risks associated with a research protocol are described in detail in the informed consent document, which participants are asked to sign before participating in research. Also, a member of the research team explains the major risks of participating in a study and will answer any questions you have about the study. Before deciding to participate, carefully consider possible risks and benefits.

Potential Benefits

Well-designed and well-executed clinical trials provide the best approach for participants to:

- Play an active role in their healthcare.
- Gain access to new research treatments before they are widely available.
- Receive regular and careful medical attention from a research team that includes doctors and other health professionals.
- Help others by contributing to medical research.

Potential Risks

Risks to participating in clinical trials include the following:

- There may be unpleasant, serious, or even life-threatening side effects to experimental treatment.
- The study may require more time and attention than standard treatment would, including visits to the study site, more blood tests, more treatments, hospital stays, or complex dosage requirements.

Chapter 14

Healthcare Quality Issues

Chapter Contents

Section 14.1

Understanding Healthcare Quality

This section includes text excerpted from "Guide to Health Care Quality," Agency for Healthcare Research and Quality (AHRQ), U.S. Department of Health and Human Services (HHS), September 2005. Reviewed January 2017.

You Deserve Quality Healthcare

Getting quality healthcare can help you stay healthy and recover faster when you become sick. However, we know that often, people do not get high-quality care.

What exactly is healthcare quality? We know that quality means different things to different people. Some people think that getting quality healthcare means seeing the doctor right away, being treated courteously by the doctor's staff, or having the doctor spend a lot of time with them. While these things are important to all of us, clinical quality of care is even more important. Think of it like this: getting quality healthcare is like taking your car to a mechanic. The people in the shop can be friendly and listen to your complaints, but the most important thing is whether they fix the problem with your car. Healthcare providers, the government, and many other groups are working hard to improve healthcare quality. You also have a role to play to make sure you and your family members receive the best quality care possible.

Be Active: Take Charge of Your Healthcare

The single, most important thing you can do to ensure you get high quality healthcare is to find and use health information and take an active role in making decisions about your care. Here are some steps you can take to improve your care:

- Work together with your doctor and other members of the healthcare team to make decisions about your care.

- Be sure to ask questions.

- Ask your doctor what the scientific evidence has to say about your condition.

- Do your homework; go online or to the library to find out more information about your condition.

- Find and use quality information in making healthcare choices. Be sure the information comes from a reliable source.

Talking with Your Doctor

Here are some examples of questions to ask your doctor. It is not a complete list. You will probably have many other questions. You should keep asking questions until you understand what is wrong with you and what you need to do to get better.

Understand your diagnosis:

- What is wrong with me?

- What do I need to do to get better?

- Where can I get more information about my condition?

If you need a lab test, an X-ray, or another kind of test, ask your doctor:

- How will the test be done?

- How accurate will the results be?

- What are the benefits and risks of the test?

- When and how will I receive the results?

- What should I do if I don't receive the results?

If you receive a prescription for a new medicine:

- What is the name of the medicine?

- What is it supposed to do?

- When should I take the medicine, and how much should I take?

- Does the medicine have any side effects?

If you need surgery:

- What kind of operation do I need?

- Why do I need an operation?

- What are the benefits and risks of the operation?

- How long will it take to recover?

- What will happen if I don't have the operation?

- Are there any other treatments I could have instead of an operation?

- Where can I get a second opinion?

Making Strategic Choices

Research has shown that science-based measures can be used to assess quality for various conditions and for specific types of care. For example, quality healthcare is:

- Doing the right thing (getting the healthcare services you need).

- At the right time (when you need them).

- In the right way (using the appropriate test or procedure).

- To achieve the best possible results.

- Providing quality healthcare also means striking the right balance of services by:

- Avoiding underuse (for example, not screening a person for high blood pressure).

- Avoiding overuse (for example, performing tests that a patient doesn't need).

- Eliminating misuse (for example, providing medications that may have dangerous interactions).

- We would like to think that every doctor, nurse, pharmacist, hospital, and other provider gives high-quality care, but we know this is not always the case. Quality varies depending on where you live. Quality can vary from one State to another, and it can vary from one doctor's office across the street to another. Healthcare quality varies widely and for many reasons.

For example, timely receipt of clot-busting drugs can save lives for patients suffering heart attacks. The national standard for providing clot-busting drugs is within 30 minutes of a patient's arrival at the hospital. But we know that this varies widely across States, from a low of 20 minutes in one State to a high of 140 minutes in another.

Efforts to Improve Healthcare Quality

Improving healthcare quality is a team effort, and it is ongoing on many levels. To succeed, every part of the healthcare system must become involved, including government and nongovernment organizations, doctors, nurses, pharmacists, hospitals, other providers, and you, the patient.

One way to assess and track quality of care is by using measures that are based on the latest scientific evidence. A healthcare measure clearly defines which healthcare services should be provided to patients who have or are at risk for certain conditions. Measures also set standards for screening, immunizations, and other preventive care.

There are two types of measures: clinical measures and consumer ratings. Because measures are intended to set general standards for a broad population, they may or may not apply to you. Always check with your doctor about your level of risk for a particular condition and which types of screening and tests you should have.

Clinical Measures

Clinical measures can be used to assess quality of care and patient satisfaction. Examples are provided here of measures that can be used to assess care quality for three of the most common conditions: diabetes, heart disease, and cancer.

Diabetes

Diabetes is the leading cause of blindness, leg amputation not resulting from trauma, and kidney disease. Diabetes increases the risk of complications in pregnant women, and it is a risk factor for heart disease and stroke. People who have diabetes are two to four times as likely to die from heart disease or stroke as those without diabetes.

The following five measures can be used to assess quality of care for diabetes. If you have diabetes, you should receive the following tests and exams:

- Regular hemoglobin A1C (blood glucose) testing.

- Regular cholesterol testing.

- Annual retinal eye exam.

- Annual foot exam.

- Flu shot each year.

Heart Disease

Heart disease—or cardiovascular disease—is a collection of diseases of the heart and blood vessels that includes heart attack, stroke, and heart failure. Heart disease is the number one cause of death in the United States. Maintaining control of blood pressure and cholesterol can help you prevent heart attack and stroke.

The following are examples of measures that can be used to assess care for heart disease.

For adults age 18 and older:

* Blood pressure measurement.

* Cholesterol testing.

In general:

* If you smoke, being advised to stop smoking.

* If you suffer a heart attack, receiving aspirin within 24 hours of hospital admission and being prescribed beta-blocker therapy at hospital discharge.

Cancer

Cancer is the Nation's second leading cause of death, after heart disease. Screening to permit early detection holds the most promise for successful cancer treatment.

Talk to your doctor about screening tests for all of these cancers, especially if other members of your family have had these cancers or if you smoke.

The following are examples of quality measures for several types of cancer screening.

Breast and cervical cancer

* Mammography exam for women age 40 and older.

* Pap smear testing for women age 18 and older.

Colorectal cancer. Men and women age 50 and older should receive the following tests:

* Fecal occult blood testing (a test to detect blood in the stool).

* Flexible sigmoidoscopy/colonoscopy exam. Check with your doctor about how often you should have this screening.

Finding Quality Information

Today, you can find a great deal of information about healthcare quality, both online and in print. New tools and resources for assessing and improving healthcare quality are being developed.

Report Cards

Reports cards and other quality reports include consumer ratings, clinical performance measures, or both. They can help you select the right treatment and the right healthcare provider based on what is most important to you. You may be able to get quality reports from:

- **Your employer:** Ask your personnel office for information on health plans.

- **Health plans:** Ask the plan's customer service office about quality reports.

- **Other healthcare providers:** Hospitals, nursing homes, and community health clinics may have quality reports.

Several government agencies publish quality reports and other types of quality information. For example, the Centers for Medicare and Medicaid Services (CMS) has detailed information on the past performance of every Medicare and Medicaid certified nursing home in the country. This tool is available online at www.medicare.gov/hospitalcompare/search.html.

Accreditation

Accreditation is another indicator that can be used to judge quality. Accreditation is a "seal of approval" given by a private, independent group. Healthcare organizations—such as hospitals—must meet national standards, including clinical performance measures, in order to be accredited.

Accreditation reports present quality information on hospitals, nursing homes, and other healthcare facilities. For example, the Joint Commission on Accreditation of Healthcare Organizations (JCAHO) prepares a performance report on each hospital that it surveys.

Another group, the National Committee for Quality Assurance (NCQA), rates health plans like Health Maintenance Organization's (HMO). NCQA's Health Plan Report Card presents accreditation results for hundreds of health plans across the country.

If you need help in finding quality reports, accreditation reports, or other types of quality information, check with your local library or your local or State health department. You can find your State health department listed in the blue pages of your phone book.

Consumer Ratings

Consumer ratings tell you what other people like you think about their healthcare. Some consumer ratings focus on health plans. For example, a survey called Consumer Assessment of Healthcare Providers and Systems (CAHPS®) asks people about the quality of care in their own health plans. Their answers can help you decide whether you want to join one of those plans. It will ask patients about their experiences with hospital care.

Choosing Quality Healthcare

Here are some tips for making quality a key factor in the healthcare decisions you make about health plans, doctors, treatments, hospitals, and long-term care.

Look for a health plan that:

- Has been given high ratings by its members on the things that are important to you.

- Has the doctors and hospitals you want or need.

- Provides the benefits (covered services) you need.

- Provides services where and when you need them.

- Has a documented history of doing a good job of preventing and treating illness.

Look for a doctor who:

- Has received high ratings for quality of care.

- Has the training and experience to meet your needs.

- Will work with you to make decisions about your healthcare.

If you become ill, make sure you understand:

- Your diagnosis.

- How soon you need to be treated.

- Your treatment choices, including the benefits and risks of each treatment.

- How much experience your doctor has in treating your condition.

  Look for a hospital that:

- Is accredited by the Joint Commission on Accreditation of Healthcare Organizations (JCAHO).

- Is rated highly by the State and by consumer groups or other organizations.

- Has a lot of experience and success in treating your condition.

- Monitors quality of care and works to improve quality.

In choosing a nursing home or other long-term care facility, look for one that:

- Has been found by State agencies and other groups to provide quality care.

- Provides a level of care, including staff and services that will meet your needs.

Section 14.2

Identifying Quality Laboratory Services

This section includes text excerpted from "Laboratory Quality Assurance and Standardization Programs," Centers for Disease Control and Prevention (CDC), July 29, 2014.

More than a billion laboratory tests that identify and measure chemicals, such as lead or cholesterol, are performed each year in the United States. Such test results have a significant influence on medical decisions.

Given the importance of laboratory test results, the Centers for Disease Control and Prevention's (CDC) National Center for Environmental Health (NCEH) has programs to help assure the quality of

101

these data so patients and healthcare providers (as well as researchers and public health officials) can be confident that laboratory test results they receive are accurate. These CDC programs focus specifically on laboratory tests that are related to chronic diseases, newborn screening disorders, nutritional status, and environmental exposures.

Quality Assurance

Laboratory Quality Assurance (QA) encompasses a range of activities that enable laboratories to achieve and maintain high levels of accuracy and proficiency despite changes in test methods and the volume of specimens tested. A good QA system does these four things:

- Establishes standard operating procedures (SOPs) for each step of the laboratory testing process, ranging from specimen handling to instrument performance validation;

- Defines administrative requirements, such as mandatory record-keeping, data evaluation, and internal audits to monitor adherence to SOPs;

- Specifies corrective actions, documentation, and the persons responsible for carrying out corrective actions when problems are identified; and

- Sustains high-quality employee performance.

Laboratory Standardization

Laboratory Standardization is achieved when test results with the same high levels of accuracy and precision can be reproduced across measurement systems, laboratories, and over time. Standardization depends on a rigorous process using:

- Reference material—a sample of the analyte with a precisely known composition, which can be used to calibrate laboratory instruments and validate test protocols;

- A reference measurement procedure (RMP)—the "gold standard" measurement system for a particular analyte; and

- Secondary measurement procedures—validated using reference material and RMP. These procedures may be less sophisticated than the RMP, but they are usually more easily implemented by a larger number of laboratories.

Well-executed standardization programs greatly improve the quality of laboratory measurements that are used to detect signs of illnesses and to guide interventions to prevent or treat illnesses. Standardization also ensures the production of credible and comparable data across laboratories—a boon to epidemiologists and researchers who may need to pool data from multiple sources.

CDC offers customized QA and standardization programs to help laboratories improve the quality and reliability of their measurement procedures. The specific CDC services that are offered are:

- Reference materials

- Proficiency testing

- Training

- Guidelines

- Consultations

Each CDC laboratory QA and standardization program is voluntary and most are free of charge.

Section 14.3

Patient Safety in Ambulatory Care

This section includes text excerpted from "Patient Safety in Ambulatory Care," Agency for Healthcare Research and Quality (AHRQ), U.S. Department of Health and Human Services (HHS), July 2016.

Factors Influencing Safety in Ambulatory Care

Ensuring patient safety outside of the hospital setting poses unique challenges for both providers and patients. A recent article proposed a model for patient safety in chronic disease management, modified from the original Chronic Care Model (CCM). This model broadly encompasses three concepts that influence safety in ambulatory care:

- the role of patient and caregiver behaviors

- the role of provider–patient interactions
- the role of the community and health system
- specific types of errors can be linked to each of these three concepts

Types of Safety Events in Ambulatory Care

Since face-to-face interactions between providers and patients in the ambulatory setting are limited and occur weeks to months apart, patients must assume a much greater role in and responsibility for managing their own health. This elevates the importance of including the patient as a partner and ensuring that patients understand their illnesses and treatments.

The need for outpatients to self-manage their own chronic diseases requires that they monitor their symptoms and, in some cases, adjust their own lifestyle or medications. For example, a patient with diabetes must measure her own blood sugars and perhaps adjust her insulin dose based on blood sugar values and dietary intake. A patient's inability or failure to perform such activities may compromise safety in the short term and clinical outcomes in the long term. Patients must also understand how and when to contact their caregivers outside of routine appointments, and they must often play a role in ensuring their own care coordination (e.g., by keeping an updated list of medications).

The nature of interactions between patients and providers—and between different providers—may also be a source of adverse events. Patients consistently voice concerns about coordination of care, particularly when one patient sees multiple physicians, and indeed communication between physicians in the outpatient setting is often suboptimal. Poorly handled care transitions (e.g., when a patient is discharged from the hospital or when care is transferred from one physician to another) also place patients at high risk for preventable adverse events. When a clinician is not immediately available—for example, after hours—patients may have to rely on telephone advice for acute illnesses, an everyday practice that has its own inherent risks.

Underlying health system flaws have been documented to increase the risk for medical errors, particularly medication errors and diagnostic errors, issues that are certainly germane to ambulatory safety. Medication errors are very common in ambulatory care, with one landmark study finding that more than 4.5 million ambulatory care visits occur every year due to adverse drug events. Likewise, prescribing errors are startlingly common in ambulatory practice. Because the likelihood of a medication error is linked to a patient's understanding of the indication, dosage schedule, proper administration, and potential adverse effects, low health literacy and poor patient education contribute to elevated error risk.

The fragmentation of ambulatory care in outpatient settings increases the challenge of making a timely and accurate diagnosis. Indeed, a recent study estimated that 5 percent of adults in the United States experience a missed or delayed diagnosis each year. Recent data suggests that timely information availability and managing test results contribute to delayed and missed diagnoses in outpatient care. Although use of electronic health records in the ambulatory setting is growing, many practices still lack reliable systems for following up on test results—a problem that has been implicated in missed and delayed diagnoses.

Finally, while an increasing amount of attention has been devoted to measuring and improving the culture of safety in acute care settings, less is known about safety culture in office practice. Burnout and work dissatisfaction, particularly among primary care physicians, may adversely affect the quality of care.

Improving Safety in Ambulatory Care

Improving outpatient safety will require both structural reform of office practice functions as well as engagement of patients in their own safety. While Electronic Health Records (EHRs) hold great promise for reducing medication errors and tracking test results, these systems have yet to reach their full potential. Coordinating care between different physicians remains a significant challenge, especially if the doctors do not work in the same office or share the same medical record system. Efforts are being made to increase use of EHRs in ambulatory care, and physicians believe that use of EHRs leads to higher quality and improved safety.

Patient engagement in outpatient safety involves two related concepts: first, educating patients about their illnesses and medications, using methods that require patients to demonstrate understanding (such as "teach-back"); and second, empowering patients and caregivers to act as a safety "double-check" by providing access to advice and test results and encouraging patients to ask questions about their care. Success has been achieved in this area for patients taking high-risk medications, even in patients with low health literacy at baseline.

Current Context

Although efforts to improve safety have largely focused on hospital care, The Joint Commission now publishes National Patient Safety Goals focused on ambulatory care. The Agency for Healthcare Research and Quality (AHRQ) is also leading efforts to improve ambulatory quality and safety through programs and research funding.

Chapter 15

Hospitalization

Chapter Contents

Section 15.1

Choosing a Hospital

This section includes text excerpted from "Guide to Choosing a Hospital," Centers for Medicare and Medicaid Services (CMS), May 2010. Reviewed January 2017.

Most people check restaurant ratings or read consumer reviews before they make a choice. Shouldn't you also check the quality of the hospitals you rely on when you need medical care?

In an emergency, your life may depend on getting to the nearest hospital. When you can plan ahead, you and your doctor should discuss which hospital will best meet your healthcare needs. Information is available to help you make an informed choice. Whether you have Medicare or another type of insurance, this section can help you find and use information about hospital quality.

Steps to Choosing a Hospital

When you're sick, you may go to the closest hospital or the hospital where your doctor practices. But which hospital is the best for your individual needs? Research now shows that some hospitals do a better job taking care of patients with certain conditions than other hospitals.

When you have a life-threatening emergency, always go to the nearest hospital. Understanding your choices will help you have a more informed discussion with your doctor or other healthcare provider.

Before You Get Started

Make the most of your appointments with your doctor or other healthcare provider to learn about your condition and healthcare needs:

- Before your appointment, make a list of things you want to talk about (such as recent symptoms, drug side effects, or other general health questions). Bring this list to your appointment.

- Bring any prescription drugs, over-the-counter drugs, vitamins, and supplements to your appointment and review them with your doctor or provider.

- During your appointment, take notes. Then, take a moment to repeat back to the doctor or provider what you were told. Ask any questions you may have.

- Consider bringing along a trusted family member or friend.

- Ask if there's any written information about your condition that you can take with you.

- Call the office if you have questions when you get home.

Steps to Choosing a Hospital Checklist

Step One: Learn about the care you need and your hospital choices.

Talk to your doctor/healthcare provider about the following:

- Find out which hospitals they work with.

- Ask which hospitals they think give the best care for your condition (for example, have enough staffing, coordinate care, promote medication safety, and prevent infection).

- Ask how well these hospitals check and improve their quality of care. Do the hospitals participate in Medicare?

Based on your condition, ask your doctor/healthcare provider questions such as:

- Which hospitals have the best experience with your condition?

- Should you consider a specialty hospital, teaching hospital (usually part of a university), community hospital, or one that does research or has clinical trials related to your condition?

- If you need a surgeon or other type of specialist, what is his or her experience and success treating your condition?

- Who will be responsible for your overall care while you're in the hospital?

- Will you need care after leaving the hospital and, if so, what kind of care? Who will arrange this care?

- Are there any alternatives to hospital care?

Step Two: Think about your personal and financial needs.
Check your hospital insurance coverage:

- Do you need permission from your health plan (like a pre-authorization or a referral) before you're admitted for hospital care?

- If you need care that's not emergency care, do you have to use certain hospitals? Do you have to see certain surgeons or specialists?

- Do you have to pay more to use a hospital (surgeon or specialist) that doesn't participate in your plan?

- Do you need to meet certain requirements to get care after you leave the hospital?

- If you don't have insurance, call the hospital before you're admitted, and ask to speak to someone about setting up a payment plan or other resources to help with payment.

Think about your preferences:

- Do you want a hospital near family members or friends?

- Does the hospital have convenient visiting hours and other rules that are important to you? For example, can a relative or someone helping with your care stay overnight in the room with you?

Step Three: Find and compare hospitals based on your condition and needs.
Use the **Hospital Compare** web tool at www.medicare.gov/hospitalcompare/search.aspx to do the following and more:

- Find hospitals by name, city, county, state, or Zone Improvement Plan (ZIP) code.

- Check the results of patient surveys (what patients said about their hospital experiences).

- Compare the results of certain measures of quality that show how well these hospitals treat certain conditions.

- Search online for other sources to compare the quality of the hospitals you're considering. Some states have laws that require hospitals to report data about the quality and cost of their care and post the data online.

Step Four: Discuss your hospital options, and choose a hospital.

- Talk with family members or friends about the hospitals you're comparing.

- Talk to your doctor or healthcare provider how the hospital information you gathered applies to you.

- Choose the hospital that's best for you.

Hospital Quality Quick Check

Look for a hospital that:

- Has the best experience with your condition.

- Checks and improves the quality of its care.

- Performs well on measures of quality, including a national patient survey, that are published on the Hospital Compare web tool. Visit www.medicare.gov/hospitalcompare/search.aspx.

- Participate in Medicare.

- Meets your needs in terms of location and other factors, like visiting hours.

- Is covered by your health plan.

Section 15.2

Basics of a Hospital Stay

This section includes text excerpted from "Hospitalization Happens: A Guide to Hospital Visits for Individuals with Memory Loss," National Institute on Aging (NIA), National Institutes of Health (NIH), August 11, 2016.

Before a Hospital Stay

If your relative is going to the hospital for a planned stay, you have time to prepare and get more information from your doctor. Ask your doctor if the procedure can be done as an outpatient visit. If not, ask if tests can be done before going to the hospital to shorten the hospital

111

stay. Ask if your doctor plans to talk with other doctors. If so, find out if your care partner can see these specialists before going into the hospital.

Build a team for care and support during a hospital stay. Develop roles for each person (spokesperson, hands-on caregivers, comfort people, home and personal affairs manager, communication center person). Do not try to do it alone. Now may be the time to have one-on-one caregivers on site if money or resources permit. They can help make sure medications and/or physical restraints are not used to control behaviors that can be managed with redirection or distraction.

Before your hospital visit, prepare a list of questions and concerns for your doctor.

Before Going to the Hospital

- If your insurance allows, ask if a private room is available. It will be more quiet and calm. Request a reclining chair or bed for you or a companion/respite provider.

- Shortly before going to the hospital, decide the best way to tell your care partner that the two of you are going to spend a short time in the hospital.

- Involve your care partner in the planning process as much as possible.

- Do not talk about the hospital stay in front of your care partner as if he or she is not there! This can be upsetting and embarrassing.

- Plan ahead. Make a schedule with family, friends and/or a professional respite care provider to take turns staying with your care partner while in the hospital. This is particularly important if your relative needs continuous supervision.

During the Hospital Stay

- Ask the hospital staff to avoid using physical restraints.

- Have a family member, trusted friend or hired caregiver with your care partner at all times if possible—even during medical tests. This may be hard to do, but it will help keep your care partner calm and less frightened, making the hospital stay easier.

- Use a "telephone tree," email or online tools to keep others posted of progress. This can greatly reduce stress and make sure that you do not receive calls just as you get your care partner settled down. You may need to turn the ringer on the phone down or off during rest times.

- Ask doctors to limit the questions directed to your relative, who may not be able to answer accurately. Instead, arrange to answer questions from the doctor in private, outside your care partner's room.

- Modify the hospital room for best performance.

- Help your relative fill out menu requests. Open food containers and remove trays. Assist with eating as needed.

- Remind your care partner to drink fluids. Offer fluids regularly and have him or her make frequent trips to the bathroom.

- Assume your care partner will experience difficulty finding the bathroom and/or using a call button, bed adjustment buttons or the phone.

- Communicate with your care partner in the way he or she will best understand or respond.

- Recognize that an unfamiliar place, medicines, invasive tests and surgery will make a person with dementia more confused. Your relative will likely need more assistance with personal care activities.

- Take deep breaths and schedule breaks for yourself.

- Be aware of acute or sudden confusion or delirium, which can be caused by serious medical problems such as fever, infection, medications and/or dehydration. Inform the doctor as soon as possible if your care partner seems suddenly worse or different. Make sure you advocate for the person you are caring for—others may not recognize the difference in your relative's condition.

Section 15.3

Medicare and Hospital Expenses

This section includes text excerpted from "Are You a Hospital
Inpatient or Outpatient?" Centers for Medicare
and Medicaid Services (CMS), May 2014.

If You Have Medicare—Ask!

Did you know that even if you stay in a hospital overnight, you might
still be considered an "outpatient?" Your hospital status (whether the
hospital considers you an "inpatient" or "outpatient") affects how much
you pay for hospital services (like X-rays, drugs, and lab tests) and
may also affect whether Medicare will cover care you get in a skilled
nursing facility (SNF) following your hospital stay.

- You're an inpatient starting when you're formally admitted to a
  hospital with a doctor's order. The day before you're discharged
  is your last inpatient day.

- You're an outpatient if you're getting emergency department
  services, observation services, outpatient surgery, lab tests,
  X-rays, or any other hospital services, and the doctor hasn't
  written an order to admit you to a hospital as an inpatient. In
  these cases, you're an outpatient even if you spend the night at
  the hospital.

Observation services are hospital outpatient services given to help
the doctor decide if the patient needs to be admitted as an inpatient or
can be discharged. Observation services may be given in the emergency
department or another area of the hospital.

The decision for inpatient hospital admission is a complex medical
decision based on your doctor's judgment and your need for medically
necessary hospital care. An inpatient admission is generally appropriate when you're expected to need 2 or more midnights of medically
necessary hospital care, but your doctor must order such admission
and the hospital must formally admit you in order for you to become
an inpatient.

Read on to understand the differences in Original Medicare coverage for hospital inpatients and outpatients, and how these rules apply to some common situations. If you have a Medicare Advantage Plan (like an HMO or PPO), your costs and coverage may be different. Check with your plan.

What Do I Pay as an Inpatient?

Medicare Part A (Hospital Insurance) covers inpatient hospital services. Generally, this means you pay a one-time deductible for all of your hospital services for the first 60 days you're in a hospital.

Medicare Part B (Medical Insurance) covers most of your doctor services when you're an inpatient. You pay 20 percent of the Medicare-approved amount for doctor services after paying the Part B deductible.

What Do I Pay as an Outpatient?

Part B covers outpatient hospital services. Generally, this means you pay a copayment for each individual outpatient hospital service. This amount may vary by service.

The copayment for a single outpatient hospital service can't be more than the inpatient hospital deductible. However, your total copayment for all outpatient services may be more than the inpatient hospital deductible.

Part B also covers most of your doctor services when you're a hospital outpatient. You pay 20 percent of the Medicare-approved amount after you pay the Part B deductible.

Generally, prescription and over-the-counter drugs you get in an outpatient setting (like an emergency department), sometimes called "self-administered drugs," aren't covered by Part B. Also, for safety reasons, many hospitals have policies that don't allow patients to bring prescription or other drugs from home.

If you have Medicare prescription drug coverage (Part D), these drugs may be covered under certain circumstances. You'll likely need to pay out-of-pocket for these drugs and submit a claim to your drug plan for a refund. Call your drug plan for more information.

Here are some common hospital situations and a description of how Medicare will pay. Remember, you pay deductibles, coinsurance, and copayments.

Table 15.1. Common Hospital Situations and Medicare

Situation	Inpatient or outpatient	Part A pays	Part B pays
You're in the emergency department (ED) (also known as the emergency room or "ER") and then you're formally admitted to the hospital with a doctor's order	Outpatient until you're formally admitted as an inpatient based on your doctor's order. Inpatient following such admission.	Your inpatient hospital stay	Your doctor services
You visit the ED and are sent to the intensive care unit (ICU) for close monitoring. Your doctor expects you to be sent home the next morning unless your condition worsens. Your condition resolves and you're sent home the next day.	Outpatient	Nothing	Your doctor services
You come to the ED with chest pain and the hospital keeps you for 2 nights. One night is spent in observation and the doctor writes an order for inpatient admission on the second day	Outpatient until you're formally admitted as an inpatient based on your doctor's order. Inpatient following such admission.	Your inpatient hospital stay	Doctor services and hospital outpatient services (for example, ED visit, observation services, lab tests, or EKGs)

Table 15.1. Continued

Situation	Inpatient or outpatient	Part A pays	Part B pays
You go to a hospital for outpatient surgery, but they keep you overnight for high blood pressure. Your doctor doesn't write an order to admit you as an inpatient. You go home the next day.	Outpatient	Nothing	Doctor services and hospital outpatient services (for example, surgery, lab tests, or intravenous medicines)
Your doctor writes an order for you to be admitted as an inpatient, and the hospital later tells you it's changing your hospital status to outpatient. Your doctor must agree, and he hospital must tell you in writing– while you're still a hospital patient before you're discharged–that your hospital status changed	Outpatient	Nothing	Doctor services and hospital outpatient services

Even if you stay overnight in a regular hospital bed, you might be an outpatient. Ask the doctor or hospital.

How Would My Hospital Status Affect the Way Medicare Covers My Care in a Skilled Nursing Facility (SNF)?

Medicare will only cover care you get in a SNF if you first have a "qualifying inpatient hospital stay."

- A qualifying inpatient hospital stay means you've been a **hospital inpatient (you were formally admitted to the**

117

hospital after your doctor writes an inpatient admission order) for at least 3 days in a row (counting the day you were admitted as an inpatient, but not counting the day of your discharge).

- If you don't have a 3-day inpatient hospital stay and you need care after your discharge from a hospital, ask if you can get care in other settings (like home healthcare) or if any other programs (like Medicaid or Veterans' benefits) can cover your SNF care. **Always ask your doctor or hospital staff if Medicare will cover your SNF stay.**

How Would Hospital Observation Services Affect My SNF Coverage?

Your doctor may order "observation services" to help decide whether you need to be admitted to a hospital as an inpatient or can be discharged. During the time you're getting observation services in a hospital, you're considered an outpatient. This means you can't count this time towards the 3-day inpatient hospital stay needed for Medicare to cover your SNF stay.

Here are some common hospital situations that may affect your SNF coverage:

Table 15.2. Common Hospital Situations That Affect SNF Coverage

Situation	Is my SNF stay covered?
You came to the ED and were formally admitted to the hospital with a doctor's order as an inpatient for 3 days. You were discharged on the 4th day.	Yes. You met the 3-day inpatient hospital stay requirement for a covered SNF stay.
You came to the ED and spent one day getting observation services. Then, you were formally admitted to the hospital as an inpatient for 2 more days.	No. Even though you spent 3 days in the hospital, you were considered an outpatient while getting ED and observation services. These days don't count toward the 3-day inpatient hospital stay requirement.

Any days you spend in a hospital as an outpatient (before you're formally admitted as an inpatient based on the doctor's order) aren't counted as inpatient days. An inpatient stay begins on the day you're formally admitted to a hospital with a doctor's order. That's your first inpatient day. The day of discharge doesn't count as an inpatient day.

What Are My Rights?

No matter what type of Medicare coverage you have, you have certain guaranteed rights. As a person with Medicare, you have the right to all of these:

- Have your questions about Medicare answered.

- Learn about all of your treatment choices and participate in treatment decisions.

- Get a decision about healthcare payment or services, or prescription drug coverage.

- Get a review of (appeal) certain decisions about healthcare payment, coverage of services, or prescription drug coverage.

- File complaints (sometimes called "grievances"), including complaints about the quality of your care.

Where Can I Get More Help?

- If you need help understanding your hospital status, speak to your doctor or someone from the hospital's utilization or discharge planning department.

- For more information about coverage of self-administered drugs, view the publication "How Medicare Covers Self-administered Drugs Given in Hospital Outpatient Settings" by visiting Medicare.gov/publications, or call 1-800-MEDICARE for a free copy.

- To ask questions or report complaints about the quality of care of a Medicare-covered service, call your Quality Improvement Organization (QIO). Visit Medicare.gov/contacts, or call 1-800-MEDICARE to get the phone number.

- To ask questions or report complaints about the quality of care or the quality of life in a nursing home, call your State Survey Agency. Visit Medicare.gov/contacts, or call 1-800-MEDICARE to get the phone number.

Chapter 16

Surgery

Chapter Contents

Section 16.1

What You Need to Know about Surgery

This section includes text excerpted from "Considering Surgery?"
National Institute on Aging (NIA), National Institutes of Health
(NIH), May 2008. Reviewed January 2017.

Deciding to have surgery can be hard, but it may be easier once
you know why you need surgery. Talk with your surgeon about the
operation. It may help to take a member of your family or a friend
with you. Don't hesitate to ask the surgeon any questions you might
have. For example, do the benefits of surgery outweigh the risks? Risks
may include infections, bleeding a lot, or a reaction to the anesthesia
(medicine that puts you to sleep).

Questions to Ask

Your surgeon should be willing to answer your questions. If you
don't understand the answers, ask the surgeon to explain more clearly.
Answers to the following questions will help you make an informed
decision about your treatment:

- What is the surgery? Do I need it now, or can I wait?

- Can another treatment be tried instead of surgery?

- How will the surgery affect my health and lifestyle?

- What kind of anesthesia will be used? What are the side effects
  and risks of having anesthesia?

- Will I be in pain? How long will the pain last?

- When will I be able to go home after the surgery?

- What will the recovery be like? How long will it take to feel
  better?

- What will happen if I don't have the surgery?

- Is there anything else I should know about this surgery?

Choosing a Surgeon

Your primary care doctor may suggest a surgeon to you. Your state or local medical society can tell you about your surgeon's training. Try to choose a surgeon who operates often on medical problems like yours.

Getting a Second Opinion

Getting a second opinion means asking another doctor about your surgical plan. It is a common medical practice. Most doctors think it's a good idea. With a second opinion, you will get expert advice from another surgeon who knows about treating your medical problem. A second opinion can help you make a good decision.

Informed Consent

Before having any surgery, you will be asked to sign a consent form. This form says that the surgeon has told you about the operation, the risks involved, and what results to expect. It's important to talk about all your concerns before signing this form. Your surgeon should be willing to take the time needed to make sure you know what is likely to happen before, during, and after surgery.

Outpatient Surgery

Outpatient surgery, sometimes called same-day surgery, is common for many types of operations. Outpatient surgery can be done in a special part of the hospital or in a surgical center. You will go home within hours after the surgery. Outpatient surgery can cost less than an overnight hospital stay. Your doctor will tell you if outpatient surgery is right for you.

Planning for Surgery

There are many steps you can take to make having surgery a little easier.

Before surgery:

- Make sure you have your pre-operation tests and screenings, such as blood tests and X-rays.

- Be sure you have all your insurance questions answered.

- Make plans for any medical equipment or help with healthcare you will need when you go home.

- Arrange for an adult to drive you home and stay with you for the first 24 hours after surgery.

- Get written instructions about your care, a phone number to call if you have a problem, and prescription medicines you'll need at home.

The day of surgery:

- Leave your jewelry at home.

- Don't wear make-up or contact lenses to surgery.

Following surgery:

- Make sure you follow all your doctor's directions once you're home.

- Go for your scheduled post-operative check-up.

- Ask your doctor when you can return to your normal activities.

Paying for Surgery

The total cost of any surgery includes many different bills. Your surgeon can tell you how much he or she charges. You may also be billed by other doctors, such as the anesthesiologist. There will be hospital charges as well. To find out what the hospital will cost, call the hospital's business office.

For information about Medicare benefits, call the toll-free customer service line at 800-633-4227. If you have secondary or supplemental health insurance, check to see what part of the costs it will pay. Talk to your surgeon if you can't afford the surgery.

In Case of Emergency Surgery

An accident or sudden illness may result in emergency surgery. That's why you should always carry the following information with you:

- your doctor's name and phone number

- family names and phone numbers

- ongoing medical problems

- medicines you take, including prescription and over-the-counter drugs
- allergies to medicines
- health insurance information and policy numbers

Section 16.2

Wrong-Site Surgery

This section includes text excerpted from "Wrong-Site, Wrong-Procedure, and Wrong-Patient Surgery," Agency for Healthcare Research and Quality (AHRQ), U.S. Department of Health and Human Services (HHS), July 2016.

Few medical errors are as vivid and terrifying as those that involve patients who have undergone surgery on the wrong body part, undergone the incorrect procedure, or had a procedure intended for another patient. These "wrong-site, wrong-procedure, wrong-patient errors" (WSPEs) are rightly termed never events—errors that should never occur and indicate serious underlying safety problems.

Wrong-site surgery may involve operating on the wrong side, as in the case of a patient who had the right side of her vulva removed when the cancerous lesion was on the left, or the incorrect body site. One example of surgery on the incorrect site is operating on the wrong level of the spine, a surprisingly common issue for neurosurgeons. A classic case of wrong-patient surgery involved a patient who underwent a cardiac procedure intended for another patient with a similar last name.

While much publicity has been given to these high-profile cases of WSPEs, these errors are in fact relatively rare. A seminal study estimated that such errors occur in approximately 1 of 112,000 surgical procedures, infrequent enough that an individual hospital would only experience one such error every 5–10 years. However, this estimate only included procedures performed in the operating room; if procedures performed in other settings (for example, ambulatory surgery or interventional radiology) are included, the rate of such errors may be significantly higher. One study using Veterans Affairs (VA) data found that fully half of WSPEs occurred during procedures outside of the operating room.

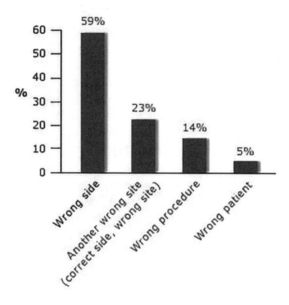

Figure 16.1. *Types of Wrong-Site Surgery Observed by Orthopedic Surgeons*

Preventing Wrong-Site, Wrong-Procedure, and Wrong-Patient Surgery

Early efforts to prevent WSPEs focused on developing redundant mechanisms for identifying the correct site, procedure, and patient, such as "sign your site" initiatives, that instructed surgeons to mark the operative site in an unambiguous fashion. However, it soon became clear that even this seemingly simple intervention was problematic. An analysis of the United Kingdom's efforts to prevent WSPEs found that, although dissemination of a site-marking protocol did increase use of preoperative site marking, implementation and adherence to the protocol differed significantly across surgical specialties and hospitals, and many clinicians voiced concerns about unintended consequences of the protocol. In some cases, there was even confusion over whether the marked site indicates the area to be operated on, or the area to be avoided. Site marking remains a core component of the Joint Commission's Universal Protocol to prevent WSPEs.

Root cause analyses of WSPEs consistently reveal communication issues as a prominent underlying factor. The concept of the surgical time out—a planned pause before beginning the procedure in order to review important aspects of the procedure with all involved personnel—was developed to improve communication in the operating room and prevent WSPEs. The Universal Protocol also specifies use of a timeout prior to all procedures. Although initially designed for operating room procedures, timeouts are now required before any invasive procedure. Comprehensive efforts to improve surgical safety have incorporated timeout principles into surgical safety checklists; while these checklists have been proven to improve surgical and postoperative safety, the low baseline incidence of WSPEs makes it difficult to establish that a single intervention can reduce or eliminate WSPEs.

It is worth noting, however, that many cases of WSPEs would still occur despite full adherence to the Universal Protocol. Errors may happen well before the patient reaches the operating room, a timeout may be rushed or otherwise ineffective, and production pressures may contribute to errors during the procedure itself. Ultimately, preventing WSPEs depends on the combination of system solutions, strong teamwork and safety culture, and individual vigilance.

In February 2009, the Centers for Medicare and Medicaid Services (CMS) announced that hospitals will not be reimbursed for any costs associated with WSPEs. (CMS has not reimbursed hospitals for additional costs associated with many preventable errors since 2007.)

Section 16.3

Anesthesia Basics

This section includes text excerpted from "Anesthesia
Fact Sheet," National Institute of General Medical
Sciences (NIGMS), June 22, 2016.

What Is Anesthesia?

Anesthesia is a medical treatment that prevents patients from feeling pain during surgery. Anesthesia has made possible countless procedures that improve human health, longevity and quality of life. Every year, millions of Americans safely undergo surgery with anesthesia, although some risks exist.

Anesthesia consists of several components, including sedation, unconsciousness, immobility, analgesia (lack of pain) and amnesia (lack of memory). Scientists have developed drugs called anesthetics that target each of these elements.

Most anesthetics fall into one of two broad categories: general or local/regional.

What Is General Anesthesia?

General anesthesia affects the entire body. It is used when it is important for a patient to be unconscious. Many major, life-saving procedures like open-heart surgery, brain surgery or organ transplantation would be impossible without general anesthesia.

General anesthetics are either delivered intravenously or breathed in as a gas. Intravenous anesthetics act quickly and disappear rapidly from the bloodstream, so patients can go home sooner after surgery. Inhaled anesthetics may take longer to wear off.

Although general anesthetics are usually considered quite safe for most patients, they can pose risks, particularly for elderly patients, those with certain genetic variations, and those with some chronic, systemic diseases, such as diabetes. In addition, some patients, especially the elderly and children, may have lingering effects for several days after general anesthesia. Fortunately, serious side effects—such as dangerously low blood pressure—are much less common than they once were.

What Are Local and Regional Anesthesia?

Doctors use local and regional anesthetics to block pain in a part of the body. Local anesthetics affect a small part of the body, such as a single tooth. Regional anesthetics affect larger areas, such as everything below the waist.

With local and regional anesthetics, patients can remain conscious and comfortable during surgery. But, like all drugs, these anesthetics can have side effects, and delivering them to the right spot is sometimes difficult.

How Does Anesthesia Work?

For many decades after anesthetics became a routine part of surgery, practically nothing was known about how they work. Virtually all scientists believed that anesthetics blocked nerve cell signaling by disrupting fatty molecules in the membranes that envelop cells. This theory, first put forward in the early 1900s, dominated research on anesthetics for much of the 20th century. Anesthetics are difficult to work with in the laboratory, and the lack of tools to study them at the molecular level contributed to this period of slow scientific progress.

Today, advances in cell biology, genetics and molecular biology have transformed anesthesiology into an active area of research. Scientists no longer think that anesthetics work by acting on fatty molecules in cell membranes. The bulk of the evidence now supports the idea that the drugs interfere with nerve signals by targeting specific protein molecules embedded in nerve cell membranes. Researchers also believe that inhaled and intravenous anesthetics each act on a different set of molecules to bring about their characteristic effects.

How Was Surgery Performed before Anesthesia Was Available?

Prior to the 1840s, doctors and dentists did not routinely use anesthesia when operating on patients. Most doctors attempted surgery only when it was absolutely necessary to save a person's life, and operations were largely limited to amputations and removal of external growths. Although alcohol, opium or other botanicals sometimes helped alleviate the agony, most surgical patients remained conscious and endured excruciating pain.

When Did Doctors and Dentists Begin Using Anesthesia?

In 1846, a dentist publicly demonstrated that ether, a colorless liquid that vaporizes quickly, would put patients to sleep during surgery. The practice began to spread. Doctors and dentists soaked a sponge or a cloth with ether and had patients breathe in the fumes through an inhaler.

The fumes knocked the person out, but there was no way to control the amount inhaled. If patients inhaled too little, they could wake up during surgery and flail about in pain; if they inhaled too much, they might never wake. To make matters worse, ether is highly flammable, and a spark in the operating room could cause a dangerous explosion. Despite the problems with ether, its use enabled surgeons to perform internal procedures that would have been too painful or complicated to conduct on conscious patients.

The introduction of less flammable anesthetic gases made operating rooms safer, and the discovery of intravenous anesthetic agents such as sodium thiopental made it possible for surgeons to control the dose. But well into the 1950s, doctors still usually sedated their patients using some type of anesthetic gas and monitored them with nothing more sophisticated than a stethoscope. Dangerous side effects were common and included heart rhythm and breathing problems, lowered blood pressure, nausea and vomiting.

How Are Anesthesiologists Trained?

Like all medical doctors, anesthesiologists earn an undergraduate degree (often in a life sciences field) and a medical degree (M.D. or D.O.). Then they must complete a 4-year residency program in anesthesiology. Many choose to complete an additional 1-year fellowship in a specialty such as pain management, pediatric anesthesiology or critical care medicine.

What Do Anesthesiologists Do during Surgery?

Anesthesiologists carefully monitor patients throughout surgery using electronic devices that continually display vital signs. Major advances in monitoring include the continuous measurement of blood pressure, blood oxygen levels, heart function and respiratory patterns. These advances have dramatically improved the safety of general anesthesia and make it possible to operate on many patients who were previously considered too sick to undergo surgery.

What Do Anesthesiologists Do Outside of the Operating Room?

The role of the anesthesiologist has expanded to include caring for patients during postoperative recovery. Anesthesiologists also provide anesthesia for nonsurgical procedures such as endoscopy and various cardiac interventions, as well as during labor and delivery. As experts in pain management, anesthesiologists may manage pain clinics or advise other specialists on how to manage pain.

What New Advancements in Anesthesia Are on the Horizon?

As scientists learn more about the molecular mechanisms by which anesthetics cause their various effects, they will be able to design agents that are more targeted, more effective and safer, with fewer side effects.

Observations of the short and long-term effects of anesthetics on subsets of the population, such as the elderly or cancer survivors, will reveal whether certain anesthetics are better than others for members of those groups. Research on how a person's genetic makeup influences the way he or she responds to anesthetics will enable doctors to further tailor anesthesia to individual patients.

How Does Anesthesia Research Contribute to Other Fields of Science and Medicine?

Knowledge of how anesthetics affect pain and consciousness helps scientists gain a better understanding of the mechanisms that underlie these physiological states. Understanding these mechanisms could lead to new ways to alleviate pain and to new treatments for conditions associated with a decrease or loss of consciousness, such as epilepsy and coma. Studies of anesthesia may also provide insights into the nature of consciousness itself.

Part Three

Health Literacy and Making Informed Health Decisions

Chapter 17

Understanding Health Literacy

What Is Health Literacy?

The Patient Protection and Affordable Care Act (PPACA) of 2010, Title V, defines health literacy as the degree to which an individual has the capacity to obtain, communicate, process, and understand basic health information and services to make appropriate health decisions.

Health Literacy Capacity and Skills

Capacity is the potential a person has to do or accomplish something. Health literacy skills are those people use to realize their potential in health situations. They apply these skills either to make sense of health information and services or provide health information and services to others.

This chapter contains text excerpted from the following sources: Text beginning with the heading "What Is Health Literacy?" is excerpted from "Learn about Health Literacy," Centers for Disease Control and Prevention (CDC), September 30, 2015; Text beginning with the heading "Health Literacy Affects Everyone" is excerpted from "Understanding Health Literacy," Centers for Disease Control and Prevention (CDC), September 2, 2015; Text under the heading "How FDA Promotes Health Literacy" is excerpted from "Making Decisions for Your Health: Getting the Info You Need," U.S. Food and Drug Administration (FDA), October 2016.

Anyone who needs health information and services also needs health literacy skills to:

- Find information and services.

- Communicate their needs and preferences and respond to information and services.

- Process the meaning and usefulness of the information and services.

- Understand the choices, consequences, and context of the information and services.

- Decide which information and services match their needs and preferences so they can act.

Anyone who provides health information and services to others, such as a doctor, nurse, dentist, pharmacist, or public health worker, also needs health literacy skills to:

- Help people find information and services.

- Communicate about health and healthcare.

- Process what people are explicitly and implicitly asking for.

- Understand how to provide useful information and services.

- Decide which information and services work best for different situations and people so they can act.

Researchers can choose from many different types of health literacy skill measures.

Health Literacy Affects Everyone

Health literacy is important for everyone because, at some point in our lives, we all need to be able to find, understand, and use health information and services.

Taking care of our health is part of everyday life, not just when we visit a doctor, clinic, or hospital. Health literacy can help us prevent health problems and protect our health, as well as better manage those problems and unexpected situations that happen.

Even people who read well and are comfortable using numbers can face health literacy issues when:

- They aren't familiar with medical terms or how their bodies work.

- They have to interpret statistics and evaluate risks and benefits that affect their health and safety.

- They are diagnosed with a serious illness and are scared and confused.

- They have health conditions that require complicated self-care.

- They are voting on an issue affecting the community's health and relying on unfamiliar technical information.

Why Do We Have a Health Literacy Problem in the United States and Many Other Countries?

When organizations or people create and give others health information that is too difficult for them to understand, we create a health literacy problem. When we expect them to figure out health services with many unfamiliar, confusing or even conflicting steps, we also create a health literacy problem.

How Can We Help People Now?

We can help people use the health literacy skills they have. How? We can:

- create and provide information and services people can understand and use most effectively with the skills they have

- work with educators and others to help people become more familiar with health information and services and build their health literacy skills over time

- build our own skills as communicators of health information

Limited Health Literacy Reports and Evidence

People need information they can understand and use to make the best decisions for their health. "Limited health literacy" happens when people's literacy and numeracy skills are poorly matched with the technical, complex, and unfamiliar information that organizations make available or health services are too complex and difficult to understand and use effectively.

Several reports document that limited health literacy affects many types of health conditions, diseases, situations, and outcomes, including health status and costs.

Are Limited Health Literacy and Limited Literacy the Same Problem?

No, but they are related. People's reading, writing, and numbers skills are only a part of health literacy. People do need strong literacy and numeracy skills to make it easier to understand and use health information and services. But, research shows that many health and healthcare activities are unfamiliar, complicated, and technical to most people.

How FDA Promotes Health Literacy

Promoting health literacy is important to U.S. Food and Drug Administration (FDA) which communicates complex science and health topics every day. And it's a key part of the agency's effort to help the public make better informed decisions about the use of FDA-regulated products. The agency aims to provide clear and accurate information to patients and to healthcare professionals in several ways. For example, FDA strives to:

- **Use plain language for clear communications.** FDA first identifies its audience. Then the agency sends communication materials with well-organized messages that use clear sentences and common words. This easy-to-understand language is especially important for popular FDA webpages, such as those that discuss seasonal flu and vaccines for children, and in FDA-approved patient package inserts (consumer-friendly summaries of patient information), instructions for use, and Medication Guides (paper handouts that come with many prescription medicines). FDA uses best practices in the principles of plain language in other communications, including videos and posts on Twitter and Facebook.

  In addition, FDA uses Drug Safety Communications to let healthcare professionals and consumers know about newly observed potential risks of FDA-approved drugs and to offer advice on how these drugs may be best used in light of this new information. And when a drug or device is identified as unsafe, FDA informs consumers about market recalls and withdrawals.

- **Create special initiatives.** Many FDA Offices and Centers use special initiatives to promote health literacy, says Duckhorn. For instance, FDA's Center for Drug Evaluation and Research offers free online resources that teach you how to buy and use medicines safely. The Center for Food Safety and Applied Nutrition offers tips on how to use the Nutrition Facts Label. Plus, the Office of Health and Constituent Affairs (OHCA) operates a web portal called the FDA Patient Network. The Patient Network gives you access to health resources (including a newsletter) and can help you better understand the medical product regulation process.

- **Translate materials.** "For people who speak English as a second language or not at all, understanding important health information can be an overwhelming challenge and an enormous barrier to health literacy," says Jonca Bull, M.D., Assistant Commissioner for Minority Health. To that end, FDA offers safety updates and other materials for people with limited English skills. For example, the agency translates FDA Consumer Updates (like this one) into Spanish. It offers free health publications in multiple languages, such as Arabic and Tagalog. "In addition, we recently piloted a campaign on health fraud for people who have limited English proficiency by translating a Consumer Update and an accompanying video in several different languages," Bull says.

Chapter 18

Understanding Health Communication and Health Information Technology (IT)

All people have some ability to manage their health and the health of those they care for. However, with the increasing complexity of health information and healthcare settings, most people need additional information, skills, and supportive relationships to meet their health needs.

Disparities in access to health information, services, and technology can result in lower usage rates of preventive services, less knowledge of chronic disease management, higher rates of hospitalization, and poorer reported health status.

Both public and private institutions are increasingly using the Internet and other technologies to streamline the delivery of health information and services. This results in an even greater need for health professionals to develop additional skills in the understanding and use of consumer health information.

This chapter contains text excerpted from the following sources: Text in this chapters begins with excerpts from "Health Communication and Health Information Technology," Office of Disease Prevention and Health Promotion (ODPHP), U.S. Department of Health and Human Services (HHS), January 1, 2017; Text under the heading "Ways to Improve Health Literacy" is excerpted from "National Action Plan to Improve Health Literacy," Office of Disease Prevention and Health Promotion (ODPHP), U.S. Department of Health and Human Services (HHS), January 10, 2017.

The increase in online health information and services challenges users with limited literacy skills or limited experience using the Internet. For many of these users, the Internet is stressful and overwhelming—even inaccessible. Much of this stress can be reduced through the application of evidence-based best practices in user-centered design.

In addition, despite increased access to technology, other forms of communication are essential to ensuring that everyone, including non-Web users, is able to obtain, process, and understand health information to make good health decisions. These include printed materials, media campaigns, community outreach, and interpersonal communication.

Emerging Issues in Health Communication and Health Information Technology

During the coming decade, the speed, scope, and scale of adoption of health IT will only increase. Social media and emerging technologies promise to blur the line between expert and peer health information. Monitoring and assessing the impact of these new media, including mobile health, on public health will be challenging.

Equally challenging will be helping health professionals and the public adapt to the changes in healthcare quality and efficiency due to the creative use of health communication and health IT. Continual feedback, productive interactions, and access to evidence on the effectiveness of treatments and interventions will likely transform the traditional patient-provider relationship. It will also change the way people receive, process, and evaluate health information. Capturing the scope and impact of these changes—and the role of health communication and health IT in facilitating them—will require multidisciplinary models and data systems.

Such systems will be critical to expanding the collection of data to better understand the effects of health communication and health IT on population health outcomes, healthcare quality, and health disparities.

Ways to Improve Health Literacy

- The National Action Plan to Improve Health Literacy seeks to engage organizations, professionals, policymakers, communities, individuals, and families in a linked, multi-sector effort to improve health literacy. The Action Plan is based on 2 core principles:

- All people have the right to health information that helps them make informed decisions

- Health services should be delivered in ways that are easy to understand and that improve health, longevity, and quality of life

- The Action Plan contains 7 goals that will improve health literacy and strategies for achieving them:

  1. Develop and disseminate health and safety information that is accurate, accessible, and actionable.

  2. Promote changes in the healthcare system that improve health information, communication, informed decision-making, and access to health services.

  3. Incorporate accurate, standards-based, and developmentally appropriate health and science information and curricula in child care and education through the university level.

  4. Support and expand local efforts to provide adult education, English language instruction, and culturally and linguistically appropriate health information services in the community.

  5. Build partnerships, develop guidance, and change policies.

  6. Increase basic research and the development, implementation, and evaluation of practices and interventions to improve health literacy.

  7. Increase the dissemination and use of evidence-based health literacy practices and interventions.

Many of the strategies highlight actions that particular organizations or professions can take to further these goals. It will take everyone working together in a linked and coordinated manner to improve access to accurate and actionable health information and usable health services. By focusing on health literacy issues and working together, we can improve the accessibility, quality, and safety of healthcare; reduce costs; and improve the health and quality of life of millions of people in the United States.

Chapter 19

How to Find Medical Information

Using Trusted Resources

Health information, whether in print or online, should come from a trusted, credible source. Government agencies, hospitals, universities, and medical journals and books that provide evidence-based information are sources you can trust. Too often, other sources can provide misleading or incorrect information. If a source makes claims that are too good to be true, remember—they usually are.

There are many websites, books, and magazines that provide health information to the public, but not all of them are trustworthy. Use the details provided below to safeguard yourself when reviewing sources of health information.

Websites

Online sources of health information should make it easy for people to learn who is responsible for posting the information. They should make clear the original source of the information, along with the medical credentials of the people who prepare or review the posted material.

This chapter includes text excerpted from "Managing Cancer Care," National Cancer Institute (NCI), March 10, 2015.

Use the following questions to determine the credibility of health information published online.

- **Who manages this information?**

  The person or group that has published health information online should be identified somewhere.

- **Who is paying for the project, and what is their purpose?**

  You should be able to find this information in the "About Us" section.

- **What is the original source of the information that they have posted?**

  If the information was originally published in a research journal or a book, they should say which one(s) so that you can find it.

- **How is information reviewed before it gets posted?**

  Most health information publications have someone with medical or research credentials (e.g., someone who has earned Doctor of Medicine (M.D.), Doctor of Osteopathic Medicine (D.O.), or Doctor of Philosophy (Ph.D.) review the information before it gets posted, to make sure it is correct.

- **How current is the information?**

  Online health information sources should show you when the information was posted or last reviewed.

- **If they are asking for personal information, how will they use that information and how will they protect your privacy?**

  This is very important. Do not share personal information until you understand the policies under which it will be used and you are comfortable with any risk involved in sharing your information online.

Books

A number of books have been written about disease treatments and complementary and alternative medicine (CAM). Some books contain trustworthy content, while others do not.

It's important to know that information is always changing and that new research results are reported every day. Be aware that if a book is written by only one person, you may only be getting that one person's view.

If you go to the library, ask the staff for suggestions. Or if you live near a college or university, there may be a medical library available. Local bookstores may also have people on staff who can help you. If you find a book online, look very carefully at the author's credentials, background, and expertise. Questions you may want to ask yourself are:

- Is the author an expert on this subject?
- Do you know anyone else who has read the book?
- Has the book been reviewed by other experts?
- Was it published in the past 5 years?
- Does the book offer different points of view, or does it seem to hold one opinion?
- Has the author researched the topic in full?
- Are the references listed in the back?

Magazines

If you want to look for articles you can trust, search online medical journal databases or ask your librarian to help you look for medical journals, books, and other research that has been done by experts.

Articles in popular magazines are usually not written by experts. Rather, the authors speak with experts, gather information, and then write the article. If claims are made in a magazine, remember:

- The authors may not have expert knowledge in this area.
- They may not say where they found their information.
- The articles have not been reviewed by experts.
- The publisher may have ties to advertisers or other organizations. Therefore, the article may be one-sided in the information or view(s) it presents.

When you read these articles, you can use the same process that the magazine writer uses:

- Speak with experts
- Ask lots of questions
- Then decide if the therapy is right for you

147

Chapter 20

How to Evaluate Health Information Found on the Internet

There are thousands of medical websites. Some provide reliable health information. Some do not. Some of the medical news is current. Some of it is not. Choosing which websites to trust is an important part of using the Internet.

How Do I Find Reliable Health Information Online?

As a rule, health websites sponsored by Federal Government agencies are good sources of information. You can reach all Federal websites by visiting www.usa.gov. Large professional organizations and well-known medical schools may also be good sources of health information.

How Do I Navigate Health Websites?

The home page is like a lobby to other areas of the website; however, it may not be the first page you see. The first page you see depends on the link you click to get to the website, for example, from a search engine.

Even if you don't start on the homepage, you can still use the website menu. Usually, you can find the menu at the top of a page or along

This chapter includes text excerpted from "Online Health Information: Can You Trust It?" National Institute on Aging (NIA), National Institutes of Health (NIH), January 27, 2016.

the left side. No matter where you start, you should be able to spot the name of the sponsor or owner of the site right away.

Where Can I Find Reliable Health Information Online?

Sometimes, it's hard to know where to begin to look for trustworthy health information. The National Institutes of Health (NIH) website, www.nih.gov, is a good place to start for reliable health information. Here are a few other helpful websites hosted by NIH:

- National Institute on Aging (NIA) (www.nia.nih.gov) has a variety of resources about health and aging, including information about Alzheimer disease.

- NIHSeniorHealth.gov (www.nihseniorhealth.gov) is a website with health and wellness information designed specifically for older people.

- MedlinePlus (www.medlineplus.gov), a website from the National Library of Medicine (NLM), has dependable information about more than 700 health-related topics.

- National Heart, Lung, and Blood Institute (NHLBI) (www.nhlbi. nih.gov) has information about managing heart disease and other topics.

- National Institute on Deafness and Other Communication Disorders (NIDCD) (www.nidcd.nih.gov) has information about hearing loss and deafness.

- National Institute of Dental and Craniofacial Research (NIDCR) (www.nidcr.nih.gov) offers, for example, tips on taking care of dentures.

Questions to Ask before Trusting a Website

As you search online, you are likely to find websites for many health agencies and organizations that are not well-known. By answering the following questions you should be able to find more information about these websites. A lot of these details might be found under the heading "About Us."

1. Who sponsors/hosts the website? Is that information easy to find? Websites cost money. Is the source of funding (sponsor) clear? Sometimes the website address is helpful. For example:

    - .gov identifies a U.S. government agency

- .edu identifies an educational institution, like a school, college, or university

- .org usually identifies nonprofit organizations (such as professional groups; scientific, medical, or research societies; advocacy groups)

- .com identifies commercial websites (such as businesses, pharmaceutical companies, and sometimes hospitals)

2. Is it clear how you can reach the sponsor? Trustworthy websites will have contact information for you to use to reach the site's sponsor or authors. An email address, toll-free phone number, and/or mailing address might be listed at the bottom of every page or on a separate "About Us" or "Contact Us" page.

3. Who wrote the information? Authors and contributors are often but not always identified. For example, most government sites have many authors and contributors and, rather than list the names of the people, they will often credit a department. A contributor's connection to the website, and any financial interest he or she has in the information on the website, should be clear.

   Be careful about testimonials. Personal stories may be helpful and comforting, but not everyone experiences health problems the same way. Also, there is a big difference between a website developed by a single person interested in a topic and a website developed using strong scientific evidence (that is, information gathered from research). No information should replace seeing a doctor or other health professional.

4. Who reviews the information? Does the website have editors? Read the "About Us" page to see if experts check the information before putting it online. Find out if the list includes actual experts in the field. Dependable websites tell you where the health information came from and how it has been reviewed.

5. When was the information written? Look for websites that stay current on their health information. You don't want to make decisions about your care based on out-of-date information. Often the bottom of the page will have a date. Pages on the same site may be updated at different times. Some may be updated more often than others. Older information isn't

useless. Many websites provide older articles as historical background.

6. Is your privacy protected? Does the website clearly state a privacy policy? Take time to read the website's privacy policy, which can usually be found at the bottom of the page or on a separate page titled "About Us," "Privacy Policy," or "Our Policies." If the website says something like, "We share information with companies that can provide you with products," that's a sign your information isn't private.

   BE CAREFUL about sharing your Social Security number. Find out why your number is needed, how it will be used, and what will happen if you do not share your number. Some websites, like for your health insurance, might need your Social Security number to process claims.

7. Are your privacy rights, as a consumer, protected when making an online purchase? If you are asked for personal information, be sure to find out how the information will be used. Contact the website sponsor by phone or mail, or use the "Contact Us" feature on the website. Be careful when buying things online. Websites without security may not protect your credit card or bank account information. Look for information saying that a website has a "secure server" before buying anything online. Secure websites that collect personal information have an "s" after "http" in the start of their website address (https://) and often require that you create a username and password.

8. Does the website offer quick and easy solutions to your health problems? Are miracle cures promised? Be careful of websites or companies that claim any one remedy will cure a lot of different illnesses. Question dramatic writing or amazing cures. Make sure you can find other websites with the same information. Even if the website links to a trustworthy source, it doesn't mean that the site has the other organization's endorsement or support—any website can link to another without permission.

Trust Yourself and Talk to Your Doctor

Use common sense and good judgment when looking at health information online. There are websites on nearly every health topic, and many have no rules overseeing the quality of the information provided. Take a deep breath and think a bit before acting on any health information you find online. Don't count on any one website and check your sources. And, remember to talk with your doctor about what you learn online before making any changes in your healthcare.

A Quick Checklist

You can use the following checklist to help make sure that the health information you are reading online can be trusted. You might want to keep this checklist by your computer.

1. Is the sponsor/owner of the website a Federal agency, medical school, or large professional or nonprofit organization, or is it related to one of these?

2. If not sponsored by a Federal agency, medical school, or large professional or nonprofit organization, does the website reference one of these trustworthy sources for its health information?

3. Is the mission or goal of the sponsor clear?

4. Can you see who works for the agency or organization and who authored the information? Is there a way to contact the sponsor of the website?

5. When was the information written or, webpage last updated?

6. Is your privacy protected?

7. Does the website offer unbelievable solutions to your health problem(s)? Are quick, miracle cures promised?

Chapter 21

Mobile Health Applications

The widespread adoption and use of mobile technologies is opening new and innovative ways to improve health and healthcare delivery.

Mobile applications (apps) can help people manage their own health and wellness, promote healthy living, and gain access to useful information when and where they need it. These tools are being adopted almost as quickly as they can be developed. According to industry estimates by 2018, 50 percent of the more than 3.4 billion smartphone and tablet users will have downloaded mobile health applications. These users include healthcare professionals, consumers, and patients.

The U.S. Food and Drug Administration (FDA) encourages the development of mobile medical apps that improve healthcare and provide consumers and healthcare professionals with valuable health information. The FDA also has a public health responsibility to oversee the safety and effectiveness of medical devices—including mobile medical apps.

The FDA issued the *Mobile Medical Applications Guidance for Industry and Food and Drug Administration Staff* on September 25, 2013 (updated February 2015), which explains the agency's oversight of mobile medical apps as devices and our focus only on the apps that present a greater risk to patients if they don't work as intended and on apps that cause smartphones or other mobile platforms to impact the functionality or performance of traditional medical devices.

This chapter includes text excerpted from "Mobile Medical Applications," U.S. Food and Drug Administration (FDA), September 22, 2015.

What Are Mobile Medical Apps?

Mobile apps are software programs that run on smartphones and other mobile communication devices. They can also be accessories that attach to a smartphone or other mobile communication devices, or a combination of accessories and software.

Mobile medical apps are medical devices that are mobile apps, meet the definition of a medical device and are an accessory to a regulated medical device or transform a mobile platform into a regulated medical device.

Consumers can use both mobile medical apps and mobile apps to manage their own health and wellness, such as to monitor their caloric intake for healthy weight maintenance. For example, the National Institutes of Health's (NIH) *LactMed* app provides nursing mothers with information about the effects of medicines on breast milk and nursing infants.

Other apps aim to help healthcare professionals improve and facilitate patient care. The Radiation Emergency Medical Management (REMM) app gives healthcare providers guidance on diagnosing and treating radiation injuries. Some mobile medical apps can diagnose cancer or heart rhythm abnormalities, or function as the "central command" for a glucose meter used by an insulin-dependent diabetic patient.

How Will the FDA Regulate Mobile Medical Apps?

The FDA will apply the same risk-based approach the agency uses to assure safety and effectiveness for other medical devices. The guidance document provides examples of how the FDA might regulate certain moderate-risk (Class II) and high-risk (Class III) mobile medical apps.

Mobile Medical Apps That the FDA Will Regulate

The FDA is taking a tailored, risk-based approach that focuses on the small subset of mobile apps that meet the regulatory definition of "device" and that:

- are intended to be used as an accessory to a regulated medical device, or

- transform a mobile platform into a regulated medical device

Mobile apps span a wide range of health functions. While many mobile apps carry minimal risk, those that can pose a greater risk to patients will require FDA review.

For a list of what is considered a mobile medical application, manufacturers and developers of mobile applications can search FDA's database of existing classification by type of mobile medical application (for example diagnostic). Approved/cleared mobile medical applications will also be listed in FDA's *510(k)* and *PMA* (Premarket approval) databases and on the FDA's *Registration and Listing Database.*

Mobile Apps for Which the FDA Intends to Exercise Enforcement Discretion

For many mobile apps that meet the regulatory definition of a "device" but pose minimal risk to patients and consumers, the FDA will exercise enforcement discretions and will not expect manufacturers to submit premarket review applications or to register and list their apps with the FDA. This includes mobile medical apps that:

- Help patients/users self-manage their disease or condition without providing specific treatment suggestions;

- Provide patients with simple tools to organize and track their health information;

- Provide easy access to information related to health conditions or treatments;

- Help patients document, show or communicate potential medical conditions to healthcare providers;

- Automate simple tasks for healthcare providers; or

- Enable patients or providers to interact with Personal Health Records (PHR) or Electronic Health Record (EHR) systems.

Does the FDA Regulate Mobile Devices and Mobile App Stores?

FDA's mobile medical apps policy does not regulate the sale or general consumer use of smartphones or tablets. FDA's mobile medical apps policy does not consider entities that exclusively distribute mobile apps, such as the owners and operators of the "iTunes App store" or the "Google Play store," to be medical device manufacturers. FDA's mobile medical apps policy does not consider mobile platform manufacturers to be medical device manufacturers just because their mobile platform could be used to run a mobile medical app regulated by FDA.

Does the Guidance Apply to Electronic Health Records?

FDA's mobile medical app policy does not apply to mobile apps that function as an electronic health record system or personal health record system.

Chapter 22

Electronic Health Records (EHRs)

Chapter Contents

Section 22.1

EHRs Basics

This section includes text excerpted from "Learn EHR Basics,"
HealthIT.gov, Office of the National Coordinator for Health
Information Technology (ONC), May 21, 2014.

What Are Electronic Health Records (EHRs)?

Electronic Health Records (EHRs) are, at their simplest, digital
(computerized) versions of patients' paper charts. But EHRs, when
fully up and running, are so much more than that.

EHRs are real-time, patient-centered records. They make information
available instantly, "whenever and wherever it is needed." And they bring
together in one place everything about a patient's health. EHRs can:

- Contain information about a patient's medical history, diagnoses, medications, immunization dates, allergies, radiology
  images, and lab and test results

- Offer access to evidence-based tools that providers can use in
  making decisions about a patient's care

- Automate and streamline providers' workflow

- Increase organization and accuracy of patient information

- Support key market changes in payer requirements and consumer expectations

One of the key features of an EHR is that it can be created, managed,
and consulted by authorized providers and staff across more than one
healthcare organization. A single EHR can bring together information
from current and past doctors, emergency facilities, school and workplace clinics, pharmacies, laboratories, and medical imaging facilities.

What Is Meaningful Use?

As you get involved with electronic health records, one of the
things you'll hear about is the concept of "meaningful use"—part of

the standards and criteria developed in the health field to encourage a smooth, productive transition to EHRs.

"Meaningful use" refers to the use of certified EHR technologies by healthcare providers in ways that measurably improve healthcare quality and efficiency. The ultimate goal is to bring about healthcare that is:

- Patient-centered
- Evidence-based
- Prevention-oriented
- Efficient
- Equitable

Health Information Privacy and Security

The need for privacy and security is at the forefront of the health movement. Like paper medical records, electronic records must always be private and secure. EHRs can help protect patient information through:

- Access controls to make sure only those who are authorized can access health information
- Audit functions that track who has accessed what pieces of health information
- Internet-based portals that allow patients to access their own health records, see who else has viewed their records, and check the accuracy of the records

Electronic Health Record Incentive

As America moves toward broad adoption of health, Medicare and Medicaid EHR incentive programs can help providers with the transition. Incentive payments include:

- Up to $44,000 for eligible professionals in the Medicare EHR Incentive Program.
- Up to $63,000 for eligible professionals in the Medicaid EHR Incentive Program.
- A base payment of $2 million for eligible hospitals and critical access hospitals, depending on certain criteria.

Section 22.2

Benefits of EHRs

This section includes text excerpted from "Benefits of Electronic
Health Records (EHRs)," HealthIT.gov, Office of the National
Coordinator for Health Information Technology (ONC), July 30, 2015.

Our world has been radically transformed by digital technology–
smart phones, tablets, and web-enabled devices have transformed
our daily lives and the way we communicate. Medicine is an informa-
tion-rich enterprise. A greater and more seamless flow of information
within a digital healthcare infrastructure, created by electronic health
records (EHRs), encompasses and leverages digital progress and can
transform the way care is delivered and compensated. With EHRs,
information is available whenever and wherever it is needed.

The Health Information Technology for Economic and Clinical
Health (HITECH) Act, a component of the American Recovery and
Reinvestment Act (ARRA) of 2009, represents the Nation's first substantial commitment of Federal resources to support the widespread
adoption of EHRs. As of August 2012, 54 percent of the Medicare-and
Medicaid-eligible professionals had registered for the meaningful use
incentive program.

Healthcare Quality and Convenience

EHRs can improve healthcare quality. EHRs can also make healthcare more convenient for providers and patients.

Snapshot of improved healthcare quality and convenience for
providers:

- Quick access to patient records from inpatient and remote locations for more coordinated, efficient care

- Enhanced decision support, clinical alerts, reminders, and medical information

- Performance-improving tools, real-time quality reporting

- Legible, complete documentation that facilitates accurate coding
and billing

- Interfaces with labs, registries, and other EHRs

- Safer, more reliable prescribing

Snapshot of improved healthcare quality and convenience for patients:

- Reduced need to fill out the same forms at each office visit

- Reliable point-of-care information and reminders notifying providers of important health interventions

- Convenience of e-prescriptions electronically sent to pharmacy

- Patient portals with online interaction for providers

- Electronic referrals allowing easier access to follow-up care with specialists

EHRs improve information availability. With EHRs, patients' health information is available in one place, when and where it is needed. Providers have access to the information they need, at the time they need it to make a decision.

EHRs can be the foundation for quality improvements. Reliable access to complete patient health information is essential for safe and effective care. EHRs place accurate and complete information about patients' health and medical history at providers' fingertips. With EHRs, providers can give the best possible care, at the point of care. This can lead to a better patient experience and, most importantly, better patient outcomes.

Practices also report that they utilize extracted reports on patient and disease registries to track patient care as well as facilitate quality improvement discussions during clinical meetings.

EHRs support provider decision making. EHRs can help providers make efficient, effective decisions about patient care, through:

- Improved aggregation, analysis, and communication of patient information

- Clinical alerts and reminders

- Support for diagnostic and therapeutic decisions

- Built-in safeguards against potential adverse events

- Healthcare convenience matters

Providers with busy practices—and patients with busy lives—appreciate convenience in their healthcare transactions. EHRs can help. For example, with e-prescribing, patients can have their prescriptions ordered and ready even before they leave the provider's office. Providers and their staff can often file insurance claims immediately from the provider's office. And providers may be able to access patient files or submit prescriptions remotely—from home or while on vacation.

Patient Participation

Providers and patients who share access to electronic health information can collaborate in informed decision making. Patient participation is especially important in managing and treating chronic conditions such as asthma, diabetes, and obesity.

How EHRs Foster Patient Participation

EHRs can help providers:

- **Ensure high-quality care.** With EHRs, providers can give patients full and accurate information about all of their medical evaluations. Providers can also offer follow-up information after an office visit or a hospital stay, such as self-care instructions, reminders for other follow-up care, and links to web resources.

- **Create an avenue for communication with their patients.** With EHRs, providers can manage appointment schedules electronically and exchange e-mail with their patients. Quick and easy communication between patients and providers may help providers identify symptoms earlier. And it can position providers to be more proactive by reaching out to patients.

Personal Health Records

A personal health record, or PHR, is an electronic application used by patients to maintain and manage their own health information (or that of others for whom they are authorized to do so). A PHR differs from an EHR in that patients themselves usually set up and access the PHR. Patients can use a PHR to keep track of information from doctor visits, record other health-related information, and link to health-related resources. PHRs can increase patient participation in their own care. They can also help families become more engaged in the healthcare of family members.

164

- With **standalone PHRs**, patients fill in the information from their own records and memories, and the information is stored on patients' computers or the Internet.

- **Tethered** or **connected PHRs** are linked to a specific healthcare organization's EHR system or to a health plan's information system. The patient accesses the information through a secure portal.

With tethered/connected PHRs, patients can log on to their own records and see, for example, the trend of their lab results over the last year. That kind of information can motivate patients to take medications and keep up with lifestyle changes that have improved their health. Ideally, patients will be able to link their PHRs with their doctors' EHRs, creating their own healthcare "hubs." Most doctors are not ready for that kind of change quite yet, but it is a worthy goal.

The Patient's Perspective

Information technology is at the heart of modern life. It touches different people in different ways. Some are comfortable with new technologies; others may be intimidated, at least at first. EHRs, PHRs, and other health IT developments tend to make many patients more active participants in their own healthcare. As providers adopt new technologies such as EHRs, it's important to keep the patient's perspective in mind.

Medical Practice Efficiencies and Cost Savings

Many healthcare providers have found that electronic health records (EHRs) help improve medical practice management by increasing practice efficiencies and cost savings.

A national survey of doctors who are ready for meaningful use offers important evidence:

- 79 percent of providers report that with an EHR, their practice functions more efficiently

- 82 percent report that sending prescriptions electronically (e-prescribing) saves time

- 68 percent of providers see their EHR as an asset with recruiting physicians

- 75 percent receive lab results faster

- 70 percent report enhances in data confidentiality

Based on the size of a health system and the scope of their implementation, benefits for large hospitals can range from $37M to $59M over a five-year period in addition to incentive payments.

Savings are primarily attributed to automating several time-consuming paper-driven and labor-intensive tasks:

- Reduced transcription costs

- Reduced chart pull, storage, and re-filing costs

- Improved and more accurate reimbursement coding with improved documentation for highly compensated codes

- Reduced medical errors through better access to patient data and error prevention alerts

- Improved patient health/quality of care through better disease management and patient education

Electronic Health Records Create More Efficient Practices

EHR-enabled medical practices report:

- Improved medical practice management through integrated scheduling systems that link appointments directly to progress notes, automate coding, and managed claims

- Time savings with easier centralized chart management, condition-specific queries, and other shortcuts

- Enhanced communication with other clinicians, labs, and health plans through:

- Easy access to patient information from anywhere

- Tracking electronic messages to staff, other clinicians, hospitals, labs, etc.

- Automated formulary checks by health plans

- Order and receipt of lab tests and diagnostic images

- Links to public health systems such as registries and communicable disease databases

Electronic Health Records Reduce Duplication of Testing

Because EHRs contain all of a patient's health information in one place, it is less likely that providers will have to spend time ordering—and reviewing the results of—unnecessary or duplicate tests and medical procedures. Less utilization means fewer costs.

Patient Participation

Providers and patients who share access to electronic health information can collaborate in informed decision making. Patient participation is especially important in managing and treating chronic conditions such as asthma, diabetes, and obesity.

How EHRs Foster Patient Participation

Electronic health records (EHRs) can help providers:

- Ensure high-quality care. With EHRs, providers can give patients full and accurate information about all of their medical evaluations. Providers can also offer follow-up information after an office visit or a hospital stay, such as self-care instructions, reminders for other follow-up care, and links to web resources.

- Create an avenue for communication with their patients. With EHRs, providers can manage appointment schedules electronically and exchange e-mail with their patients. Quick and easy communication between patients and providers may help providers identify symptoms earlier. And it can position providers to be more proactive by reaching out to patients.

Improved Diagnostics and Patient Outcomes

When healthcare providers have access to complete and accurate information, patients receive better medical care. Electronic health records (EHRs) can improve the ability to diagnose diseases and reduce—even prevent—medical errors, improving patient outcomes. A national survey of doctors who are ready for meaningful use offers important evidence:

- 94 percent of providers report that their EHR makes records readily available at point of care.

- 88 percent report that their EHR produces clinical benefits for the practice.

- 75 percent of providers report that their EHR allows them to deliver better patient care.

EHRs Can Aid In Diagnosis

With EHRs, providers can have reliable access to a patient's complete health information. This comprehensive picture can help providers diagnose patients' problems sooner.

EHRs Can Reduce Errors, Improve Patient Safety, and Support Better Patient Outcomes

How? EHRs don't just contain or transmit information; they "compute" it. That means that EHRs manipulate the information in ways that make a difference for patients. For example:

- A qualified EHR not only keeps a record of a patient's medications or allergies, it also automatically checks for problems whenever a new medication is prescribed and alerts the clinician to potential conflicts.

- Information gathered by a primary care provider and recorded in an EHR tells a clinician in the emergency department about a patient's life-threatening allergy, and emergency staff can adjust care appropriately, even if the patient is unconscious.

- EHRs can expose potential safety problems when they occur, helping providers avoid more serious consequences for patients and leading to better patient outcomes.

- EHRs can help providers quickly and systematically identify and correct operational problems. In a paper-based setting, identifying such problems is much more difficult, and correcting them can take years.

Risk Management and Liability Prevention

EHRs may improve risk management by:

- Providing clinical alerts and reminders

- Improving aggregation, analysis, and communication of patient information

- Making it easier to consider all aspects of a patient's condition

- Supporting diagnostic and therapeutic decision making

- Gathering all relevant information (lab results, etc.) in one place

- Support for therapeutic decisions

- Enabling evidence-based decisions at point of care

- Preventing adverse events

- Providing built-in safeguards against prescribing treatments that would result in adverse events

- Enhancing research and monitoring for improvements in clinical quality

Certified EHRs may help providers prevent liability actions by:

- Demonstrating adherence to the best evidence-based practices

- Producing complete, legible records readily available for the defense (reconstructing what actually happened during the point of care)

- Disclosing evidence that suggests informed consent

EHRs Can Improve Public Health Outcomes

EHRs can also have beneficial effects on the health of groups of patients. Providers who have electronic health information about the entire population of patients they serve can look more meaningfully at the needs of patients who:

- Suffer from a specific condition

- Are eligible for specific preventive measures

- Are currently taking specific medications

This EHR function helps providers identify and work with patients to manage specific risk factors or combinations of risk factors to improve patient outcomes. For example, providers might wish to identify:

- How many patients with hypertension have their blood pressure under control

- How many patients with diabetes have their blood sugar measurements in the target range and have had appropriate screening tests

This EHR function also can detect patterns of potentially related adverse events and enable at-risk patients to be notified quickly.

Better Patient Outcomes with EHRs

Using EHR Prompts and Reminders to Improve Quality of Patient Care

High Patient Satisfaction

- 92 percent were happy their doctor used e-prescribing.

- 90 percent reported rarely or only occasionally going to the pharmacy and having prescription not ready.

- 76 percent reported it made obtaining medications easier.

- 63 percent reported fewer medication errors.

High Provider Satisfaction

- Reduced overall rate of after-hours clinic calls.

Using EHRs to Improve Quality of Care

Improved Quality of Care Screenings

- Breast cancer

- Diabetes

- Chlamydia

- Colorectal cancer

Increase in Services

- Blood pressure control for patients with hypertension

- Breast cancer screenings

- Recording of body mass index and blood testing for patients with diabetes

Section 22.3

Blue Button and Using Your Health Records

This section includes text excerpted from "Your Health Records,"
HealthIT.gov, Office of the National Coordinator for Health
Information Technology (ONC), October 30, 2015.

How to Begin Downloading and Using Your Health Records

Get started by finding out if your doctor, hospital, drug store, lab, or health insurance company offers Blue Button. Although Blue Button is in its early stages, it is expanding rapidly.

Go to the Blue Button Connector

Today, millions of Americans have access to their health records through their healthcare providers or health insurance company, along with Medicare beneficiaries, veterans, and uniformed service members.

In 2014, Office of the National Coordinator for Health Information Technology (ONC) did an early launch of the online Blue Button Connector tool to help consumers find out which healthcare providers offer electronic access to their health records, what to do with them, and useful tools to help meet their health needs and lifestyle. Various Blue Button capable products and tools will be featured to help patients better navigate online resources tailored to help them manage their health needs. ONC continues to improve and populate the site and will rely on you to help.

Ask Your Healthcare Providers

More and more healthcare providers are giving patients easy-to-use tools to securely access, reliably download, and easily share their own health records. If you do not see your healthcare providers listed on the Blue Button Connector, it is encouraged to ask them if they offer a way for you to view and download your health records online so you have this information available when you need it.

171

Look for the Blue Button Logo

Healthcare organizations who participate in Blue Button display the logo as a symbol that you can easily access your health records here! Look for this symbol:

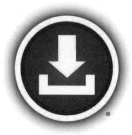

Figure 22.1. *Blue Button Logo*

About Blue Button

The Blue Button symbol signifies that a site has functionality for customers to go online and download health records. You can use your health data to improve your health, and to have more control over your personal health information and your family's healthcare.

- Do you want to feel more in control of your health and your personal health information? Do you have a health issue?

- Are you caring for an elderly parent?

- Are you changing doctors?

- Do you need to find the results of a medical test or a complete and current list of your medications?

Blue Button may be able to help. Look for the Blue Button symbol and take action using your personal health information.

Frequently Asked Questions on Blue Button

How Does the Blue Button Work?

The Blue Button enables you to securely access your personal health data online by clicking on a "Blue Button" logo or icon. You may have access to your claims and personal health information that is maintained by your doctors, hospitals, health plans, and others, depending on the tools and data they are offering. Patients can securely access their health data and then choose to download that data to their computer, thumb drive or smartphone without using any special software, or share that data with individuals they trust—whether it's their other physicians or family members.

Is There a Cost to Use the Blue Button?

There should not be a cost. Ask your healthcare provider or health plan if they offer a way for you to view, download, and share your health information online.

What Kind of Technology Do I Need to Access the Blue Button?

Remember that unless you are a veteran, Medicare beneficiary or service member or your health plan, healthcare provider (doctor or hospital) or other entities where you seek care use Blue Button, it may not yet be available to you. You shouldn't need any special technology to take advantage of Blue Button's ability to make it easier for you to view, download and share your personal health data with others you trust. However, you may want to consider using a personal health record to store and manage all your health information in one place. Increasingly, more health plans, healthcare providers, nursing homes, pharmacies, laboratories and other institutions that have your health information on file are offering you a portal or personal health record—a place for you to store and manage your health information online. You can also sign up to get one on your own.

Can I Sign Up for Blue Button Today?

It depends if your healthcare provider, health plan (insurer), or other entity that manages your health data (e.g., pharmacy, lab, etc.) offers a way for you to get secure access to your health information online so you can view and download that information and share it with others you trust. The best way to find out is to ask. If you are a Medicare beneficiary, a veteran or an active service member you can get secure, electronic access to your health data today by clicking the Blue Button in the patient portal. Increasingly, more doctors, health plans and hospital websites are offering patients portals through which patients can view and download their health information.

If I Don't Have Access to Blue Button Now, Why Should I Care about This?

Even if you don't have access to Blue Button through your health plan, doctor or other healthcare provider such as pharmacies, nursing homes and labs, you still have a legal right to see and get a copy of your health records. You should be able to get your health records from most doctors, hospitals and other healthcare providers, as well as from your health plan (insurer) in the form that fits your needs—either electronically or in a paper form—as long as your health plan or provider is able to do so. Having electronic access to your health record allows you to have the information you need at your fingertips to share with other doctors or in case of an emergency. More healthcare providers and health plans are adopting Blue Button, which means more people are gaining a convenient and secure way to access to their health information on demand, rather than having to ask for that information from their provider or health plan. As more providers adopt electronic health records and meet the meaningful use requirements that support patients and families having access to their health information online, more patients will be able to have the information they need to play a more active role in their healthcare. To meet "Meaningful Use" requirements, more doctors will be using electronic health records and providing patients with easy, electronic access to that information. And more and more, that information is getting converted from paper records into a digital health format, allowing for more information to be integrated into the Blue Button.

Does My Doctor Have to Use the Blue Button?

Your doctor is not required to offer Blue Button. However, there are financial incentives available from the federal government to encourage healthcare providers to adopt electronic health record systems (EHRs) and to use these systems in a way that improves your care. As part of meeting the requirements for receiving these payments, doctors must provide patients with an electronic copy of their health record. Over time, these requirements will also require providers to provide you with a way to view, download and share your health information online.

What If My Doctor Doesn't Want to Use Blue Button?

Although your doctor may not want to offer you with a way to securely access your health record online, they are required by law to provide you with a way to view and get a copy of your medical records (called right to access).

Does Blue Button Let Other People Get Access to My Health Records?

Blue Button puts the information others hold about you in your hands. You decide how to use it. Using Blue Button does not give anyone else access to your health records unless you choose to share it. Healthcare providers, such as doctors and hospitals, are accountable for the privacy and security of patients' health records by a law called "The Health Insurance Portability and Accountability Act (HIPAA)." Healthcare providers are required by HIPAA to set up physical, administrative and technical safeguards to protect your health records. This may include "access controls" like passwords and PIN numbers (Personal Identification Number) to help limit who has access to your information; "encryption" so your health information can't be read or understood except by someone who is approved to view it; and an "audit trail" so there is a record of who has looked at your information and what changes were made to it and when. Once you download your health records from your healthcare provider or health insurance company's website via Blue Button, it is your responsibility to protect that information.

How Safe Is It to Log Into Blue Button or Use It to Transmit My Health Records?

To ensure that your health records are kept private and secure, only you or someone who has your permission can access your health records through Blue Button. Since this requires that you log in to your healthcare provider's or health insurance company's website or patient portal (a place for you to store and manage your health records online), you will likely be able to secure your health records with a username and password. The specific privacy and security safeguards associated with Blue Button vary depending on the organization that is offering it. Read the privacy policy on the site you are using for details.

To maximize the security of your information, it is recommended that you use an encrypted "Direct" health email address. The Direct Project offers easy and secure messaging, enabling healthcare providers and hospitals to send your health records to you, including summaries of your recent visits, or reminders about preventive or follow-up care. Some Personal Health Records can provide you with a Direct Address that you can use to receive such messages. Direct Project messages are secure, which means that unlike email, they can be used by your healthcare provider to send your information securely to you and to other healthcare providers who are participating in your care. See if your healthcare provider and your personal health record provider support the Direct Project.

Once you download your health records, it is recommended that you protect that information by either securing it with a password or encrypting it (translating it into a secret code).

Chapter 23

Creating a Personal Health Record

What Is a Personal Health Record (PHR)?

A personal health record (PHR) is another health IT term you may have heard already. A PHR is a lot like an electronic health record (EHR), except you set up and control the information yourself. You don't have to wait for your doctor to build an electronic system into his or her practice. One of your healthcare or health insurance providers may already offer a PHR for you to use. You can also create a PHR through other software and online services.

Much like the EHR, the PHR can be an electronic storage center for your most important health information, such as:

- emergency contacts

- allergies

This chapter contains text excerpted from the following sources: Text under the heading "What Is a Personal Health Record (PHR)?" is excerpted from "Basics of Health IT," HealthIT.gov, Office of the National Coordinator for Health Information Technology (ONC), May 2, 2016; Text under the heading "Are There Different Types of Personal Health Records (PHRs)?" is excerpted from "Frequently Asked Questions," HealthIT.gov, Office of the National Coordinator for Health Information Technology (ONC), March 3, 2016; Text under the heading "What Are the Benefits of Personal Health Records?" is excerpted from "Frequently Asked Questions," HealthIT.gov, Office of the National Coordinator for Health Information Technology (ONC), March 3, 2016.

- illnesses or conditions

- medications

- immunization dates

- lab and test results

Your PHR may also have its own "apps"—programs that are used on smartphones—that can help you, improve your health by linking with other devices such as a web-enabled digital scale or pedometer.

Ideally, you should be able to link your PHR with your doctor's EHR, making it a personal healthcare "hub," although most doctors may not be technologically ready for this quite yet. PHRs can be maintained in a variety of formats, such as a USB "memory stick" or on a password-protected Internet site.

The advantage of a PHR is that it's all about you. You decide whether to create one in the first place, and what to put in it. Most of what you do for your health occurs outside the doctor's office and you can use your PHR to record that information. You can include:

- Over-the-counter (OTC) medications

- Exercise habits

- Sleep patterns

It can even reflect your preferences and values on sensitive issues, such as end-of-life care. It's your record: you know better than anyone else what your record should contain.

Are There Different Types of Personal Health Records (PHRs)?

Yes, there are two main kinds of personal health records (PHRs).

- **Standalone Personal Health Records:** With a standalone PHR, patients fill in information from their own records, and the information is stored on patients' computers or the Internet. In some cases, a standalone PHR can also accept data from external sources, including providers and laboratories. With a standalone PHR, patients could add diet or exercise information to track progress over time. Patients can decide whether to share the information with providers, family members, or anyone else involved in their care.

- **Tethered/Connected Personal Health Records:** A tethered, or connected, PHR is linked to a specific healthcare organization's electronic health record (EHR) system or to a health plan's information system. With a tethered PHR, patients can access their own records through a secure portal and see, for example, the trend of their lab results over the last year, their immunization history, or due dates for screenings.

What Are the Benefits of Personal Health Records?

Personal health records (PHRs) can help your patients better manage their care. Having important health information—such as immunization records, lab results, and screening due dates—in electronic form makes it easy for patients to update and share their records. PHRs can:

- **Improve patient engagement:** Much of what your patients do for their health happens outside clinical settings. When your patients can track their health over time and have information and tools to manage their health, they can be more engaged in their health and healthcare.

- **Coordinate and combine information from multiple providers:** PHRs can promote better healthcare by helping your patients manage information from various providers and improve care coordination.

- **Help to ensure patient information is available:** Online PHRs can ensure your patients' information is available in emergencies and when your patients are traveling.

- **Reduce administrative costs:** Your organization can reduce administrative costs by using a PHR to provide patients with easy access to electronic prescription refill and appointment scheduling applications. With PHRs, your staff can spend less time searching for patient-requested information and responding to patient questions.

- **Enhance provider-patient communication:** Many PHRs allow direct, secure communication between patients and providers. PHRs can make communicating with your patients faster and easier. With open lines of communication, you can be informed and intervene earlier if health problems arise and improve the provider-patient relationship.

- **Encourage family health management:** Having a system for tracking and updating healthcare information can help caregivers; such as those caring for young children, elderly parents, or spouses, manage your patients' care and coordinate with you to improve healthcare quality.

Chapter 24

Questions for the Doctor

Your Health Depends on Good Communication

Asking questions and providing information to your doctor and other care providers can improve your care. Talking with your doctor builds trust and leads to better results, quality, safety, and satisfaction. Quality healthcare is a team effort. You play an important role. One of the best ways to communicate with your doctor and healthcare team is by asking questions. Because time is limited during medical appointments, you will feel less rushed if you prepare your questions before your appointment.

Your Doctor Wants Your Questions

Doctors know a lot about a lot of things, but they don't always know everything about you or what is best for you. Your questions give your doctor and healthcare team important information about you, such as your most important healthcare concerns. That is why they need you to speak up.

This chapter includes text excerpted from "Questions to Ask Your Doctor," Agency for Healthcare Research and Quality (AHRQ), U.S. Department of Health and Human Services (HHS), September 2012. Reviewed January 2017.

Ten Questions You Should Know

A simple question can help you feel better, let you take better care of yourself, or save your life. The questions below can get you started.

1. What is the test for?
2. How many times have you done this procedure?
3. When will I get the results?
4. Why do I need this treatment?
5. Are there any alternatives?
6. What are the possible complications?
7. Which hospital is best for my needs?
8. How do you spell the name of that drug?
9. Are there any side effects?
10. Will this medicine interact with medicines that I'm already taking?

Questions to Ask before Your Appointment

You can make sure you get the best possible care by being an active member of your healthcare team. Being involved means being prepared and asking questions. Asking questions about your diagnoses, treatments, and medicines can improve the quality, safety, and effectiveness of your healthcare. Taking steps before your medical appointments will help you to make the most of your time with your doctor and healthcare team.

Prepare Your Questions

Time is limited during doctor visits. Prepare for your appointment by thinking about what you want to do during your next visit. Do you want to:

- Talk about a health problem?
- Get or change a medicine?
- Get medical tests?
- Talk about surgery or treatment options?

Write down your questions to bring to your appointment. The answers can help you make better decisions, get good care, and feel better about your healthcare.

Questions to Ask during Your Appointment

During your appointment, make sure to ask the questions you prepared before your appointment. Start by asking the ones that are most important to you.

- To get the most from your visit, tell the nurse or person at the front desk that you have questions for your doctor. If your doctor does not ask you if you have questions, ask your doctor when the best time would be to ask them.

Understand the Answers and next Steps

Asking questions is important but so is making sure you hear—and understand—the answers you get. Take notes. Or bring someone to your appointment to help you understand and remember what you heard. If you don't understand or are confused, ask your doctor to explain the answer again.

- It is very important to understand the plan or next steps that your doctor recommends. Ask questions to make sure you understand what your doctor wants you to do.

- The questions you may want to ask will depend on whether your doctor gives you a diagnosis; recommends a treatment, medical test, or surgery; or gives you a prescription for medicine.

- Questions could include:
    - What is my diagnosis?
    - What are my treatment options? What are the benefits of each option? What are the side effects?
    - Will I need a test? What is the test for? What will the results tell me?
    - What will the medicine you are prescribing do? How do I take it? Are there any side effects?
    - Why do I need surgery? Are there other ways to treat my condition? How often do you perform this surgery?
    - Do I need to change my daily routine?

Questions to Ask during Your Appointment

After you meet with your doctor, you will need to follow his or her instructions to keep your health on track. Your doctor may have you fill a prescription or make an another appointment for tests, lab work, or a follow-up visit. It is important for you to follow your doctor's instructions. It also is important to call your doctor if you are unclear about any instructions or have more questions.

Prioritize Your Questions

- Create a list of follow-up questions to ask if you:
- Have a health problem
- Need to get or change a medicine
- Need a medical test
- Need to have surgery

Other Times to Call Your Doctor

- There are other times when you should follow up on your care and call your doctor. Call your doctor:
- If you experience any side effects or other problems with your medicines.
- If your symptoms get worse after seeing the doctor.
- If you receive any new prescriptions or start taking any over-the-counter medicines.
- To get results of any tests you've had. Do not assume that no news is good news.
- To ask about test results you do not understand.

Your questions help your doctor and healthcare team learn more about you. Your doctor's answers to your questions can help you make better decisions, receive a higher level of care, avoid medical harm, and feel better about your healthcare. Your questions can also lead to better results for your health.

Chapter 25

Health Information Privacy Rule

Most of us believe that our medical and other health information is private and should be protected, and we want to know who has this information. The Privacy Rule, a Federal law, gives you rights over your health information and sets rules and limits on who can look at and receive your health information. The Privacy Rule applies to all forms of individuals' protected health information, whether electronic, written, or oral. The Security Rule is a Federal law that requires security for health information in electronic form.

What Information Is Protected

- Information your doctors, nurses, and other healthcare providers put in your medical record.

- Conversations your doctor has about your care or treatment with nurses and others.

- Information about you in your health insurer's computer system.

- Billing information about you at your clinic.

- Most other health information about you held by those who must follow these laws.

This chapter includes text excerpted from "Your Rights under HIPAA," U.S. Department of Health and Human Services (HHS), July 26, 2013. Reviewed January 2017.

How This Information Is Protected

- Covered entities must put in place safeguards to protect your health information and ensure they do not use or disclose your health information improperly.

- Covered entities must reasonably limit uses and disclosures to the minimum necessary to accomplish their intended purpose.

- Covered entities must have procedures in place to limit who can view and access your health information as well as implement training programs for employees about how to protect your health information.

- Business associates also must put in place safeguards to protect your health information and ensure they do not use or disclose your health information improperly.

What Rights Does the Privacy Rule Give Me over My Health Information?

Health insurers and providers who are covered entities must comply with your right to:

- Ask to see and get a copy of your health records.

- Have corrections added to your health information.

- Receive a notice that tells you how your health information may be used and shared.

- Decide if you want to give your permission before your health information can be used or shared for certain purposes, such as for marketing.

- Get a report on when and why your health information was shared for certain purposes.

- If you believe your rights are being denied or your health information isn't being protected, you can:

  - File a complaint with your provider or health insurer

  - File a complaint with HHS

You should get to know these important rights, which help you protect your health information. You can ask your provider or health insurer questions about your rights.

Who Can Look at and Receive Your Health Information

The Privacy Rule sets rules and limits on who can look at and receive your health information. To make sure that your health information is protected in a way that does not interfere with your healthcare, your information can be used and shared:

- For your treatment and care coordination.

- To pay doctors and hospitals for your healthcare and to help run their businesses.

- With your family, relatives, friends, or others you identify who are involved with your healthcare or your healthcare bills, unless you object.

- To make sure doctors give good care and nursing homes are clean and safe.

- To protect the public's health, such as by reporting when the flu is in your area.

- To make required reports to the police, such as reporting gunshot wounds.

Your health information cannot be used or shared without your written permission unless this law allows it. For example, without your authorization, your provider generally cannot:

- Give your information to your employer.

- Use or share your information for marketing or advertising purposes or sell your information.

Who Must Follow These Laws

Entities that must follow the HIPAA regulations are called "covered entities."

Covered entities include:

- **Health Plans,** including health insurance companies, Health Maintenance Organizations (HMO), company health plans, and certain government programs that pay for healthcare, such as Medicare and Medicaid.

- **Most Healthcare Providers**—those that conduct certain business electronically, such as electronically billing your health insurance—including most doctors, clinics, hospitals, psychologists, chiropractors, nursing homes, pharmacies, and dentists.

- **Healthcare Clearinghouses**—entities that process nonstandard health information they receive from another entity into a standard (i.e., standard electronic format or data content), or vice versa.

In addition, business associates of covered entities must follow parts of the HIPAA regulations.

Often, contractors, subcontractors, and other outside persons and companies that are not employees of a covered entity will need to have access to your health information when providing services to the covered entity. These entities are called "business associates." Examples of business associates include:

- Companies that help your doctors get paid for providing healthcare, including billing companies and companies that process your healthcare claims.

- Companies that help administer health plans.

- People like outside lawyers, accountants, and Information Technology (IT) specialists.

- Companies that store or destroy medical records.

Covered entities must have contracts in place with their business associates, ensuring that they use and disclose your health information properly and safeguard it appropriately. Business associates must also have similar contracts with subcontractors. Business associates (including subcontractors) must follow the use and disclosure provisions of their contracts and the Privacy Rule, and the safeguard requirements of the Security Rule.

Who Is Not Required to Follow These Laws

Many organizations that have health information about you do not have to follow these laws. Examples of organizations that do not have to follow the Privacy and Security Rules include:

- Life insurers

- Employers

- Workers compensation carriers

188

- Most schools and school districts
- Many state agencies like child protective service agencies
- Most law enforcement agencies
- Many municipal offices

Chapter 26

Patient's Rights and Responsibilities

Chapter Contents

Section 26.1

Patient's Rights and Responsibilities under the Affordable Care Act (ACA)

This section includes text excerpted from "Health Coverage Rights and Protections," Centers for Medicare and Medicaid Services (CMS), November 21, 2015.

The healthcare law offers rights and protections that make coverage more fair and easy to understand. Some rights and protections apply to plans in the health insurance marketplace or other individual insurance, some apply to job-based plans, and some apply to all health coverage. The protections outlined below may not apply to grandfathered health insurance plans.

How the Healthcare Law Protects You

- Requires insurance plans to cover people with pre-existing health conditions, including pregnancy, without charging more.

- Provides free preventive care.

- Gives young adults more coverage options.

- Ends lifetime and yearly dollar limits on coverage of essential health benefits.

- Helps you understand the coverage you're getting.

- Holds insurance companies accountable for rate increases.

- Makes it illegal for health insurance companies to cancel your health insurance just because you get sick.

- Protects your choice of doctors.

- Protects you from employer retaliation.

Additional Rights and Benefits

- Breastfeeding equipment and support.

- Health insurance plans must provide breastfeeding support, counseling, and equipment for the duration of breastfeeding. These services may be provided before and after birth.

- Your health insurance plan must cover the cost of a breast pump. It may be either a rental unit or a new one you'll keep. Your plan may have guidelines on whether the covered pump is manual or electric, the length of the rental, and when you'll receive it (before or after birth).

- Birth control methods and counseling.

U.S. Department of Food and Drug Administration (FDA)-approved contraceptive methods prescribed by a woman's doctor are covered, including:

- Barrier methods, like diaphragms and sponges.

- Hormonal methods, like birth control pills and vaginal rings.

- Implanted devices, like intrauterine devices (IUDs)..

- Emergency contraception, like Plan B® and ella®.

- Sterilization procedures.

- Patient education and counseling.

- Mental health and substance abuse services.

All plans must cover:

- Behavioral health treatment, such as psychotherapy and counseling.

- Mental and behavioral health inpatient services.

- Substance use disorder (commonly known as substance abuse) treatment.

- The right to appeal a health plan decision.

There are two ways to appeal a health plan decision:

- Internal appeal: If your claim is denied or your health insurance coverage cancelled, you have the right to an internal appeal. You may ask your insurance company to conduct a full and fair review of its decision. If the case is urgent, your insurance company must speed up this process.

- External review: You have the right to take your appeal to an independent third party for review. This is called external review. External review means that the insurance company no longer gets the final say over whether to pay a claim.

- The right to choose an individual marketplace plan rather than the one your employer offers you.

It's against the law for your employer to fire or retaliate against you because you get a premium tax credit when you buy a health plan in the Marketplace. It's also against the law for your employer to fire or retaliate against you if you report violations of the Affordable Care Act's health insurance reforms to your employer or the government.

Section 26.2

Medicare Rights

This chapter includes text excerpted from "Your Medicare Rights," Centers for Medicare and Medicaid Services (CMS), January 29, 2015.

No matter how you get your Medicare, you have certain rights and protections designed to:

- Protect you when you get healthcare.
- Make sure you get the healthcare services that the law says you can get.
- Protect you against unethical practices.
- Protect your privacy.

Rights and Protections for Everyone with Medicare

- Be treated with dignity and respect at all times.
- Be protected from discrimination. Every company or agency that works with Medicare must obey the law, and can't treat you differently because of your race, color, national origin, disability, age, religion, or sex.
- Have your personal and health information kept private.

- Get information in a way you understand from Medicare, health-care providers, and, under certain circumstances, contractors.
- Get understandable information about Medicare to help you make healthcare decisions, including:
  - What's covered.
  - What Medicare pays.
  - How much you have to pay.
  - What to do if you want to file a complaint or appeal.
- Have your questions about Medicare answered.
- Have access to doctors, specialists, and hospitals.
- Learn about your treatment choices in clear language that you can understand, and participate in treatment decisions.
- Get healthcare services in a language you understand and in a culturally-sensitive way.
- Get Medicare-covered services in an emergency.
- Get a decision about healthcare payment, coverage of services, or prescription drug coverage.
  - When a claim is filed, you get a notice from Medicare or from your Medicare Advantage Plan (Part C), other Medicare health plan, or Medicare Prescription Drug Plan (Part D) letting you know what it will and won't cover.
  - If you disagree with the decision of your claim, you have the right to file an appeal.
- Request a review (appeal) of certain decisions about healthcare payment, coverage of services, or prescription drug coverage.
  - If you disagree with a decision about your claims or services, you have the right to appeal.
- File complaints (sometimes called "grievances"), including complaints about the quality of your care.

Your Rights in Original Medicare

If you have Original Medicare, in addition to the rights and protections for all people with Medicare, you have the right to:
- See any doctor or specialist (including women's health specialists), or go to any Medicare-certified hospital, that participates in Medicare.

- Get certain information, notices, and appeal rights that help you resolve issues when Medicare may not or doesn't pay for healthcare. Learn about notices of noncoverage.

- Request an appeal of health coverage or payment decisions.

- Buy a Medicare Supplement Insurance (Medigap policy).

Your Rights in Medicare Health Plans

If you're in a Medicare Advantage Plan (Part C) or other Medicare health plan, in addition to the rights and protections for all people with Medicare, you have the right to:

- Choose healthcare providers within the plan, so you can get the healthcare you need.

- Get a treatment plan from your doctor.

  - If you have a complex or serious medical condition, a treatment plan lets you directly see a specialist within the plan as many times as you and your doctor think you need.

  - Women have the right to go directly to a women's healthcare specialist without a referral within the plan for routine and preventive healthcare services.

- Know how your doctors are paid.

  - When you ask your plan how it pays its doctors, the plan must tell you.

  - Medicare doesn't allow a plan to pay doctors in a way that could interfere with you getting the care you need.

- Request an appeal to resolve differences with your plan.

- File a complaint (called a "grievance") about other concerns or problems with your plan.

- Get a coverage decision or coverage information from your plan before getting services.

Your Rights in Medicare Drug Plans

In addition to the rights and protections for all people with Medicare, if you have a Medicare Prescription Drug Plan you have the right to:

- Request a coverage determination or appeal to resolve differences with your plan.

- File a complaint (called a "grievance") with the plan.

- Have the privacy of your health and prescription drug information protected.

If you have Medicare prescription drug coverage, your plan will send you information that explains your rights.

Get Help with Your Rights and Protections

With Medicare, you have special rights and protections. There are resources available to you to make sure your rights are protected, including:

- The Medicare Beneficiary Ombudsman

- The Competitive Acquisition Ombudsman (CAO)

- Your State Health Insurance Assistance Program (SHIP)

- The Beneficiary and Family Centered Care Quality Improvement Organization (BFCC-QIO)

The Medicare Beneficiary Ombudsman

The Medicare Beneficiary Ombudsman helps you with Medicare-related complaints, grievances, and information requests. The Medicare Beneficiary Ombudsman makes sure information is available about:

- What you need to know to make healthcare decisions that are right for you

- Your Medicare rights and protections

- How you can get issues resolved

The Medicare Beneficiary Ombudsman also shares information with the Secretary of Health and Human Services, Congress, and other organizations about what does and doesn't work well to improve the quality of the services and care you get through Medicare.

If you've contacted 1-800-MEDICARE (1-800-633-4227) about a Medicare-related inquiry or complaint but still need help, ask the 1-800-MEDICARE representative to send your inquiry or complaint to the Medicare Ombudsman's Office. The Medicare Ombudsman's Office helps make sure that your inquiry or complaint is resolved.

The Competitive Acquisition Ombudsman (CAO)

The CAO helps review and resolve complaints about durable medical equipment (DME) from people with Medicare and suppliers in Competitive Bidding Areas. The CAO responds to individual and supplier inquiries, issues, and complaints, and helps make sure that your complaint is resolved.

If you still need help after contacting your supplier and 1-800 MEDICARE, ask the 1-800-MEDICARE representative to send your inquiry or complaint to the CAO. The CAO helps make sure that your inquiry or complaint is resolved.

State Health Insurance Assistance Program (SHIP)

SHIPs offer local, personalized counseling to people with Medicare and their families.

SHIPs provide free information and counseling to help you with:

- Your Medicare questions, including your benefits, coverage, premiums, deductibles, and coinsurance

- Complaints (Grievances)

- Appeals

- Joining or leaving a Medicare Advantage Plan (Part C) (like an HMO or PPO), any other Medicare health plan, or Medicare Prescription Drug Plan (Part D).

Beneficiary and Family Centered Care Quality Improvement Organization (BFCC-QIO)

The BFCC-QIOs review complaints and quality of care for people with Medicare to improve the effectiveness, efficiency, economy, and quality of services delivered to people with Medicare.

BFCC-QIOs provide services to help you with:

- Filing appeals in hospital and non-hospital settings if you think your coverage is ending too soon

- Complaints (Grievances)

- Quality of care reviews

- Medical necessity reviews

The State Survey Agency

State Survey Agencies oversee healthcare facilities that participate in the Medicare and/or Medicaid programs. The State Survey Agency inspects healthcare facilities and investigates complaints to ensure that health and safety standards are met. If you have a complaint about improper care or unsafe conditions in a hospital, home health agency, hospice, or nursing home, or you're concerned about the healthcare, treatment, or services that you or another person got or didn't get in a healthcare setting, you can contact your State Survey Agency.

You can contact the State Survey Agency if you have concerns about things like:

- Abuse

- Neglect

- Mistreatment

- Poor care

- Not enough staff

- Unsafe or unsanitary conditions

- Dietary problems

Your Right to Access Your Personal Health Information

By law, you or your legal representative generally have the right to view and/or get copies of your personal health information from these groups:

- Healthcare providers who treat you

- Health plans that pay for your care, including Medicare

In most cases, you also have the right to have a provider or plan send copies of your information to a third party that you choose, like these:

- Other providers who treat you

- A family member

- A researcher

- A mobile application (or "app") you use to manage your personal health information

This information includes:

- Claims and billing records

- Information related to your enrollment in health plans, including Medicare

- Medical and case management records (except psychotherapy notes)

- Any other records that contain information that doctors or health plans use to make decisions about you

You may have to fill out a health information "request" form and pay a reasonable, cost-based fee for copies. Your providers or plans are supposed to tell you about the fee when you make the request. If they don't, ask. The fee can only be for the labor to make the copies, copying supplies, and postage (if needed). In most cases, you won't be charged for viewing, searching, downloading, or sending your information through an electronic portal.

Generally, you can get your information on paper or electronically. If your providers or plans store your information electronically, they generally must give you electronic copies, if that's your preference.

You have the right to get your information in a timely manner, but it may take up to 30 days to fill the request.

Chapter 27

Informed Consent

What Is Informed Consent?

Before a person has a procedure, it is important that he or she fully understands the testing procedure, the benefits and limitations of the test, and the possible consequences of the test results. The process of educating a person about the test and obtaining permission to carry out testing is called informed consent. "Informed" means that the person has enough information to make an educated decision about testing; "consent" refers to a person's voluntary agreement to have the test done.

In general, informed consent can only be given by adults who are competent to make medical decisions for themselves. For children and others who are unable to make their own medical decisions (such as people with impaired mental status), informed consent can be given by a parent, guardian, or other person legally responsible for making decisions on that person's behalf.

Informed consent for genetic testing is generally obtained by a doctor or genetic counselor during an office visit. The healthcare provider will discuss the test and answer any questions. If the person

This chapter contains text excerpted from the following sources: Text under the heading "What Is Informed Consent" is excerpted from "What Is Informed Consent?" Genetics Home Reference (GHR), National Institutes of Health (NIH), January 3, 2017; Text under the heading "Informed Consent Standards" is excerpted from "Informed Consent," Indian Health Service (IHS), U.S. Department of Health and Human Services (HHS), April 27, 2007. Reviewed January 2017.

wishes to have the test, he or she will then usually read and sign a consent form.

Several factors are commonly included on an informed consent form:

- A general description of the test, including the purpose of the test and the condition for which the testing is being performed.

- How the test will be carried out (for example, a blood sample).

- What the test results mean, including positive and negative results, and the potential for uninformative results or incorrect results such as false positives or false negatives.

- Any physical or emotional risks associated with the test.

- Whether the results can be used for research purposes.

- Whether the results might provide information about other family members' health, including the risk of developing a particular condition or the possibility of having affected children.

- How and to whom test results will be reported and under what circumstances results can be disclosed (for example, to health insurance providers).

- What will happen to the test specimen after the test is complete.

- Acknowledgement that the person requesting testing has had the opportunity to discuss the test with a healthcare professional.

- The individual's signature, and possibly that of a witness.

The elements of informed consent may vary, because some states have laws that specify factors that must be included. (For example, some states require disclosure that the test specimen will be destroyed within a certain period of time after the test is complete).

Informed consent is not a contract, so a person can change his or her mind at any time after giving initial consent. A person may choose not to go through with genetic testing even after the test sample has been collected. A person simply needs to notify the healthcare provider if he or she decides not to continue with the testing process.

Informed Consent Standards

Courts generally use one of two informed consent standards. The older "professional disclosure" standard is followed in about half the states. This standard requires the physician to disclose to the patient everything that is customary in the profession to disclose under the same or similar circumstances. In court, plaintiffs in these states must produce an expert witness to testify that the defendant's actions fell below the standard of customary disclosure.

The newer "reasonable patient standard" has been adopted in the remaining states. Under this standard, physicians are required to tell their patients everything that would reasonably bear on a decision to submit to treatment. Because expert testimony is not needed, it is generally easier to sue on informed consent grounds in states using this standard. In the case of federal court malpractice suits, the standard of the state in which the facility is located is used.

Most courts also require proximate cause. This means that plaintiffs must also prove that a reasonable person would not have gone through with the procedure if they had been fully informed of the risks and alternatives. In the case of elective surgery, it is easier for a patient to prove that he/she would not want the procedure if additional information had been provided; for more urgent or life saving procedures, the plaintiff's argument must be much more convincing. As a general rule, the more elective the procedure (and hence the greater the number of therapeutic alternatives), the more detailed the disclosure should be.

Required Elements: No matter what standard is applicable, there are five basic elements that must be disclosed to patients in language that a lay individual reasonably can be expected to understand:

1. The diagnosis, including the disclosure of any reservations the provider has concerning the diagnosis;

2. The nature and purpose of the proposed procedure or treatment;

3. The risks and consequences of the proposed procedure or treatment. This includes only those risks and consequences of which the physician has, or reasonably should have, knowledge. It is not necessary to disclose every potential minor risk or side effect.

4. Reasonable treatment alternatives. This includes other treatment modalities that are considered to be appropriate for the situation, even though they may not be the personal preference of the disclosing physician.

5. Prognosis without treatment. The patient must be informed of the potential consequences, if he/she elects not to have the recommended procedure.

Therapeutic Privilege: Under limited circumstances, courts have recognized that a physician may be justified in withholding information if it can be shown to be in the patient's best interest. This privilege applies only when a patient is unusually sensitive, anxious, or emotional.

Patient hypersensitivity should never be presumed. There must be ample justification for withholding information and the physician should carefully document his/her reasoning in the medical record. If the physician's use of the therapeutic privilege is challenged, it must be determined whether the physician acted appropriately. The use of this therapeutic privilege should be relied upon only in rare circumstances.

Implied Consent: Consent is either expressed (verbally or written) or implied. Consent may be implied under a variety of circumstances. For example, when a patient comes to see a physician for a particular ailment, it is implied that they consent to be examined. If a patient has a fractured arm, it is implied that he consents to casting. In general, physicians can assume that most patients would readily consent to care or treatments that are customary, noninvasive, and non-experimental.

Implied consent also relates to the performance of additional procedures when medically justified. When a physician is performing a hysterectomy, for example, an incidental appendectomy cannot be performed without the patient's expressed consent to do so. However, if the appendix is diseased, it is reasonable to assume that the patient would allow the procedure, unless the patient had expressly prohibited the appendix from being removed.

The use of general or blanket consent forms is not sound practice. These types of consent forms do not represent true informed consent as they are often solicited by an admission clerk, adequate information is not given, and they are not specific to any particular treatment or procedure. Blanket consent forms only serve as evidence of the patient's voluntary submission to treatment in general, which is usually self evident (implied), but these types of forms do not demonstrate that the patient understood specific indications and risks of any proposed invasive procedures. Again, it is recommended that blanket consent forms not be used.

Who May Give Consent: If the patient is a competent adult, the authority to give consent to treatment rests exclusively with the patient, unless the patient formally delegates that authority to someone else. Through the use of a document called a "power of attorney," executed in writing, a competent adult can delegate the responsibility for healthcare decisions to another competent adult.

A power of attorney in most states becomes ineffective when the person granting it becomes incompetent. For this reason, many states now recognize a "durable power of attorney," which generally remains effective even after the person granting the power becomes incompetent. In the healthcare setting, a durable power of attorney is the preferred document. Healthcare providers should always be careful to ensure that the proposed treatment lies within the scope of the expressed authorization.

Individuals who have not attained the legal age of majority (in most states, age 18) cannot legally give consent except in the following situations:

1. The patient is an emancipated minor (e.g., the minor is married, lives away from their parent's home, or is financially independent);

2. The state has fixed a lower limit of age for certain healthcare decisions (such as in the case of abortion, pregnancy, and treatment of venereal disease);

3. The state recognizes a "mature minor" exception, which allows minors to give consent to healthcare when there is a pressing need and the parent or guardian is unavailable. It is recommended that the reader be familiar with the laws in the state in which you practice.

The law holds that the closest available relative or legal guardian can authorize necessary and reasonable care when the patient is incapable of giving consent because of age, incompetency, or incapacity. A healthcare provider acting on the reasonable belief that a person is the patient's next of kin is legally protected if the authorizing person turns out not to be a close relative.

Emergency Situations: When the need for care is urgent, the patient is unable to give consent, and it is not feasible to contact the patient's next of kin, then the law does allow the physician to proceed with life saving diagnostic and therapeutic procedures without informed consent. The emergency consent exception is based on the following concepts:

1. The healthcare provider is entitled to presume that the patient would have chosen the care others would have chosen under

similar circumstances, unless the provider has information to the contrary;

2. The exception only applies to situations where immediate action is necessary to preserve life (or in some states "to prevent serious physical harm");

3. The circumstances justifying the emergency consent exception are well documented, including all attempts to notify the next of kin before treatment is begun.

Informed Refusal: The issue of documenting informed refusal is a relatively recent development. It is clear, as noted above, that patients have both the right to determine what is done to their body, and what is not. However, a patient should be very well informed if he/she is going to refuse a well established, common procedure such as a cancer screening test. On more than one occasion when patients have sued over a delayed diagnosis of cancer, courts have held that the physician was liable because he/she failed to adequately inform a patient about the consequences of the patient's prior refusal to accept standard cancer screening procedures.

For this reason, it is becoming more common for physicians to send registered letters to patients who decline certain types of care, informing them of the consequences in detail. Alternatively there may be circumstances where it would be wise to have the patient sign a written "informed refusal" document. Is this necessary every time a patient declines a test? No, but it would seem prudent to assess each situation carefully.

Document, Document, Document: All physicians should accept the doctrine of informed consent. It has b ethical and moral backing, it emanates from the right of self-determination and the right to privacy, and healthcare providers should not expect the courts to lose interest in patient rights.

In most states, verbal consent to treatment is legally sound, but it is very difficult for the provider to prove what the patient was told in the event that an adverse outcome leads to a malpractice claim. There is no question that written documentation enhances a physician's credibility. It, therefore, makes for good defensive medicine to carefully document the informed consent process, which includes, but is not limited to, a form that details the information disclosed to the patient, signed by both the patient and provider, and witnessed by a third party. It is helpful to have a third person (preferably a healthcare provider) present at the counseling session to witness the exchange of information, help solicit and answer questions, verify that the patient understands the information, and attest that the session took place. By signing the consent form, the third party is serving as a witness, and he/ she is not liable for the quality and sufficiency of the information given.

The patient-counseling session must be documented. There should be ample written evidence that informed consent was given to the patient, and the process by which it was given. In addition to a signed consent form, a progress note should include the fact that a counseling session took place, the mode of information delivery, and any additional clinically important details not specified on the consent form.

The American College of Surgeons recommends that the following principles be adhered to when documenting informed consent:

1. There should be a clear explanation of each medical term in lay language;

2. There should be a listing of commonly occurring risks of the procedure;

3. Never describe a procedure as "simple," "uncomplicated," or "minor." The consent form should include a statement that no result has been guaranteed;

4. Avoid the use of national statistics, as the operating surgeon's own experience, may vary from the national norm;

5. Indicate on the consent form if the patient has been given an informational brochure or shown a video;

6. The patient should acknowledge on the consent form that the information disclosed has been understood, that an opportunity to ask questions has been provided, and that all questions have been answered to the patient's satisfaction;

7. The signature of both the patient and operating surgeon should be on the consent form, timed and dated;

8. The form should include a statement indicating that "unexpected risks or complications not discussed may occur," and that "unforeseen conditions may be revealed requiring the performance of additional procedures, and I authorize such procedures to be performed."

Chapter 28

Preventing Medical Errors

An Overview on Medical Errors

Medical errors can occur anywhere in the healthcare system: In hospitals, clinics, surgery centers, doctors' offices, nursing homes, pharmacies, and patients' homes. Errors can involve medicines, surgery, diagnosis, equipment, or lab reports. These tips tell what you can do to get safer care.

One in seven Medicare patients in hospitals experience a medical error. But medical errors can occur anywhere in the healthcare system: In hospitals, clinics, surgery centers, doctors' offices, nursing homes, pharmacies, and patients' homes. Errors can involve medicines, surgery, diagnosis, equipment, or lab reports. They can happen during even the most routine tasks, such as when a hospital patient on a salt-free diet is given a high-salt meal.

Most errors result from problems created by today's complex healthcare system. But errors also happen when doctors and patients have problems communicating. These tips tell what you can do to get safer care.

What You Can Do to Stay Safe

The best way you can help to prevent errors is to be an active member of your healthcare team. That means taking part in every decision

---

This chapter includes text excerpted from "20 Tips to Help Prevent Medical Errors," Agency for Healthcare Research and Quality (AHRQ), U.S. Department of Health and Human Services (HHS), December 2014.

about your healthcare. Research shows that patients who are more involved with their care tend to get better results.

Medicines

1. Make sure that all of your doctors know about every medicine you are taking. This includes prescription and over-the-counter medicines and dietary supplements, such as vitamins and herbs.

2. Bring all of your medicines and supplements to your doctor visits. "Brown bagging" your medicines can help you and your doctor talk about them and find out if there are any problems. It can also help your doctor keep your records up to date and help you get better quality care.

3. Make sure your doctor knows about any allergies and adverse reactions you have had to medicines. This can help you to avoid getting a medicine that could harm you.

4. When your doctor writes a prescription for you, make sure you can read it. If you cannot read your doctor's handwriting, your pharmacist might not be able to either.

5. Ask for information about your medicines in terms you can understand—both when your medicines are prescribed and when you get them:

    • What is the medicine for?

    • How am I supposed to take it and for how long?

    • What side effects are likely? What do I do if they occur?

    • Is this medicine safe to take with other medicines or dietary supplements I am taking?

    • What food, drink, or activities should I avoid while taking this medicine?

6. When you pick up your medicine from the pharmacy, ask: Is this the medicine that my doctor prescribed?

7. If you have any questions about the directions on your medicine labels, ask. Medicine labels can be hard to understand. For example, ask if "four times daily" means taking a dose every 6 hours around the clock or just during regular waking hours.

8. Ask your pharmacist for the best device to measure your liquid medicine. For example, many people use household teaspoons, which often do not hold a true teaspoon of liquid. Special devices, like marked syringes, help people measure the right dose.

9. Ask for written information about the side effects your medicine could cause. If you know what might happen, you will be better prepared if it does or if something unexpected happens.

Hospital Stays

10. If you are in a hospital, consider asking all healthcare workers who will touch you whether they have washed their hands. Hand washing can prevent the spread of infections in hospitals.

11. When you are being discharged from the hospital, ask your doctor to explain the treatment plan you will follow at home. This includes learning about your new medicines, making sure you know when to schedule follow-up appointments, and finding out when you can get back to your regular activities.

    It is important to know whether or not you should keep taking the medicines you were taking before your hospital stay. Getting clear instructions may help prevent an unexpected return trip to the hospital.

Surgery

12. If you are having surgery, make sure that you, your doctor, and your surgeon all agree on exactly what will be done. Having surgery at the wrong site (for example, operating on the left knee instead of the right) is rare. But even once is too often. The good news is that wrong-site surgery is 100 percent preventable. Surgeons are expected to sign their initials directly on the site to be operated on before the surgery.

13. If you have a choice, choose a hospital where many patients have had the procedure or surgery you need. Research shows that patients tend to have better results when they are treated in hospitals that have a great deal of experience with their condition.

Other Steps

14. Speak up if you have questions or concerns. You have a right to question anyone who is involved with your care.

15. Make sure that someone, such as your primary care doctor, coordinates your care. This is especially important if you have many health problems or are in the hospital.

16. Make sure that all your doctors have your important health information. Do not assume that everyone has all the information they need.

17. Ask a family member or friend to go to appointments with you. Even if you do not need help now, you might need it later.

18. Know that "more" is not always better. It is a good idea to find out why a test or treatment is needed and how it can help you. You could be better off without it.

19. If you have a test, do not assume that no news is good news. Ask how and when you will get the results.

20. Learn about your condition and treatments by asking your doctor and nurse and by using other reliable sources. Ask your doctor if your treatment is based on the latest evidence.

Chapter 29

The Partnership for Patients Program

The Partnership for Patients initiative is a public-private partnership working to improve the quality, safety and affordability of healthcare for all Americans.

Who Is in the Partnership?

Physicians, nurses, hospitals, employers, patients and their advocates, and the Federal and State governments have joined together to form the Partnership for Patients.

Key Elements of the Partnership

The Partnership for Patients aims to engage 100 percent of the nation's acute care medical centers participating in making hospital care safer, more reliable, and less costly through the achievement of two goals:

- **Making care safer**. Keep patients from getting injured or sicker. Decrease all-cause patient harm (to 97 Hospital-Acquired Conditions [HACs]/1,000 discharges) by 20 percent compared to the 2014 interim baseline (of 121 HACs/1,000 patient discharges).

This chapter includes text excerpted from "About the Partnership," Centers for Medicare and Medicaid Services (CMS), September 28, 2016.

- **Improving care transitions**. Help patients heal without complications. Decrease preventable complications during a transition from one care setting to another so that all 30-day hospital readmissions would be reduced by 12 percent as a population-based measure (readmissions per 1,000 people).

What Is the Partnership About?

The **Hospital Improvement Innovation Network (HIINs)** hospitals across the country are critical partners in this work. Through the Partnership for Patients, national, regional, or state hospital associations, quality improvement organizations, and health system organizations serve as Hospital Improvement Innovation Networks. On May 25, 2016, the Centers for Medicare and Medicaid Services (CMS) posted a request for proposals for Hospital Improvement Innovation Network (HIINs) contracts to continue the success achieved in improving patient safety.

On September 28, 2016 the Centers for Medicare and Medicaid Services (CMS) awarded contracts to 16 Hospital Improvement Innovation Networks as a part of the integration of the Partnership for Patients (PfP) Hospital Engagement Networks (HEN) into the Quality Improvement Network-Quality Improvement Organization (QIN-QIO) program to prepare for the continuation of the Partnership for Patients. The Hospital Improvement Innovation Networks (HIINs) will build upon the collective momentum of the PfP's Hospital Improvement Innovation Networks and Quality Improvement Organizations (QIO) to reduce patient harm and re-admissions. The HIINs also represent the integration of the work previously done by the HENs in support of the QIO and quality improvement efforts for the Medicare population.

The community-based care transitions program. Another major Partnership for Patients network includes the 46 sites awarded to participate in the Community-based Care Transitions Program (CCTP). These sites each constitute a collaborative community effort including community-based organizations such as social service providers or Area Agencies on Aging (AAAs), multiple hospital partners, nursing homes, home health agencies, pharmacies, primary care practices, and other types of health and social service providers serving patients in that community. Through the program, these sites are testing models for improving care transitions from the hospital to other settings and for reducing readmissions for high-risk Medicare beneficiaries.

Patient and family engagement. The relationship between healthcare professionals and their patients and families is critically important to the Partnership. It is a key part of keeping patients from getting injured or sicker in the hospital and helping patients heal without complication through improved transitions across healthcare settings and reduced re-admissions.

Where Partnerships Are in Action

The nationwide Partnership for Patients initiative aims to save lives by averting hospital acquired conditions and improving the transition of care from care setting to another through reducing readmissions. At the core of this initiative are 16 Hospital Improvement Innovation Networks (HIINs), which partner with more than 4,000 hospitals, working with healthcare providers and institutions, to identify best practices and solutions to reducing hospital acquired conditions and readmissions. Also, the Community-based Care Transitions Program (CCTP) aims to further improve the quality of care for Medicare beneficiaries while improving care transitions from inpatient hospital settings and document measurable savings to the Medicare program.

Chapter 30

Healthcare Fraud

What Is Healthcare Fraud?

Healthcare fraud occurs when an individual, a group of people, or a company knowingly mis-represents or mis-states something about the type, the scope, or the nature of the medical treatment or service provided, in a manner that could result in unauthorized payments being made. Examples of healthcare fraud include:
Billing for services not rendered or goods not provided;

- Falsifying certificates of medical necessity and billing for services not medically necessary;

- Billing separately for services that should be included in single service fees;

- Falsifying plans of treatment or medical records to justify payments;

This chapter contains text excerpted from the following sources: Text under the heading "What Is Healthcare Fraud?" is excerpted from "Health Care Fraud," U.S. Department of Justice (DOJ), August 25, 2016; Text under the heading "Fighting Healthcare Fraud" is excerpted from "Health Care Fraud Unit," U.S. Department of Justice (DOJ), December 30, 2016; Text under the heading "Types of Healthcare Fraud" is excerpted from "Common Types of Health Care Fraud," Centers for Medicare and Medicaid Services (CMS), July 2016; Text beginning with the heading "Protect Yourself from Healthcare Fraud" is excerpted from "Protect Yourself from Marketplace Fraud," HealthCare.gov, Centers for Medicare and Medicaid Services (CMS), January 19, 2014.

- Misrepresenting diagnoses or procedures to maximize payments;

- Misrepresenting charges or entitlements to payments in cost reports; and

- Soliciting "kickbacks" for the provision of various services or goods.

Healthcare fraud may be perpetrated against all types of health insurers and health insurance companies, including Medicare, Medicaid, Blue Cross Blue Shield, workers compensation, and other private entities.

Medicare services are divided into Part A and Part B coverage. Part A coverage includes hospital care, home healthcare, and skilled nursing care; Part B coverage includes physician services, laboratory tests and X-rays, outpatient services, and medical supplies.

Fighting Healthcare Fraud

Healthcare fraud costs the United States tens of billions of dollars each year. Some estimates put the figure close to $100 billion a year. It is a rising threat, with national healthcare expenditures estimated to exceed $3 trillion in 2014. Healthcare fraud schemes continue to grow in complexity and seriousness. The dedicated efforts of law enforcement are a major component of the fight against healthcare fraud.

The Health Insurance Portability and Accountability Act of 1996 (HIPAA) established a national Health Care Fraud and Abuse Control Program (HCFAC or the Program) under the joint direction of the Attorney General and the Secretary of the U.S. Department of Health and Human Services (HHS), designed to coordinate Federal, state and local law enforcement activities with respect to healthcare fraud and abuse. In its seventeenth year of operation, the Program's continued success confirms the soundness of a collaborative approach to identify and prosecute the most egregious instances of healthcare fraud, to prevent future fraud and abuse, and to protect program beneficiaries.

Types of Healthcare Fraud

Fraud, waste, and abuse pose major risks for the Medicaid program. Providers who engage in fraud and abuse are subject to sanctions under a number of Federal and State laws. Sanctions under Federal law, for example, can take the form of administrative, civil, and criminal penalties. These penalties range from monetary fines and damages to prison time and exclusion from the Federal healthcare programs, including Medicaid. Becoming familiar with common types of fraud, waste, and abuse, will better position providers to ensure they are not involved in such conduct. Providers will also be better equipped to identify and report others who may be engaged in fraud, waste, and abuse.

This chapter provides a brief overview of some common types of Medicaid fraud, waste, and abuse involving providers. Although the examples involve violation of Federal laws, many States have similar laws against fraud, waste, and abuse. This list is not intended to be complete.

- **Medical identity theft.** Medical identity theft involves the misuse of a person's medical identity to wrongfully obtain healthcare goods, services, or funds. Specifically, medical identity theft has been defined as "the appropriation or misuse of a patients' or providers' unique medical identifying information to obtain or bill public or private payers for fraudulent medical goods or services." Stolen physician identifiers can be used to fill fraudulent prescriptions, refer patients for unnecessary additional services or supplies, or bill for services that were never provided.

  Some people use beneficiary medical identifiers to fraudulently bill services or items not provided, or to enable an ineligible person to receive services by impersonating a beneficiary. Providers should take steps to protect their identifying information and that of their patients from unauthorized use.

- **Billing for unnecessary services or items.** Under Section 1902(a)(30)(A) of the Social Security Act, States are required to "provide such methods and procedures relating to the utilization of, and the payment for, care and services available under the plan ... as may be necessary to safeguard against unnecessary utilization of such care and services." States may "place appropriate limits on a service based on such criteria as medical necessity." Providers are responsible for ensuring authorized services meet the definition of medical necessity in the States where they practice. Intentional billing of unnecessary services or items can lead to the serious consequences mentioned earlier.

- **Billing for services or items not furnished.** To be covered by Medicaid, the billed service or supply must be provided. Some providers bill Medicaid for a covered service or item but do not deliver the service or item. These providers may create

219

false records in an attempt to justify the bills. For example, a physician might sign charts and submit bills for examinations and tests that never took place. Providers should only bill for the medically necessary or otherwise authorized services or items provided to beneficiaries and should ensure that proper documentation is in place. Healthcare professionals should exercise appropriate caution when evaluating offers of payment in exchange for reviewing medical records written by others.

- **Upcoding.** Upcoding is a term that is not defined in the regulations but is generally understood as billing for services at a higher level of complexity than the service actually provided or documented in the file. For example, a supplier of durable medical equipment might bill for motorized scooters while supplying less expensive manual wheelchairs. As another example, a physician might bill simple office visits at the higher rate for complex visits. These practices are illegal. Providers should only bill for the level of services or items provided.

- **Unbundling.** According to the Federal Bureau of Investigation, unbundling "is the practice of submitting bills in a fragmented fashion in order to maximize the reimbursement for various tests or procedures that are required to be billed together at a reduced cost." For example, a laboratory might receive an order for a panel of blood tests on a patient. Instead of billing for the panel, the laboratory might attempt to increase its income by billing for each test separately. This is like ordering a value meal at a fast-food restaurant and then being charged the higher individual prices for each item. Providers who bill Medicaid are responsible for knowing which procedures are subject to bundling requirements and billing accordingly.

- **Kickbacks.** Kickbacks can be defined as offering, soliciting, paying, or receiving remuneration (in kind or in cash) to induce, or in return for referral of patients or the generation of business involving any item or service for which payment may be made under Federal healthcare programs. Rewarding sources of new business may be acceptable in some industries, but not when Federal healthcare programs and beneficiaries are involved. For example, it would be illegal for a physician to accept payments from a medical imaging facility for referring patients. Kickbacks in healthcare can lead to overutilization, increased program costs, corruption of medical decision-making, patient steering, and unfair competition.

Specific examples of provider prosecutions and settlements resulting from these types of fraud are updated frequently and posted on the U.S. Department of Health and Human Services (HHS), Office of Inspector General (OIG) website.

Protect Yourself from Healthcare Fraud

When you apply for health coverage through the Health Insurance Marketplace, you can protect yourself from fraud by following a few simple guidelines.

After you complete an application, you may get a phone call from the Marketplace to verify or ask for more information.

Be Informed about Your Healthcare Choices

- Spend some time with HealthCare.gov to learn the basics about getting health coverage. It's the official Marketplace website.

- Compare insurance plans carefully before making your decision. If you have questions, contact the Health Insurance Marketplace call center at 1-800-318-2596. TTY users should call 1-855-889-4325.

- Look for official government seals, logos, or web addresses (which end in ".gov") on materials you see in print or online.

- Know the Marketplace Open Enrollment dates. No one can enroll you in a health plan in the Marketplace until Open Enrollment begins or after it ends unless you have special circumstances.

Protect Your Private Healthcare and Financial Information

Never give your financial information, like your banking, credit card, or account numbers, to someone who calls or comes to your home uninvited, even if they say they are from the Marketplace.

Never give your personal health information, like your medical history or specific treatments you've received, to anyone who asks you for it. (If you apply for certain Marketplace exemptions, you may be asked for medical documentation.)

Ask Questions and Verify the Answers You Get

- The Marketplace has trained assisters in every state to help you at no cost. You should never be asked to pay for services or help to apply for Marketplace coverage. Find a free, trained local assister.

- Ask questions if any information is unclear.

- Write down and keep a record of the name of a salesperson or anyone who may assist you, who he or she works for, telephone number, street address, mailing address, email address, and website.

- Double check any information that is confusing or sounds fishy. Check out HealthCare.gov to verify things or call the Marketplace at 1-800-318-2596 (TTY: 1-855-889-4325).

If You Get a Call from the Marketplace

After you apply you may get a phone call from the Marketplace asking you to verify or provide more information.

Follow these tips to help prevent fraud. If your phone has caller ID, check the number. The display may show one of these:

- Health Insurance MP

- InsMarketplace

- 701-264-3124

- 844-477-7500

The customer service representative will say they are calling from the Marketplace and provide a first name and agent ID number. Write them down.

A Marketplace representative may leave a message on your answering machine. If this happens, you won't be able to call back. If the Marketplace can't reach you after 3 tries, you'll get a letter in the mail telling you what to do next.

The Marketplace representative may ask you the following:

- To verify your identity, using information you provided on your application, including your full name and address.

- To provide or verify your Social Security number, application ID, policy ID, user ID, date of birth, or phone number.

- To verify or provide income, household, and employment information, but NOT personal financial information, like a bank name and account number. They will also not ask about any personal health information, like your medical history or conditions. (If you're applying for certain Marketplace exemptions, you may be asked to provide medical documentation.)

If you don't want to answer over the phone, ask the representative to mail you a letter with instructions for completing your application.

In certain cases, the Marketplace may request additional documentation. If you need to mail any information to the:

Health Insurance Marketplace

465 Industrial Blvd.

London, KY 40750-0001

Don't mail any information to a different address. The Zone Improvement Plan (ZIP) code may end with 4 extra numbers the representative provides.

When to Report Suspected Fraud

It's time to take action if:

- Someone other than the insurance company you've chosen contacts you about health insurance and asks you to pay—or asks for your financial or personal health information

- Someone you don't know contacts you about getting health insurance and asks you to pay—or asks you for your personal financial or health information

- Someone contacts you and claims to be from the government or Medicare—and asks you to pay for a new "Obamacare" insurance card

- You give your personal health, bank account, or credit card information to someone who calls you and says they're from the government

How to Report Suspected Fraud

You can report suspected fraud one of two ways:

1. If you suspect identity theft, or feel like you gave your personal information to someone you shouldn't have, use the Federal

Trade Commission's (FTC) online Complaint Assistant. You should also contact your local police department.

2. Call the Health Insurance Marketplace call center at 1-800-318-2596 (TTY: 1-855-889-4325). Explain what happened and your information will be handled appropriately.

Part Four

Prescription (Rx) and Over-the-Counter (OTC) Medications

Chapter 31

Understanding Medications and What They Do

Your pharmacist can help you learn how to use your prescription and nonprescription (over-the-counter) medicines safely and to increase the benefits and decrease the risks. You can also use these tips when talking with your other healthcare professionals.

Tell your pharmacist

- everything you use. Keep a record and give it to your pharmacist. Make sure you put all the prescription and nonprescription medicines, vitamins, herbals, and other supplements you use. Your pharmacist will use this to keep his/her records up-to-date and help you use medicine safely.

- if you've had any allergic reactions or problems with medicines, medicines with dietary supplements, medicines with food, or medicines with other treatments.

This chapter contains text excerpted from the following sources: Text in this chapter begins with excerpts from "Stop—Learn—Go—Tips for Talking with Your Pharmacist to Learn How to Use Medicines Safely," U.S. Food and Drug Administration (FDA), August 30, 2013. Reviewed January 2017; Text under the heading "General Drug Categories" is excerpted from "General Drug Categories," U.S. Food and Drug Administration (FDA), December 7, 2015; Text under the heading "The Drug Facts Label" is excerpted from "Checklist for Choosing Over-the-Counter (OTC) Medicine for Children," U.S. Food and Drug Administration (FDA), July 17, 2008. Reviewed January 2017.

- anything that could affect your use of medicine, such as, if you have trouble swallowing, reading labels, remembering to use medicine, or paying for medicine.

- before you start using something new. Your pharmacist can help you avoid medicines, supplements, foods, and other things that don't mix well with your medicines.

- if you are pregnant, might become pregnant, or if you are breast feeding.

Ask your pharmacist

- What are the brand and generic (non-brand) names?

- What is the active ingredient? Can I use a generic?

- What is this for, and how is it going to help me?

- How and when should I use it? How much do I use?

- How long should I use it? Can I stop using the medicine or use less if I feel better?

- What should I do if I ...miss a dose? ....use too much?

- Will this take the place of anything else I am using?

- When will the medicine start working? How should I expect to feel?

- Are there any special directions for using this?

- Should I avoid any other medicines, dietary supplements, drinks, foods, activities, or other things?

- Is there anything I should watch for, like allergic reactions or side effects? What do I do if I get any?

- Will I need any tests to check the medicine's effects (blood tests, X-rays, other)? When will I need those?

- How and where should I keep this medicine?

- Is there a medication guide or other patient information for this medicine?

- Where and how can I get more written information?

After you have the medicine, and before you leave the pharmacy

- Look to be sure you have the right medicine. If you've bought the medicine before, make sure this medicine has the same shape, color, size, markings, and packaging. Anything different? Ask your pharmacist. If it seems different when you use it, tell your pharmacist, doctor, or other healthcare professional.

- Be sure you know the right dose for the medicine and you know how to use it. Any questions? Ask your pharmacist.

- Make sure there is a measuring spoon, cup, or syringe for liquid medicine. If the medicine doesn't come with a special measuring tool, ask your pharmacist about one. (Spoons used for eating and cooking may give the wrong dose. Don't use them.)

- Be sure you have any information the pharmacist can give you about the medicine. Read it and save it.

- Get the pharmacy phone number, so you can call back.

General Drug Categories

Analgesics: Drugs that relieve pain. There are two main types: non-narcotic analgesics for mild pain, and narcotic analgesics for severe pain.

Antacids: Drugs that relieve indigestion and heartburn by neutralizing stomach acid.

Antianxiety Drugs: Drugs that suppress anxiety and relax muscles (sometimes called anxiolytics, sedatives, or minor tranquilizers).

Antiarrhythmics: Drugs used to control irregularities of heartbeat.

Antibacterials: Drugs used to treat infections.

Antibiotics: Drugs made from naturally occurring and synthetic substances that combat bacterial infection. Some antibiotics are effective only against limited types of bacteria. Others, known as broad spectrum antibiotics, are effective against a wide range of bacteria.

Anticoagulants and Thrombolytics: Anticoagulants prevent blood from clotting. Thrombolytics help dissolve and disperse blood clots and may be prescribed for patients with recent arterial or venous thrombosis.

Anticonvulsants: Drugs that prevent epileptic seizures.

Antidepressants: There are three main groups of mood-lifting antidepressants: tricyclics, monoamine oxidase inhibitors, and selective serotonin reuptake inhibitors (SSRIs).

Antidiarrheals: Drugs used for the relief of diarrhea. Two main types of antidiarrheal preparations are simple adsorbent substances and drugs that slow down the contractions of the bowel muscles so that the contents are propelled more slowly.

Antiemetics: Drugs used to treat nausea and vomiting.

Antifungals: Drugs used to treat fungal infections, the most common of which affect the hair, skin, nails, or mucous membranes.

Antihistamines: Drugs used primarily to counteract the effects of histamine, one of the chemicals involved in allergic reactions.

Antihypertensives: Drugs that lower blood pressure. The types of antihypertensives currently marketed include diuretics, beta-blockers, calcium channel blocker, ACE (angiotensin- converting enzyme) inhibitors, centrally acting antihypertensives and sympatholytics.

Anti-Inflammatories: Drugs used to reduce inflammation—the redness, heat, swelling, and increased blood flow found in infections and in many chronic noninfective diseases such as rheumatoid arthritis and gout.

Antineoplastics: Drugs used to treat cancer.

Antipsychotics: Drugs used to treat symptoms of severe psychiatric disorders. These drugs are sometimes called major tranquilizers.

Antipyretics: Drugs that reduce fever.

Antivirals: Drugs used to treat viral infections or to provide temporary protection against infections such as influenza.

Barbiturates: See "sleeping drugs."

Beta-Blockers: Beta-adrenergic blocking agents, or beta-blockers for short, reduce the oxygen needs of the heart by reducing heartbeat rate.

Bronchodilators: Drugs that open up the bronchial tubes within the lungs when the tubes have become narrowed by muscle spasm. Bronchodilators ease breathing in diseases such as asthma.

Cold Cures: Although there is no drug that can cure a cold, the aches, pains, and fever that accompany a cold can be relieved by aspirin or acetaminophen often accompanied by a decongestant, antihistamine, and sometimes caffeine.

Corticosteroids: These hormonal preparations are used primarily as anti-inflammatories in arthritis or asthma or as immunosuppressives, but they are also useful for treating some malignancies or compensating for a deficiency of natural hormones in disorders such as Addison disease.

Cough Suppressants: Simple cough medicines, which contain substances such as honey, glycerine, or menthol, soothe throat irritation but do not actually suppress coughing. They are most soothing when taken as lozenges and dissolved in the mouth. As liquids they are probably swallowed too quickly to be effective. A few drugs are actually cough suppressants. There are two groups of cough suppressants: those that alter the consistency or production of phlegm such as mucolytics and expectorants; and those that suppress the coughing reflex such as codeine (narcotic cough suppressants), antihistamines, dextromethorphan and isoproterenol (non-narcotic cough suppressants).

Cytotoxics: Drugs that kill or damage cells. Cytotoxics are used as antineoplastics (drugs used to treat cancer) and also as immunosuppressives.

Decongestants: Drugs that reduce swelling of the mucous membranes that line the nose by constricting blood vessels, thus relieving nasal stuffiness.

Diuretics: Drugs that increase the quantity of urine produced by the kidneys and passed out of the body, thus ridding the body of excess fluid. Diuretics reduce water logging of the tissues caused by fluid retention in disorders of the heart, kidneys, and liver. They are useful in treating mild cases of high blood pressure.

Expectorant: A drug that stimulates the flow of saliva and promotes coughing to eliminate phlegm from the respiratory tract.

Hormones: Chemicals produced naturally by the endocrine glands (thyroid, adrenal, ovary, testis, pancreas, parathyroid). In some disorders, for example, diabetes mellitus, in which too little of a particular hormone is produced, synthetic equivalents or natural hormone extracts are prescribed to restore the deficiency. Such treatment is known as hormone replacement therapy.

Hypoglycemics (Oral): Drugs that lower the level of glucose in the blood. Oral hypoglycemic drugs are used in diabetes mellitus if it cannot be controlled by diet alone, but does require treatment with injections of insulin.

Immunosuppressives: Drugs that prevent or reduce the body's normal reaction to invasion by disease or by foreign tissues.

Immunosuppressives are used to treat autoimmune diseases (in which the body's defenses work abnormally and attack its own tissues) and to help prevent rejection of organ transplants.

Laxatives: Drugs that increase the frequency and ease of bowel movements, either by stimulating the bowel wall (stimulant laxative), by increasing the bulk of bowel contents (bulk laxative), or by lubricating them (stool-softeners, or bowel movement-softeners). Laxatives may be taken by mouth or directly into the lower bowel as suppositories or enemas. If laxatives are taken regularly, the bowels may ultimately become unable to work properly without them.

Muscle Relaxants: Drugs that relieve muscle spasm in disorders such as backache. Antianxiety drugs (minor tranquilizers) that also have a muscle-relaxant action are used most commonly.

Sedatives: Same as Antianxiety drugs.

Sex Hormones (Female): There are two groups of these hormones (estrogens and progesterone), which are responsible for development of female secondary sexual characteristics. Small quantities are also produced in males. As drugs, female sex hormones are used to treat menstrual and menopausal disorders and are also used as oral contraceptives. Estrogens may be used to treat cancer of the breast or prostate, progestins (synthetic progesterone to treat endometriosis).

Sex Hormones (Male): Androgenic hormones, of which the most powerful is testosterone, are responsible for development of male secondary sexual characteristics. Small quantities are also produced in females. As drugs, male sex hormones are given to compensate for hormonal deficiency in hypopituitarism or disorders of the testes. They may be used to treat breast cancer in women, but either synthetic derivatives called anabolic steroids, which have less marked side-effects, or specific anti-estrogens are often preferred. Anabolic steroids also have a "body building" effect that has led to their (usually nonsanctioned) use in competitive sports, for both men and women.

Sleeping Drugs: The two main groups of drugs that are used to induce sleep are benzodiazepines and barbiturates. All such drugs have a sedative effect in low doses and are effective sleeping medications in higher doses. Benzodiazepines drugs are used more widely than barbiturates because they are safer, the side-effects are less marked, and there is less risk of eventual physical dependence.

Tranquilizer: This is a term commonly used to describe any drug that has a calming or sedative effect. However, the drugs that are sometimes called minor tranquilizers should be called antianxiety drugs, and the drugs that are sometimes called major tranquilizers should be called antipsychotics.

Vitamins: Chemicals essential in small quantities for good health. Some vitamins are not manufactured by the body, but adequate quantities are present in a normal diet. People whose diets are inadequate or who have digestive tract or liver disorders may need to take supplementary vitamins.

The Drug Facts Label

In the United States, each OTC medicine has a Drug Facts label. The Drug Facts label is there to help you choose the right OTC medicine and use it safely. All medicines, even OTC medicines, can cause side effects (unwanted or unexpected effects). But if the directions on the label are followed, the chance of side effects can be lowered.

These are the sections of the Drug Facts label:

The **Active ingredients/Purposes** section tells you the part of the medicine that makes it work (active ingredient), what it does (purpose), and how much of each active ingredient is in each unit (such as pill, capsule, or teaspoon). Choose a medicine that treats only the problem(s) you want to treat. Extra medicine won't help, and could cause harmful or unwanted side effects.

The **Uses** section tells you the problems the medicine will treat. The problem(s) you want to treat should match at least one of the Uses.

The **Warnings** section tells you:

- When to talk to a doctor first.

- How the medicine might make a person feel.

- When the medicine shouldn't be used.

- Things that shouldn't be done while using the medicine.

- When to stop using the medicine.

- To check with a doctor before using medicine if the person is pregnant or breastfeeding.

- To keep medicines away from children.

The **Directions** section tells you how to use the medicine safely:

- How much to use.

- How to use it.

- How often to use it (how many times per day, how many hours apart).

- How long it can be used.

The **Other Information** section tells you how to keep the medicine when it isn't being used.

The **Inactive ingredients** section tells you the parts of the medicine that aren't the active ingredient(s). These parts are added to the active ingredient(s) to help shape the form, to flavor or color the medicine, or to help the medicine last longer (preservatives). Check this section to see if there is anything that might cause an allergic reaction.

- Child's weight and age

- Use your child's weight to find the right dose of medicine on the Drug Facts label.

- If you don't know your child's weight or the Drug Facts label doesn't show a dose by weight, use her/his age to find the right dose. Never guess at a dose. If a dose for your child's weight or age is not listed on the label, ask your doctor or pharmacist what to do.

- Using more medicine than directed may raise the chance of unwanted side effects. If you think more is needed, or the medicine is needed for a longer time, talk to the doctor.

- Using less medicine than directed may not help and could cause unwanted side effects.

- Child safety caps on medicines can help keep children safer in your home. Most OTC medicines come with child safety caps. For your family's prescription medicines, you can ask your pharmacist for child safety caps.

Chapter 32

Medicines and Your Body

What Are Medicines?

Medicines are chemicals that affect the way your body works. Each medicine works in a person's body for a certain length of time. The Drug Facts label tells you how often to use a medicine based on how long the medicine works in people's bodies. What will happen depends on the medicine and how often you are using it. If you use a medicine too soon, nothing may happen if you only do it once. If you keep using a medicine too often, the medicine can build up in your body to a level that may harm you. Sometimes use of too much medicine can permanently injure your liver, kidneys, or other parts of you.

Medicines inside Our Body

Pharmacology is the scientific field that studies how the body reacts to medicines and how medicines affect the body. Scientists funded by

This chapter contains text excerpted from the following sources: Text under the heading "What Are Medicines?" is excerpted from "Medicines in My Home—Frequently Asked Questions," U.S. Food and Drug Administration (FDA), May 3, 2007. Reviewed January 2017; Text beginning with the heading "Medicines inside Our Body" is excerpted from "A Medicine's Life inside the Body," National Institute of General Medical Sciences (NIGMS), May 1, 2014; Text under the heading "Side Effects of Medicines" is excerpted from "Learning about Side Effects," U.S. Department of Food and Drug Administration (FDA), December 30, 2016; Text under the heading "How to Avoid Side Effects" is excerpted from "Side Effects," NIHSeniorHealth, National Institute on Aging (NIA), March 2016.

the National Institutes of Health (NIH) are interested in many aspects of pharmacology, including one called pharmacokinetics, which deals with understanding the entire cycle of a medicine's life inside the body. Knowing more about each of the four main stages of pharmacokinetics, collectively referred to as ADME (absorption, distribution, metabolism, and excretion), aids the design of medicines that are more effective and that produce fewer side effects.

Absorption

The first stage of ADME is A, for absorption. Medicines are absorbed when they travel from the site of administration into the body's circulation. A few of the most common ways to administer drugs are oral (such as swallowing an aspirin tablet), intramuscular (getting a flu shot in an arm muscle), subcutaneous (injecting insulin just under the skin), intravenous (receiving chemotherapy through a vein) or transdermal (wearing a skin patch). Medicines taken by mouth are shuttled via a special blood vessel leading from the digestive tract to the liver, where a large amount of the medicine is broken down. Other routes of drug administration bypass the liver, entering the bloodstream directly or via the skin or lungs.

Distribution

Once a drug gets absorbed, the next stage of ADME is D, for distribution. Most often, the bloodstream is the vehicle for carrying medicines throughout the body. During this step, side effects can occur when a drug has an effect at a site other than its target. For a pain reliever, the target organ might be a sore muscle in the leg; irritation of the stomach could be a side effect. Drugs destined for the central nervous system face a nearly impenetrable barricade called the blood-brain barrier that protects the brain from potentially dangerous substances such as poisons or viruses. Fortunately, pharmacologists have devised various ways to sneak some drugs past the blood-brain barrier. Other factors that can influence distribution include protein and fat molecules in the blood that can put drug molecules out of commission by latching onto them.

Metabolism

After a medicine has been distributed throughout the body and has done its job, the drug is broken down, or metabolized, the M in

ADME. Everything that enters the bloodstream-whether swallowed, injected, inhaled or absorbed through the skin-is carried to the body's chemical processing plant, the liver. There, substances are chemically pummeled, twisted, cut apart, stuck together and transformed by proteins called enzymes. Many of the products of enzymatic breakdown, or metabolites, are less chemically active than the original molecule. Genetic differences can alter how certain enzymes work, also affecting their ability to metabolize drugs. Herbal products and foods, which contain many active components, can interfere with the body's ability to metabolize drugs.

Excretion

The now-inactive drug undergoes the final stage of its time in the body, excretion, the E in ADME. This removal happens via the urine or feces. By measuring the amounts of a drug in urine (as well as in blood) over time, clinical pharmacologists can calculate how a person is processing a drug, perhaps resulting in a change to the prescribed dose or even the medicine. For example, if the drug is being eliminated relatively quickly, a higher dose may be needed.

Side Effects of Medicines

Side effects, also known as adverse events, are unwanted or unexpected events or reactions to a drug. Side effects can vary from minor problems like a runny nose to life-threatening events, such as an increased risk of a heart attack. Several things can affect who does and does not have a side effect when taking a drug—age, gender, allergies, how the body absorbs the drug, other drugs, vitamins and dietary supplements that you may be taking. Common side effects include upset stomach, dry mouth, and drowsiness. A side effect is considered serious if the result is: death; life-threatening; hospitalization; disability or permanent damage; or exposure prior to conception or during pregnancy caused birth defect.

Side effects can happen when you:

- start taking a new drug, dietary supplement, or vitamin/mineral

- stop taking a drug that you've been on for a while, or

- when you increase or decrease the amount of a drug that you take.

How to Avoid Side Effects

Stomach upset, including diarrhea or constipation, is a side effect common to many medications. Often, this side effect can be lessened by taking the drug with meals. Always check with your doctor, nurse, or pharmacist to see if you should take a particular medication with food.

Here are some more tips to help you avoid side effects.

- **Always inform your doctor or pharmacist** about all medicines you are already taking, including herbal products and over-the-counter medications. Be sure to include products like pain relievers, antacids, alcohol, herbal remedies, food supplements, vitamins, hormones and other substances you might not think are medicines.

- **Tell your doctor, nurse, or pharmacist about past problems** you have had with medicines, such as rashes, indigestion, dizziness, or loss of appetite.

- **Ask whether the drug may interact** with any foods or other over-the-counter drugs or supplements you are taking.

- **Read the prescription label** on the container or the drug information sheet that comes with your medication carefully and follow its directions. Make sure you understand how often, when and how much medicine to take each day.

- **If you experience side effects**, write them down so you can report them to your doctor accurately.

- **Call your doctor right away** if you have any problems with your medicines or if you are worried that the medicine might be doing more harm than good. He or she may be able to change your medicine to another one that will work just as well.

- **Don't mix alcohol and medicine** unless your doctor or pharmacist says it's okay. Some medicines may not work well or may make you sick if taken with alcohol.

Chapter 33

Pharmacogenomics: Genes Affect Individual Responses to Medicines

What Is Pharmacogenomics?

Pharmacogenomics (sometimes called pharmacogenetics) is a field of research focused on understanding how genes affect individual responses to medications. The long-term goal of pharmacogenomics is to help doctors select the drugs and dosages best suited for each person.

What Role Do Genes Play in How Medicines Work?

Just as our genes determine our hair and eye color, they are partially responsible for how our bodies respond to medications.

Genes are instructions, written in deoxyribonucleic acid (DNA), for building protein molecules. Different people can have different versions—slightly different DNA sequences—of the same gene. Some

This chapter contains text excerpted from the following sources: Text beginning with the heading "What Is Pharmacogenomics?" is excerpted from "Pharmacogenomics Fact Sheet," National Institute of General Medical Sciences (NIGMS), April 6, 2016; Text beginning with the heading "What Other Uses of Pharmacogenomics Are Being Studied?" is excerpted from "Frequently Asked Questions about Pharmacogenomics," National Human Genome Research Institute (NHGRI), May 2, 2016.

of these variations are common and some are rare. Some are relevant for health, such as those associated with a tendency to develop certain diseases.

Pharmacogenomics looks at variations in genes for proteins that influence drug responses. Such proteins include a number of liver enzymes that convert medications into their active or inactive forms. Even small differences in the genetic sequences of these enzymes can have a big impact on a drug's safety or effectiveness.

One example involves a liver enzyme known as *CYP2D6*. This enzyme acts on a quarter of all prescription drugs, including the pain-killer codeine, which it converts into the drug's active form, morphine. The *CYP2D6* gene exists in more than 160 different versions, many of which vary by only a single difference in their DNA sequence, although some have larger changes. The majority of these variants don't affect drug responses.

Some people have hundreds or even thousands of copies of the *CYP2D6* gene (typically, people have two copies of each gene). Those with extra copies of this gene manufacture an overabundance of *CYP2D6* enzyme molecules and metabolize the drug very rapidly. As a result, codeine may be converted to morphine so quickly and completely that a standard dose of the drug can be an overdose.

On the other end of the spectrum, some variants of *CYP2D6* result in a nonfunctional enzyme. People with these variants metabolize codeine slowly, if at all, so they might not experience much pain relief. For these people, doctors might prescribe a different type of pain reliever.

How Is Pharmacogenomics Affecting Drug Design, Development, and Prescribing Guidelines?

The U.S. Food and Drug Administration (FDA), which monitors the safety of all drugs in the United States, has included pharmacogenomics information on the labels of more than 150 medications. This information—which can cover dosage guidance, possible side effects or differences in effectiveness for people with certain genomic variations—can help doctors tailor their drug prescriptions for individual patients.

Pharmaceutical companies are beginning to use pharmacogenomics knowledge to develop and market drugs for people with specific genetic profiles. Studying a drug only in those likely to benefit from it could speed up and streamline its development and maximize its therapeutic benefit.

Additionally, if scientists can identify the genetic basis for certain serious side effects, drugs could be prescribed only to people who are not at risk for them. As a result, potentially lifesaving medications, which otherwise might be taken off the market because they pose a risk for some people, could still be available to those who could benefit from them.

How Is Pharmacogenomics Affecting Medical Treatment?

Currently, doctors base the majority of their drug prescriptions on clinical factors, such as a patient's age, weight, sex, and liver and kidney function. For a small subset of drugs, researchers have identified genetic variations that influence how people respond. In these cases, doctors can use the pharmacogenomics information to select the best medication and identify people who need an unusually high or low dose.

What Other Uses of Pharmacogenomics Are Being Studied?

Much research is underway to understand how genomic information can be used to develop more personalized and cost-effective strategies for using drugs to improve human health.

In 2007, the FDA revised the label on the common blood-thinning drug warfarin (Coumadin) to explain that a person's genetic makeup might influence response to the drug. Some doctors have since begun using genetic information to adjust warfarin dosage. Still, more research is needed to conclusively determine whether warfarin dosing that includes genetic information is better than the current trial-and-error approach.

The FDA also is considering genetic testing for another blood-thinner, clopidogrel bisulfate (Plavix), used to prevent dangerous blood clots. Researchers have found that Plavix may not work well in people with a certain genetic variant.

Cancer is another very active area of pharmacogenomics research. Studies have found that the chemotherapy drugs, gefitinib (Iressa) and erlotinib (Tarceva), work much better in lung cancer patients whose tumors have a certain genetic change. On the other hand, research has shown that the chemotherapy drugs cetuximab (Erbitux) and panitumumab (Vecitibix) do not work very well in the 40 percent of colon cancer patients whose tumors have a particular genetic change.

Pharmacogenomics may also help to quickly identify the best drugs to treat people with certain mental health disorders. For example, while some patients with depression respond to the first drug they are given, many do not, and doctors have to try another drug. Because each drug takes weeks to take its full effect, patients' depression may grow worse during the time spent searching for a drug that helps.

Recently, researchers identified genetic variations that influence the response of depressed people to citalopram (Celexa), which belongs to a widely used class of antidepressant drugs called selective serotonin re-uptake inhibitors (SSRIs). Clinical trials are now underway to learn whether genetic tests that predict SSRI response can improve patients' outcomes.

Can Pharmacogenomics Be Used to Develop New Drugs?

Yes. Besides improving the ways in which existing drugs are used, genome research will lead to the development of better drugs. The goal is to produce new drugs that are highly effective and do not cause serious side effects.

Until recently, drug developers usually used an approach that involved screening for chemicals with broad action against a disease. Researchers are now using genomic information to find or design drugs aimed at subgroups of patients with specific genetic profiles. In addition, researchers are using pharmacogenomics tools to search for drugs that target specific molecular and cellular pathways involved in disease.

Pharmacogenomics may also breathe new life into some drugs that were abandoned during the development process. For example, development of the beta-blocker drug bucindolol (Gencaro) was stopped after two other beta-blocker drugs won FDA approval to treat heart failure. But interest in Gencaro revived after tests showed that the drug worked well in patients with two genetic variants that regulate heart function. If Gencaro is approved by the FDA, it could become the first new heart drug to require a genetic test before prescription.

Chapter 34

Using Medicines Safely

Medicines can help you feel better and get well when you are sick. But if you don't follow the directions, medicines can hurt you.

You can lower your chances of side effects from medicines by carefully following the directions on the medicine label or from your pharmacist, doctor, or nurse. Side effects may be mild, like an upset stomach. Other side effects—like damage to your liver—can be more serious.

Take these simple steps to avoid problems with medicines.

- Follow the directions on the medicine label carefully.

- If you don't understand the directions, ask your doctor, nurse, or pharmacist to explain them to you.

- Keep a list of all the medicines, vitamins, minerals, and herbs you use. Share this information with your doctor.

- Store your medicines in a cool, dry place where children and pets can't see or reach them.

This chapter contains text excerpted from the following sources: Text in this chapter begins with excerpts from "Use Medicines Safely," Office of Disease Prevention and Health Promotion (ODPHP), U.S. Department of Health and Human Services (HHS), August 29, 2016; Text beginning with the heading "Managing the Benefits and Risks of Medicines" is excerpted from "Think It Through: A Guide to Managing the Benefits and Risks of Medicines," U.S. Food and Drug Administration (FDA), March 25, 2016.

There Are Different Types of Medicine

The two categories of medicine are prescription and over-the-counter (OTC).

Prescription Medicines

Prescription medicines are medicines you can get only with a prescription (order) from your doctor. You get these medicines from a pharmacy. Prescription medicines shouldn't be used by anyone except the person whose name is on the prescription. Get rid of expired (out-of-date) or unused prescription medicines. Ask your pharmacist how to get rid of medicines safely. Sometimes you can choose between a generic medicine and a brand name medicine. Generic and brand name medicines work the same way, but generic medicine usually costs less. Talk to your doctor, pharmacist, or insurance company for more information about generic medicines.

Over-the-Counter Medicines

Over-the-counter medicines are medicines you can buy at a store without a prescription. Some examples of OTC medicines include:

- Cold and flu medicines
- Pain medicines like aspirin, acetaminophen, and ibuprofen
- Allergy medicines
- Sleep aids
- Toothpaste with fluoride

Drug Facts Label

All OTC medicines come with a Drug Facts label. The information on this label can help you choose the right OTC medicine for your symptoms. The Drug Facts label also gives you instructions for using the medicine safely. OTC medicines can cause side effects or harm if you use too much or don't use them correctly. Following the directions on the Drug Facts label will lower your chances of side effects. Your doctor, nurse, or pharmacist can also help you choose OTC medicines and can answer any questions you may have.

Take Action!

Prevent problems and mistakes with your medicines.

Follow the Directions Carefully

Be sure to read the directions carefully when taking prescription or OTC medicines. If you notice unpleasant side effects after taking medicine, like feeling dizzy or having an upset stomach, call your doctor or nurse.

Talk to Your Doctor

Before you use any new prescription medicines, tell your doctor:

- About other medicines you use–both prescription and OTC medicines

- About any vitamins, minerals, or herbs you use

- If you are allergic to any medicines

- If you've had side effects after using any medicines

- If you are pregnant or breastfeeding, because some medicines may harm your baby

- If you have any questions or concerns about the new medicine

Be sure to keep taking prescription medicines until your doctor tells you it is okay to stop—even if you are feeling better. It's also a good idea to talk to your doctor before you stop taking a prescription medicine—even if you're worried it's making you feel worse.

Ask Questions to Make Sure You Understand

To use a medicine safely, you need to know:

- The name of the medicine

- Why you are using the medicine

- How to use the medicine the right way

- If there are any medicines you shouldn't take with this one

Ask your doctor or nurse questions to be sure you understand how to use your medicines. Take notes to help you remember the answers. You can even ask to record the instructions on your phone. You can also ask a pharmacist if you forget how to use a medicine or you don't understand the directions. Use these tips to talk with a pharmacist about your medicines.

Keep Track of Your Medicines

- Make a list of the medicines you use. Write down how much you use and when you use each medicine.

- Take the list with you whenever you go to a medical appointment. You may also want to make a copy to give to a family member or friend in case you have a medical emergency.

- Read and save any information that comes with your medicine.

- Keep your medicine in the box or bottle it came in so you have all of the information from the label.

- Pay attention to the color and shape of your pills. If they look different when you get a refill, ask your pharmacist to double-check that you have the right medicine.

Put Your Medicines in a Safe Place

Medicines that are stored correctly last longer and work better.

- Check for storage instructions on the medicine label—for example, some medicines need to be stored in the refrigerator.

- Store medicines that don't have special storage instructions in a cool, dry place. Medicines can break down quickly in places that are damp and warm, like the kitchen or bathroom.

- Keep medicines away from children and pets. A locked box, cabinet, or closet is best. Get more tips for how to keep medicines away from children.

- Get rid of expired (out-of-date) medicines and medicines you no longer use. Follow these instructions to get rid of old or extra medicines safely.

Call the Poison Control Center (PCS) 1-800-222-1222 right away if a child or someone else accidentally uses your medicine.

Managing the Benefits and Risks of Medicines

Although medicines can make you feel better and help you get well, it's important to know that ALL medicines, both prescription and over-the-counter, have risks as well as benefits.

The benefits of medicines are the helpful effects you get when you use them, such as lowering blood pressure, curing infection or relieving pain. The risks of medicines are the chances that something unwanted or unexpected could happen to you when you use them. Risks could be less serious things, such as an upset stomach, or more serious things, such as liver damage.

When a medicine's benefits outweigh its known risks, the U.S. Food and Drug Administration (FDA) considers it safe enough to approve. But before using any medicine—as with many things that you do every day—you should think through the benefits and the risks in order to make the best choice for you.

There are several types of risks from medicine use:

- The possibility of a harmful interaction between the medicine and a food, beverage, dietary supplement (including vitamins and herbals), or another medicine. Combinations of any of these products could increase the chance that there may be interactions.

- The chance that the medicine may not work as expected.

- The possibility that the medicine may cause additional problems.

For example, every time you get into a car, there are risks—the possibility that unwanted or unexpected things could happen. You could have an accident, causing costly damage to your car, or injury to yourself or a loved one. But there are also benefits to riding in a car: you can travel farther and faster than walking, bring home more groceries from the store, and travel in cold or wet weather in greater comfort.

To obtain the benefits of riding in a car, you think through the risks. You consider the condition of your car and the road, for instance, before deciding to make that trip to the store.

The same is true before using any medicine. Every choice to take a medicine involves thinking through the helpful effects as well as the possible unwanted effects.

How Do You Lower the Risks and Obtain the Full Benefits?

Car

- Wear a seatbelt.
- Drive defensively.
- Obey the speed limit and traffic laws.

- Avoid alcohol or medicines that could affect your driving ability.

- Keep your car in good repair.

Medicine

- Talk to your doctor, pharmacist, or other healthcare professionals.

- Know your medicines.

- Read the label and follow directions.

- Avoid interactions.

- Monitor the medicine's effects.

Weighing the Risks, Making the Choice

The benefit/risk decision is sometimes difficult to make. The best choice depends on your particular situation.

You must decide what risks you can and will accept in order to get the benefits you want. For example, if facing a life-threatening illness, you might choose to accept more risk in the hope of getting the benefits of a cure or living a longer life. On the other hand, if you are facing a minor illness, you might decide that you want to take very little risk. In many situations, the expert advice of your doctor, pharmacist, or other healthcare professionals can help you make the decision.

Here Are Some Specific Ways to Lower the Risks and Obtain the Full Benefits of Medicines

Talk with your doctor, pharmacist, or other healthcare professionals

- Keep an up-to-date, written list of all of the medicines (prescription and over-the-counter) and dietary supplements, including vitamins and herbals, that you use—even those you only use occasionally.

- Share this list with all of your healthcare professionals.

- Tell about any allergies or sensitivities that you may have.

- Tell about anything that could affect your ability to take medicines, such as difficulty swallowing or remembering to take them.

- Tell if you are or might become pregnant, or if you are nursing a baby.

- Always ask questions about any concerns or thoughts that you may have.

Know your medicines—prescription and over-the-counter (OTC)

- The brand and generic names.
- What they look like.
- How to store them properly.
- When, how, and how long to use them.
- How and under what conditions you should stop using them.
- What to do if you miss a dose.
- What they are supposed to do and when to expect results.
- Side effects and interactions.
- Whether you need any tests or monitoring.
- Always ask for written information to take with you.

Read the label and follow directions

- Make sure you understand the directions; ask if you have questions or concerns.
- Always double check that you have the right medicine.
- Keep medicines in their original labeled containers, whenever possible.
- Never combine different medicines in the same bottle.
- Read and follow the directions on the label and the directions from your doctor, pharmacist, or other healthcare professional. If you stop the medicine or want to use the medicine differently than directed, consult with your healthcare professional.

Avoid interactions

- Ask if there are interactions with any other medicines or dietary supplements (including vitamins or herbal supplements), beverages, or foods.
- Use the same pharmacy for all of your medicine needs, whenever possible.
- Before starting any new medicine or dietary supplement (including vitamins or herbal supplements), ask again if there are possible interactions with what you are currently using.

249

Monitor your medicines' effects—and the effects of other products that you use

- Ask if there is anything you can do to minimize side effects, such as eating before you take a medicine to reduce stomach upset.

- Pay attention to how you are feeling; note any changes. Write down the changes so that you can remember to tell your doctor, pharmacist, or other healthcare professional.

- Know what to do if you experience side effects and when to notify your doctor. Know when you should notice an improvement and when to report back.

Chapter 35

Over-the-Counter (OTC) Medicines

Over-the-counter medicine is also known as OTC or nonprescription medicine. All these terms refer to medicine that you can buy without a prescription. They are safe and effective when you follow the directions on the label and as directed by your healthcare professional.

The information in this chapter will help you to work with your healthcare professionals to choose and use over-the-counter medicine wisely.

Choosing the Right Over-the-Counter Medicine

American medicine cabinets contain a growing choice of nonprescription, over-the-counter (OTC) medicines to treat an expanding range of ailments. OTC medicines often do more than relieve aches, pains and itches. Some can prevent diseases like tooth decay, cure diseases like athlete's foot and, with a doctor's guidance, help manage recurring conditions like vaginal yeast infection, migraine and minor pain in arthritis.

This chapter contains text excerpted from the following sources: Text in this chapter begins with excerpts from "Understanding Over-the-Counter Medicines," U.S. Food and Drug Administration (FDA), August 26, 2016; Text beginning with the heading "Choosing the Right Over-the-Counter Medicine" is excerpted from "Over-the-Counter Medicines: What's Right for You?" U.S. Food and Drug Administration (FDA), September 3, 2013. Reviewed January 2017.

The U.S. Food and Drug Administration (FDA) determines whether medicines are prescription or nonprescription. The term prescription (Rx) refers to medicines that are safe and effective when used under a doctor's care. Nonprescription or OTC drugs are medicines FDA decides are safe and effective for use without a doctor's prescription.

FDA also has the authority to decide when a prescription drug is safe enough to be sold directly to consumers over the counter. This regulatory process allowing Americans to take a more active role in their healthcare is known as Rx-to-OTC switch. As a result of this process, more than 700 products sold over the counter today use ingredients or dosage strengths available only by prescription 30 years ago.

Increased access to OTC medicines is especially important for our maturing population. Two out of three older Americans rate their health as excellent to good, but four out of five report at least one chronic condition.

Fact is, today's OTC medicines offer greater opportunity to treat more of the aches and illnesses most likely to appear in our later years. As we live longer, work longer, and take a more active role in our own healthcare, the need grows to become better informed about self-care.

The best way to become better informed—for young and old alike—is to read and understand the information on OTC labels. Next to the medicine itself, label comprehension is the most important part of self-care with OTC medicines.

With new opportunities in self-medication come new responsibilities and an increased need for knowledge. FDA and the Consumer Healthcare Products Association (CHPA) have prepared the following information to help Americans take advantage of self-care opportunities.

OTC Know-How: It's on the Label

You wouldn't ignore your doctor's instructions for using a prescription drug; so don't ignore the label when taking an OTC medicine. Here's what to look for:

- PRODUCT NAME

- "ACTIVE INGREDIENTS": therapeutic substances in medicine

- "PURPOSE": product category (such as antihistamine, antacid, or cough suppressant)

- "USES": symptoms or diseases the product will treat or prevent

- "WARNINGS": when not to use the product, when to stop taking it, when to see a doctor, and possible side effects

- "DIRECTIONS": how much to take, how to take it, and how long to take it

- "OTHER INFORMATION": such as storage information

- "INACTIVE INGREDIENTS": substances such as binders, colors, or flavoring

You can help yourself read the label too. Always use enough light. It usually takes three times more light to read the same line at age 60 than at age 30. If necessary, use your glasses or contact lenses when reading labels. Always remember to look for the statement describing the tamper-evident feature(s) before you buy the product and when you use it. When it comes to medicines, more does not necessarily mean better. You should never misuse OTC medicines by taking them longer or in higher doses than the label recommends. Symptoms that persist are a clear signal it's time to see a doctor.

Be sure to read the label each time you purchase a product. Just because two or more products are from the same brand family doesn't mean they are meant to treat the same conditions or contain the same ingredients. Remember, if you read the label and still have questions, talk to a doctor, nurse, or pharmacist.

Drug Interactions: A Word to the Wise

Although mild and relatively uncommon, interactions involving OTC drugs can produce unwanted results or make medicines less effective. It's especially important to know about drug interactions if you're taking Rx and OTC drugs at the same time.

Some drugs can also interact with foods and beverages, as well as with health conditions such as diabetes, kidney disease, and high blood pressure.

Here are a few drug interaction cautions for some common OTC ingredients:

- Avoid alcohol if you are taking antihistamines, cough-cold products with the ingredient dextromethorphan, or drugs that treat sleeplessness.

- Do not use drugs that treat sleeplessness if you are taking prescription sedatives or tranquilizers.

- Check with your doctor before taking products containing aspirin if you're taking a prescription blood thinner or if you have diabetes or gout.

- Do not use laxatives when you have stomach pain, nausea, or vomiting.

- Unless directed by a doctor, do not use a nasal decongestant if you are taking a prescription drug for high blood pressure or depression, or if you have heart or thyroid disease, diabetes, or prostate problems.

This is not a complete list. Read the label! Drug labels change as new information becomes available. That's why it's important to read the label each time you take medicine.

Time for a Medicine Cabinet Checkup?

- Be sure to look through your medicine supply at least once a year.

- Always store medicines in a cool, dry place or as stated on the label.

- Throw away any medicines that are past the expiration date.

- To make sure no one takes the wrong medicine, keep all medicines in their original containers.

Pregnancy and Breast-Feeding

Drugs can pass from a pregnant woman to her unborn baby. A safe amount of medicine for the mother may be too much for the unborn baby. If you're pregnant, always talk with your doctor before taking any drugs, Rx or OTC.

Although most drugs pass into breast milk in concentrations too low to have any unwanted effects on the baby, breast-feeding mothers still need to be careful. Always ask your doctor or pharmacist before taking any medicine while breast-feeding. A doctor or pharmacist can tell you how to adjust the timing and dosing of most medicines so the baby is exposed to the lowest amount possible, or whether the drugs should be avoided altogether.

Over-the-Counter Medicines for Infants and Children

OTC drugs rarely come in one-size-fits-all. Here are some tips about giving OTC medicines to children:

- Children aren't just small adults, so don't estimate the dose based on their size.

- Read the label. Follow all directions.

- Follow any age limits on the label.

- Some OTC products come in different strengths. Be aware!

- Know the difference between TBSP. (tablespoon) and TSP. (teaspoon). They are very different doses.

- Be careful about converting dose instructions. If the label says two teaspoons, it's best to use a measuring spoon or a dosing cup marked in teaspoons, not a common kitchen spoon.

- Don't play doctor. Don't double the dose just because your child seems sicker than last time.

- Before you give your child two medicines at the same time, talk to your doctor or pharmacist.

- Never let children take medicine by themselves.

- Never call medicine candy to get your kids to take it. If they come across the medicine on their own, they're likely to remember that you called it candy.

Child-Resistant Packaging

Child-resistant closures are designed for repeated use to make it difficult for children to open. Remember, if you don't re-lock the closure after each use, the child-resistant device can't do its job—keeping children out!

It's best to store all medicines and dietary supplements where children can neither see nor reach them. Containers of pills should not be left on the kitchen counter as a reminder. Purses and briefcases are among the worst places to hide medicines from curious kids. And since children are natural mimics, it's a good idea not to take medicine in front of them. They may be tempted to "play house" with your medicine later on.

If you find some packages too difficult to open—and don't have young children living with you or visiting—you should know the law allows one package size for each OTC medicine to be sold without child-resistant features. If you don't see it on the store shelf, ask.

Protect Yourself against Tampering

Makers of OTC medicines seal most products in tamper-evident packaging (TEP) to help protect against criminal tampering. TEP works by providing visible evidence if the package has been disturbed. But OTC packaging cannot be 100 percent tamper-proof. Here's how to help protect yourself:

- Be alert to the tamper-evident features on the package before you open it. These features are described on the label.

- Inspect the outer packaging before you buy it. When you get home, inspect the medicine inside.

- Don't buy an OTC product if the packaging is damaged.

- Don't use any medicine that looks discolored or different in any way.

- If anything looks suspicious, be suspicious. Contact the store where you bought the product. Take it back!

- Never take medicines in the dark.

Chapter 36

Buying Prescription Drugs

Chapter Contents

Section 36.1

Cost May Result in Underuse of Medications

This section includes text excerpted from "Effect of Financial Stress
and Positive Financial Behaviors on Cost-Related Nonadherence to
Health Regimens among Adults in a Community-Based Setting,"
Centers for Disease Control and Prevention (CDC), April 7, 2016.

One of four Americans reports financial difficulty in paying medical
bills; this difficulty has significant public health implications, especially for the 50 percent of the population that is managing chronic
illness. Seven systematic reviews concluded that several factors influence adherence to treatment, but cost to the patient is one that demon-
strates a consistent negative effect. Nearly 18 percent of chronically ill
Americans report underusing medications and delaying or not fulfilling
therapeutic recommendations because of cost, which is referred to
as cost-related nonadherence (CRN) and varies by therapeutic class
across chronic therapies. Fifty-six percent of American adults with
common chronic diseases self-report non fulfillment of medication as
a result of financial hardship.

Health insurance coverage is a strong predictor of financial burden. Nearly half of Americans have literacy challenges with health
insurance and pay more for healthcare out of pocket because of these
challenges, despite improvements as a result of the Affordable Care
Act (ACA).

Although health literacy and health insurance literacy are commonly discussed as integral for individuals to have the capacity to
obtain, process, and understand basic health information or services
and health insurance, financial literacy in the context of health has
received little attention. Financial literacy is a set of skills and knowledge that allows individuals to make informed decisions with their
financial resources, and it is associated with more frequent engagement in health-promoting behaviors.

Studies show that social determinants of health that contribute
to financial burden correlate with CRN. Therefore, financial burden
may be experienced in the context of a growing concern for financial
insecurity and may not be exclusively health-related. Given the role

that cost to the patient plays in adherence to therapeutic regimens, improving financial literacy to influence positive financial behaviors (behaviors that allow individuals to maintain financial stability with their financial resources) may have implications for CRN, and may be a necessary adjunct to policy reforms.

Few interventions have aimed to mitigate CRN beyond reducing out-of-pocket costs, which have shown modest improvements in health status. Whether positive financial behavior is protective of CRN has not been explored and may have implications for behavioral interventions to promote financial literacy, especially among people who have chronic illnesses.

Section 36.2

Saving Money on Prescription Drugs

This section includes text excerpted from "Apply Online for Extra Help with Medicare Prescription Drug Costs," U.S. Social Security Administration (SSA), March 2016.

What Is Extra Help with Medicare Prescription Drug Plan Costs?

Anyone who has Medicare can get Medicare prescription drug coverage. Some people with limited resources and income may also be able to get Extra Help to pay for the costs—monthly premiums, annual deductibles and prescription copayments—related to a Medicare prescription drug plan. The Extra Help is estimated to be worth about $4,000 per year. Many people qualify for these important savings and don't even know it.

To qualify for Extra Help:

- You must reside in one of the 50 states or the District of Columbia;

- Your resources must be limited to $13,640 for an individual or $27,250 for a married couple living together. Resources include such things as bank accounts, stocks and bonds.

Some examples where you may have higher income and still qualify for Extra Help include if you or your spouse:

- Support other family members who live with you;

- Have earnings from work; or

- Live in Alaska or Hawaii.

How Do I Apply?

Applying for Extra Help is easy. Just complete Social Security's Application for Extra Help with Medicare Prescription Drug Plan Costs (SSA-1020). Here's how:

- Apply online at www.socialsecurity.gov/extrahelp;

- Call Social Security at 1-800-772-1213 (TTY 1-800-325-0778) to apply over the phone or to request an application; or

- Apply at your local Social Security office.

After you apply, Social Security will review your application and send a letter to you to let you know if you qualify for Extra Help. Once you qualify, you can choose a Medicare prescription drug plan. If you don't select a plan, the Centers for Medicare and Medicaid Services will do it for you. The sooner you join a plan, the sooner you begin receiving benefits. If you aren't eligible for Extra Help, you still may be able to enroll in a Medicare prescription drug plan.

Late Enrollment Penalty

If you don't enroll in a Medicare prescription drug plan when you're first eligible, you may pay a late enrollment penalty if you join a plan later. You'll have to pay this penalty for as long as you have Medicare prescription drug coverage. However, you won't pay a penalty if you get Extra Help or another eligible prescription drug plan coverage.

The Medicare prescription drug plan late enrollment penalty is different than the Medicare Part B late enrollment penalty. If you don't enroll in Part B when you're first eligible for it, you may have to pay a late enrollment penalty for as long as you have Part B coverage. Also, you may have to wait to enroll, which will delay Part B coverage.

For information about enrollment periods, call 1-800-MEDICARE (1-800-633-4227; TTY 1-877-486-2048).

Why Should I Apply Online?

The online application is secure and offers several advantages. It takes you through the process step-by-step, with a series of self-help screens. The screens will tell you what information you need to complete the application and will guide you in answering the questions fully.

You can apply from any computer. You can start and stop at any time during the process, so you can leave the application and go back later to update or complete any of the required information.

Can State Agencies Help with My Medicare Costs?

When you file your application for Extra Help, you also can start your application process for the Medicare Savings Programs. These state programs provide help with other Medicare costs. Social Security will send information to your state unless you tell not to on the Extra Help application. Your state will contact you to help you apply for a Medicare Savings Program.

These Medicare Savings Programs help people with limited resources and income pay for their Medicare expenses. The Medicare Savings Programs help pay for your Medicare Part B (medical insurance) premiums. For some people, the Medicare Savings Programs may also pay for Medicare Part A (hospital insurance) premiums, if any, and Part A and B deductibles and copayments.

Medicaid or medical assistance is a joint Federal and state program that helps pay medical costs for some people who have limited resources and income. Each state has different rules about eligibility and applying for Medicaid.

Section 36.3

Purchase Prescription Medicine Online Safely

This section includes text excerpted from "The Possible Dangers
of Buying Medicines over the Internet," U.S. Food and Drug
Administration (FDA), January 16, 2015.

The U.S. Food and Drug Administration (FDA) wants to warn
consumers about the possible dangers of buying medicines over the
Internet. Some websites sell prescription and over-the-counter (OTC)
drugs that may not be safe to use and could put people's health at risk.

So how can you protect yourself? FDA says that consumers should
know how to recognize a legal Internet pharmacy and how to buy
medicines online safely.

Don't Be Deceived

Buying prescription and over-the-counter drugs on the Internet
from a company you don't know means you may not know exactly
what you're getting.

There are many websites that operate legally and offer convenience,
privacy, and safeguards for purchasing medicines. But there are also
many "rogue websites" that offer to sell potentially dangerous drugs
that have not been checked for safety or effectiveness. Though a rogue
site may look professional and legitimate, it could actually be an illegal
operation.

These rogue sites often sell unapproved drugs, drugs that contain the wrong active ingredient, drugs that may contain too much
or too little of the active ingredient, or drugs that contain dangerous
ingredients.

For example, FDA purchased and analyzed several products that
were represented online as Tamiflu (oseltamivir). One of the orders,
which arrived in an unmarked envelope with a postmark from India,
consisted of unlabeled, white tablets. When analyzed by FDA, the
tablets were found to contain talc and acetaminophen, but none of the
active ingredient oseltamivir.

262

FDA also became aware of a number of people who placed orders over the Internet for one of the following products:

- Ambien (zolpidem tartrate)
- Xanax (alprazolam)
- Lexapro (escitalopram oxalate)
- Ativan (lorazepam)

Instead of receiving the drug they ordered, several customers received products containing what was identified as foreign versions of Haldol (haloperidol), a powerful anti-psychotic drug. As a result, these customers needed emergency medical treatment for symptoms such as difficulty in breathing, muscle spasms, and muscle stiffness—all problems that can occur with haloperidol.

Other websites sell counterfeit drugs that may look exactly like real FDA-approved medicines, but their quality and safety are unknown.

Signs of an unsafe website:

- It sends you drugs with unknown quality or origin.
- It gives you the wrong drug or another dangerous product for your illness.
- It doesn't provide a way to contact the website by phone.
- It offers prices that are dramatically lower than the competition.
- It may offer to sell prescription drugs without a prescription—this is against the law!
- It may not protect your personal information.

Another way to check on a website is to look for the National Association of Boards of Pharmacy's (NABP) Verified Internet Pharmacy Practice Sites™ Seal, also known as the VIPPS® Seal.

This seal means that the Internet pharmacy is safe to use because it has met state licensure requirements, as well as other NABP criteria. Visit the VIPPS website to find legitimate pharmacies that carry the VIPPS® seal.

Know Your Medicines

Before you get any new medicine for the first time, talk to a health-care professional such as your doctor or pharmacist about any special steps you need to take to fill your prescription.

Any time you get a prescription refilled:

- check the physical appearance of the medicine (color, texture, shape, and packaging)
- check to see if it smells and tastes the same when you use it
- alert your pharmacist or whoever is providing treatment to anything that is different

Be aware that some drugs sold online:

- are too old, too strong, or too weak
- aren't FDA-approved
- aren't made using safe standards
- aren't safe to use with other medicines or products
- aren't labeled, stored, or shipped correctly
- may be counterfeit

Counterfeit Drugs

Counterfeit drugs are fake or copycat products that can be difficult to identify. The deliberate and fraudulent practice of counterfeiting can apply to both brand name and generic products, where the identity of the source is often mislabeled in a way that suggests it is the authentic approved product.

Counterfeit drugs may:

- be contaminated
- not help the condition or disease the medicine is intended to treat
- lead to dangerous side effects
- contain the wrong active ingredient
- be made with the wrong amounts of ingredients
- contain no active ingredients at all or contain too much of an active ingredient
- be packaged in phony packaging that looks legitimate

For example, counterfeit versions of the FDA-approved weight loss drug Xenical, which contains the active ingredient orlistat, recently were obtained by three consumers from two different websites.

Laboratory analysis showed that the capsules that the consumers received contained the wrong active ingredient, sibutramine.

Sibutramine is the active ingredient of a different medicine called Meridia, a prescription drug also approved by FDA to help obese people lose weight and maintain weight loss. In addition, sibutramine is classified as a controlled substance by the Drug Enforcement Administration (DEA) because of its potential for abuse and misuse.

Using medicine that contains an active ingredient that wasn't prescribed by your licensed healthcare provider may be harmful.

FDA continues to proactively protect consumers from counterfeit drugs. The agency is working with drug manufacturers, wholesalers, and retailers to identify and prevent counterfeit drugs. FDA also is exploring the use of modern technologies and other measures that will make it more difficult for counterfeit drugs to get mixed up with, or deliberately substituted for, safe and effective medicines.

How to Protect Yourself

- Only buy from state-licensed pharmacy websites located in the United States.

- Don't buy from websites that sell prescription drugs without a prescription.

- Don't buy from websites that offer to prescribe a drug for the first time without a physical exam by your doctor or by answering an online questionnaire.

- Check with your state board of pharmacy or the National Association of Boards of Pharmacy (NABP) to see if an online pharmacy has a valid pharmacy license and meets state quality standards.

- Look for privacy and security policies that are easy to find and easy to understand.

- Don't give any personal information—such as a social security number, credit card information, or medical or health history—unless you are sure the website will keep your information safe and private.

- Use legitimate websites that have a licensed pharmacist to answer your question.

- Make sure that the website will not sell your personal information, unless you agree.

Section 36.4

Truth in Advertising: Ads for Prescription Drugs

This section includes text excerpted from "Prescription
Drug Advertising," U.S. Food and Drug Administration
(FDA), June 19, 2015.

Your healthcare provider is the best source of information about
the right medicines for you. Prescription drug advertisements can
provide useful information for consumers to work with their healthcare providers to make wise decisions about treatment. The example
ads below show the correct and incorrect versions of different types
of drug ads.

Basics of Drug Advertisements

A drug is "prescription only" when medical professionals must
supervise its use because patients are not able to use the drug safely
on their own. Because of this, Congress laid out different requirements for prescription and non-prescription or "over-the-counter"
drugs. Congress also gave the U.S. Food and Drug Administration
(FDA) authority to oversee prescription drug ads. In turn, the FDA
passed regulations detailing how it would enforce those requirements. These regulations are also known as "rules." However, while
the FDA oversees ads for prescription drugs, the Federal Trade
Commission (FTC) oversees ads for over-the-counter (non-prescription) drugs.

Product Claim Advertisements

Product claim ads are the only type of ads that name a drug and
discuss its benefits and risks. However, these ads must not be false
or misleading in any way. Companies are encouraged to use understandable language throughout product claim ads that are directed
to consumers.

All product claim ads, regardless of the media in which they appear, must include certain key components within the main part of the ad:

- The name of the drug (brand and generic)

- At least one FDA-approved use for the drug

- The most significant risks of the drug

Product claim ads must present the benefits and risks of a prescription drug in a balanced fashion.

Print product claim ads also must include a "brief summary" about the drug that generally includes all the risks listed in its approved prescribing information.

- Under the Food and Drug Administration Amendments Act (FDAAA) of 2007, print advertisements need to include the following statement: "You are encouraged to report negative side effects of prescription drugs to the FDA. Visit MedWatch or call 1-800-FDA-1088."

Broadcast product claim ads (TV, radio, telephone) must include the following:

- The drug's most important risks ("major statement") presented in the audio (that is, spoken) and

- Either all the risks listed in the drug's prescribing information or a variety of sources for viewers to find the prescribing information for the drug

This means that drug companies do not have to include all of a drug's risk information in a broadcast ad. Instead, the ad may tell where viewers or listeners can find more information about the drug in the FDA-approved prescribing information. This is called the "adequate provision" requirement. For broadcast ads, it is said that including a variety of sources of prescribing information fulfills this requirement.

It is suggested that broadcast ads give the following sources for finding a drug's prescribing information:

- A healthcare provider (for example, a doctor)

- A toll-free telephone number

- The current issue of a magazine that contains a print ad

- A website address

Reminder Advertisements

Reminder ads give the name of a drug, but not the drug's uses. These ads assume that the audience already knows the drug's use.

A reminder ad does not have to contain risk information about the drug because the ad does not say what the drug does or how well it works. Unlike product claim ads, reminder ads cannot suggest, in either words or pictures, anything about the drug's benefits or risks. For example, a reminder ad for a drug that helps treat asthma should not include a drawing of a pair of lungs, because this implies what the drug does.

Reminder ads are not allowed for certain prescription drugs with serious risks. Drugs with serious risks have a special warning, often called a "boxed warning," in the drug's FDA-approved prescribing information. Because of their seriousness, the risks must be included in all ads for these drugs.

Help-Seeking Advertisements

Help-seeking ads describe a disease or condition but do not recommend or suggest a specific drug treatment. Some examples of diseases or conditions discussed in help-seeking ads include allergies, asthma, erectile dysfunction, high cholesterol, and osteoporosis. The ads encourage people with these symptoms to talk to their doctor. Help-seeking ads may include a drug company's name and may also provide a telephone number to call for more information.

When done properly, help-seeking ads are not considered to be drug ads. FTC does regulate them. If an ad recommends or suggests the use of a specific drug, however, it is considered a product claim ad that must comply with FDA rules.

Other Product Claim Promotional Materials

Other types of promotional materials than advertisements are used to promote the use of a drug. These are called "promotional labeling" and include brochures, materials mailed to consumers, and other types of materials given out by drug companies. If these materials mention the drug's benefit(s) they must also include the drug's prescribing information.

Risk Disclosure Requirements for Different Types of Advertisements

Different advertisements require different amounts of benefit and risk information.

Reminder ads do not have to include any risk information because they cannot include any claims or pictures about what a drug does or how it works. Reminder ads are only for drugs without certain specified serious risks.

Print product claim ads may make statements about a drug's benefit(s). They must present the drug's most important risks in the main part of the ad ("fair balance"). These ads generally must include every risk, but can present the less important risks in the detailed information known as the "brief summary."

Also, print product claim and reminder ads must include the following statement:

"You are encouraged to report negative side effects of prescription drugs to the FDA. Visit MedWatch or call 1-800-FDA-1088."

Broadcast product claim ads may make statements about a drug's benefit(s). They must include the drug's most important risk information ("major statement") in a way that is clear, conspicuous, and neutral. In addition, they must include either every risk or provide enough sources for the audience to obtain the drug's prescribing information ("adequate provision").

Prescription Drug Advertising: Questions to Ask Yourself

Think about the following questions when you see an ad for a prescription drug. Also, think about asking these questions when you talk to your doctor or pharmacist about a drug.

- What condition does this drug treat?

- Why do I think that I might have this condition?

- If I have the condition, am I part of the population the drug is approved to treat?

- Should I take this drug if I have a certain condition?

- Should I take this drug if I am taking certain other drugs?

- Which of the drug's possible side effects am I concerned about?

- How will this drug affect other drugs I am taking?
- Will foods, beverages (alcoholic or non-alcoholic), vitamins, or other supplements affect how this drug works?
- Are there other drugs that treat my condition?
- Is there a less costly drug I could use to treat my condition?
- What else can I do to help deal with my condition? For example, should I exercise or change my diet?
- Do other drugs for my condition have different side effects?
- How can I learn more about this condition and this drug?

Chapter 37

Facts about Generic Drugs

What Are Generic Drugs?

A generic drug is identical — or bioequivalent — to a brand name drug in dosage form, safety, strength, route of administration, quality, performance characteristics and intended use. Although generic drugs are chemically identical to their branded counterparts, they are typically sold at substantial discounts from the branded price. According to the Congressional Budget Office (CBO), generic drugs save consumers an estimated $8 to $10 billion a year at retail pharmacies. Even more billions are saved when hospitals use generics.

Drug companies must submit an abbreviated new drug application (ANDA) for approval to market a generic product. The Drug Price Competition and Patent Term Restoration Act of 1984, more commonly known as the Hatch-Waxman Act, made ANDAs possible by creating a compromise in the drug industry. Generic drug companies gained greater access to the market for prescription drugs, and innovator companies gained restoration of patent life of their products lost during FDA's approval process.

New drugs, like other new products, are developed under patent protection. The patent protects the investment in the drug's development by giving the company the sole right to sell the drug while the patent is in effect. When patents or other periods of exclusivity expire, manufacturers can apply to the FDA to sell generic versions.

This chapter includes text excerpted from "Understanding Generic Drugs," U.S. Food and Drug Administration (FDA), October 17, 2016.

The ANDA process does not require the drug sponsor to repeat costly animal and clinical research on ingredients or dosage forms already approved for safety and effectiveness. This applies to drugs first marketed after 1962.

Health professionals and consumers can be assured that FDA approved generic drugs have met the same rigid standards as the innovator drug. To gain FDA approval, a generic drug must:

- contain the same active ingredients as the innovator drug (inactive ingredients may vary)

- be identical in strength, dosage form, and route of administration

- have the same use indications

- be bioequivalent

- meet the same batch requirements for identity, strength, purity, and quality

- be manufactured under the same strict standards of FDA's good manufacturing practice regulations required for innovator products

Facts about Generic Drugs

Nearly 8 in 10 prescriptions filled in the United States are for generic drugs. The use of generic drugs is expected to grow over the next few years as a number of popular drugs come off patent through 2015. Here are some Facts about generic drugs:

- When a generic drug product is approved, it has met rigorous standards established by the FDA with respect to identity, strength, quality, purity, and potency. However, some variability can and does occur during manufacturing, for both brand name and generic drugs. When a drug, generic or brand name, is mass-produced, very small variations in purity, size, strength, and other parameters are permitted. FDA limits how much variability is acceptable.

- Generic drugs are required to have the same active ingredient, strength, dosage form, and route of administration as the brand name product. Generic drugs do not need to contain the same inactive ingredients as the brand name product.

- The generic drug manufacturer must prove its drug is the same as (bioequivalent) the brand name drug. For example, after the patient takes the generic drug, the amount of drug in the bloodstream is measured. If the levels of the drug in the bloodstream are the same as the levels found when the brand name product is used, the generic drug will work the same.

- Through review of bioequivalence data, FDA ensures that the generic product performs the same as its respective brand name product. This standard applies to all generic drugs, whether immediate or controlled release.

- All generic manufacturing, packaging, and testing sites must pass the same quality standards as those of brand name drugs, and the generic products must meet the same exacting specifications as any brand name product. In Fact, many generic drugs are made in the same manufacturing plants as brand name drug products.

Fact: Research shows that generics work just as well as brand name drugs.

A study evaluated the results of 38 published clinical trials that compared cardiovascular generic drugs to their brand name counterparts. There was no evidence that brand name heart drugs worked any better than generic heart drugs.

Fact: FDA does not allow a 45 percent difference in the effectiveness of the generic drug product.

FDA recently evaluated 2,070 human studies conducted between 1996 and 2007. These studies compared the absorption of brand name and generic drugs into a person's body. These studies were submitted to FDA to support approval of generics. The average difference in absorption into the body between the generic and the brand name was 3.5 percent. Some generics were absorbed slightly more, some slightly less. This amount of difference would be expected and acceptable, whether for one batch of brand name drug tested against another batch of the same brand, or for a generic tested against a brand name drug. In Fact, there have been studies in which brand name drugs were compared with themselves as well as with a generic. As a rule, the difference for the generic-to-brand comparison was about the same as the brand-to-brand comparison.

Any generic drug modeled after a single, brand name drug must perform approximately the same in the body as the brand name drug. There will always be a slight, but not medically important, level of natural variability–just as there is for one batch of brand name drug compared to the next batch of brand name product.

Fact: When it comes to price, there is a big difference between generic and brand name drugs. On average, the cost of a generic drug is 80 to 85 percent lower than the brand name product.

In 2010 alone, the use of FDA-approved generics saved $158 billion, an average of $3 billion every week.

Fact: Cheaper does not mean lower quality.

Generic manufacturers are able to sell their products for lower prices because they are not required to repeat the costly clinical trials of new drugs and generally do not pay for costly advertising, marketing, and promotion. In addition, multiple generic companies are often approved to market a single product; this creates competition in the marketplace, often resulting in lower prices.

Fact: FDA monitors adverse events reports for generic drugs.

The monitoring of adverse events for all drug products, including generic drugs, is one aspect of the overall FDA effort to evaluate the safety of drugs after approval. Many times, reports of adverse events describe a known reaction to the active drug ingredient.

Reports are monitored and investigated, when appropriate. The investigations may lead to changes in how a product (brand name and generic counterparts) is used or manufactured.

Fact: FDA is actively engaged in making all regulated products–including generic drugs–safer.

FDA is aware that there are reports noting that some people may experience an undesired effect when switching from brand name drug to a generic formulation or from one generic drug to another generic drug. FDA wants to understand what may cause problems with certain formulations if, in Fact, they are linked to specific generic products.

FDA is encouraging the generic industry to investigate whether, and under what circumstances, such problems occur. The agency does not have the resources to perform independent clinical studies and lacks the regulatory authority to require industry to conduct such studies. FDA will continue to investigate these reports to ensure that it has all the Facts about these treatment failures and will make recommendations to healthcare professionals and the public if the need arises.

Chapter 38

Taking Medicine

Chapter Contents

Section 38.1

Tips for Taking Medications

This section includes text excerpted from "Are You Taking
Medication as Prescribed?" U.S. Food and Drug
Administration (FDA), July 25, 2015.

Medication adherence, or taking medications correctly, is generally
defined as the extent to which patients take medication as prescribed
by their doctors. This involves factors such as getting prescriptions
filled, remembering to take medication on time, and understanding
the directions.

Common barriers to medication adherence include:

- the inability to pay for medications

- disbelief that the treatment is necessary or helping

- difficulty keeping up with multiple medications and complex
dosing schedules

- confusion about how and when to take the medication

Poor adherence can interfere with the ability to treat many diseases, leading to greater complications from the illness and a lower
quality of life for patients. Here are some examples of areas in which
medication adherence can pose challenges, along with tips for taking
medications correctly and talking with healthcare professionals about
your questions and concerns.

Taking Antibiotics

If you feel better and no longer have symptoms, you may think
your illness is cured. But if you have a bacterial infection, this can be
a dangerous assumption.

If the full course of antibiotics is not taken, a small number of bacteria are likely to still be alive. These surviving germs are likely to
have some natural resistance to the antibiotic. As they multiply and
spread, a new strain of resistant germs may begin to develop. This
may be one way that Methicillin-Resistant Staphylococcus Aureus

(MRSA) infections occur. MRSA is a type of bacteria that's resistant to certain antibiotics.

It's important to use antibiotics appropriately and to take the medication exactly as directed.

- Take all doses of the antibiotic, even if the infection is getting better.

- Don't stop taking the antibiotic unless your doctor tells you to stop.

- Don't share antibiotics with others.

- Don't save unfinished antibiotics for another time.

Taking Human Immunodeficiency Virus (HIV) / Acquired Immune Deficiency Syndrome (AIDS) Medications

People with HIV/AIDS can have a particularly difficult time taking medications as prescribed, according to Richard Klein, the HIV/AIDS program director for the Food and Drug Administration's (FDA) Office of Special Health Initiatives (OSHI).

Some of the main reasons:

- Multiple drugs may need to be taken at different times, which can be hard to remember.

- The side effects of certain drugs can sometimes make people feel worse instead of better.

- When people feel okay, they may not feel the need to take their drugs. They don't have the 'physical reminder' to take the medications.

- People may not be aware of the risks of drug resistance that can occur if they stop treatment or skip or lower doses.

When you skip doses or stop taking a prescribed medication, you may develop strains of human immunodeficiency virus (HIV) that are resistant to the medications you are taking and even to some medications you haven't taken yet. This may result in fewer treatment options should you need to change treatment regimens in the future.

FDA has given expedited reviews to several fixed dose combination medications like Atripla (a combination of efavirenz, emtricitabine and tenofovir) and Combivir (a combination of retrovir and epivir) to treat HIV. Fixed dose combination tablets contain two or more anti-HIV medications that can be from one or more drug classes.

"These fixed dose combinations are examples where the constituent drugs were already approved," says Klein, "but the agency expedited review because the combined formulations simplified dosing, and thus were likely to improve adherence." A standard drug review time is 10 months, while an expedited review of fixed dose combination tablets is generally completed within 6 months.

Tips for Consumers

Communicate with your healthcare professional. If medication side effects are bothering you, talk with your doctor or pharmacist about what you can do to lessen the problem. You might be able to switch to a different medication or your doctor may be able to adjust the timing of your dose.

Make sure you understand how long to take the medication. Some questions to ask when you're prescribed a new medication are:

- Is it necessary to empty the bottle, or can I stop taking this medication once I feel better?

- Will I need to get a refill, or can I stop treatment when the bottle is empty?

Tell your doctor if paying for prescription drugs is a problem. Your doctor may be able to prescribe a generic medication or offer other suggestions to offset the cost of a drug. Generic drugs use the same active ingredients and are shown to work the same way in the body, but they can cost 30 percent to 80 percent less. Generics also have the same risks and benefits as their brand-name counterparts.

You can also shop around your neighborhood or legitimate online pharmacies for the best prices on prescription drugs.

You can also:

- Check whether you are eligible for drug assistance programs in your state.

- Check with the pharmaceutical companies that manufacture your medicines to find out whether you qualify for assistance.

Set daily routines to take medication. It can be helpful to connect taking the medication with normal, daily activities such as eating meals or going to bed. You can also keep backup supplies of your medication at your workplace or in your briefcase or purse.

Keep medications where you'll notice them. For a medication that should be taken with food, place that medication on the dinner table or television (TV) tray, or wherever you eat on a regular basis. If there are medications you need to take in the morning, put those medications in your bathroom, next to your toothbrush or your deodorant, or something else that you use as part of your morning routine.

Use daily dosing containers. These are available at most pharmacies and allow you to keep medications in compartments that are labeled with the days of the week and various dosage frequencies.

Keep a written or computerized schedule. This can cover the medications you take, how often you take them, and any special directions. Thanks to modern technology, there are a number of devices that have been designed to help patients adhere to a prescribed medication schedule. These include medication reminder pagers and wristwatches, automatic pill dispensers, and even voice-command medication managers. Ask your pharmacist for suggestions as to which particular devices may be helpful for you.

Section 38.2

Giving Medicine to Your Child

This chapter contains text excerpted from the following sources: Text under the heading "Safety Information for Parents and Caregivers" is excerpted from "Kids Aren't Just Small Adults—Medicines, Children, and the Care Every Child Deserves," U.S. Food and Drug Administration (FDA), August 28, 2013. Reviewed January 2017; Text under the heading "Giving Cough and Cold Products to Kids" is excerpted from "Use Caution When Giving Cough and Cold Products to Kids," U.S. Food and Drug Administration (FDA), November 4, 2016.

Safety Information for Parents and Caregivers

Use care when giving any medicine to an infant or a child. Even over-the-counter (OTC) medicines that you buy are serious medicines. The following is advice for giving OTC medicine to your child, from the U.S. Food and Drug Administration (FDA) and the makers of OTC medicines:

1. **Always read and follow the Drug Facts label on your OTC medicine.** This is important for choosing and safely using all OTC medicines. Read the label every time, before you give the medicine. Be sure you clearly understand how much medicine to give and when the medicine can be taken again.

2. **Know the "active ingredient" in your child's medicine.** This is what makes the medicine work and is always listed at the top of the Drug Facts label. Sometimes an active ingredient can treat more than one medical condition. For that reason, the same active ingredient can be found in many different medicines that are used to treat different symptoms. For example, a medicine for a cold and a medicine for a headache could each contain the same active ingredient. So, if you're treating a cold and a headache with two medicines and both have the same active ingredient, you could be giving two times the normal dose. If you're confused about your child's medicines, check with a doctor, nurse, or pharmacist.

3. **Give the right medicine, in the right amount, to your child.** Not all medicines are right for an infant or a child. Medicines with the same brand name can be sold in many different strengths, such as infant, children, and adult formulas. The amount and directions are also different for children of different ages or weights. Always use the right medicine and follow the directions exactly. Never use more medicine than directed, even if your child seems sicker than the last time.

4. **Talk to your doctor, pharmacist, or nurse to find out what mixes well and what doesn't.** Medicines, vitamins, supplements, foods, and beverages don't always mix well with each other. Your healthcare professional can help.

5. **Use the dosing tool that comes with the medicine, such as a dropper or a dosing cup.** A different dosing tool, or a kitchen spoon, could hold the wrong amount of medicine.

6. Know the difference between a tablespoon (tbsp.) and a teaspoon (tsp.) Do not confuse them! A tablespoon holds three times as much medicine as a teaspoon. On measuring tools, a teaspoon (tsp.) is equal to "5 cc" or "5 mL"

7. **Know your child's weight.** Directions on some OTC medicines are based on weight. Never guess the amount of medicine to give to your child or try to figure it out from the adult

dose instructions. If a dose is not listed for your child's age or weight, call your doctor or other members of your healthcare team.

8. **Prevent a poison emergency by always using a child-resistant cap.** Re-lock the cap after each use. Be especially careful with any products that contain iron; they are the leading cause of poisoning deaths in young children.

9. **Store all medicines in a safe place.** Today's medicines are tasty, colorful, and many can be chewed. Kids may think that these products are candy. To prevent an overdose or poisoning emergency, store all medicines and vitamins in a safe place out of your child's (and even your pet's) sight and reach. If your child takes too much, call the Poison Center Hotline at 1-800-222-1222 (open 24 hours every day, 7 days a week) or call 9-1-1.

10. **Check the medicine three times.** First, check the outside packaging for such things as cuts, slices, or tears. Second, once you are at home, check the label on the inside package to be sure you have the right medicine. Make sure the lid and seal are not broken. Third, check the color, shape, size, and smell of the medicine. If you notice anything different or unusual, talk to a pharmacist or another healthcare professional.

Giving Cough and Cold Products to Kids

Children under 2 years of age should not be given any kind of cough and cold product that contains a decongestant or antihistamine because serious and possibly life-threatening side effects could occur. Reported side effects of these products included convulsions, rapid heart rates and death. What about older children? When giving cough and cold medicine to children over 2 years of age, parents and caregivers should use caution.

A meeting about the safety and effectiveness of cough and cold drug product use in children by the U.S. Food and Drug Administration (FDA) in 2007 revealed that there were many reports of harm, and even death, in children who used these products. During 2004-2005, an estimated 1,519 children less than two years of age were treated in U.S. emergency departments for adverse events, including overdoses, associated with cough and cold medications. Manufacturers voluntarily removed over-the-counter (OTC) infant cough and cold products intended for children under two years of age due to these safety concerns.

Treating Toddlers and Older Children

Cough and cold products for children older than two years of age were not affected by the voluntary removal and these products are still sold in pharmacies and other retail outlets. Manufactures also voluntarily re-labeled these cough and cold products to state: "do not use in children under four years of age."

Parents need to be aware that many OTC cough and cold products contain multiple ingredients which can lead to accidental overdosing. Reading the Drug Facts label can help parents learn about what drugs (active ingredients) are in a product.

When giving children four years of age and older a cough and cold product, remember, OTC cough and cold products can be harmful if:

- more than the recommended amount is used

- they are given too often

- more than one product containing the same drug is being used

Children should not be given medicines that are packaged and made for adults.

Other Options for Treating Colds

Here are a few alternative treatments for infants to help with cough and cold symptoms:

- A cool mist humidifier helps nasal passages shrink and allow easier breathing. Do not use warm mist humidifiers. They can cause nasal passages to swell and make breathing more difficult

- Saline nose drops or spray keep nasal passages moist and helps avoid stuffiness

- Nasal suctioning with a bulb syringe—with or without saline nose drops—works very well for infants less than a year old. Older children often resist the use of a bulb syringe

- Acetaminophen or ibuprofen can be used to reduce fever, aches and pains. Parents should carefully read and follow the product's instructions for use on the Drug Facts label

- Drinking plenty of liquids will help children stay hydrated.

Section 38.3

Over-the-Counter (OTC) Dosage Delivery Devices

This section contains text excerpted from the following sources:
Text beginning with the heading "Understanding Medication
Errors" is excerpted from "Medication Errors," U.S. Food and Drug
Administration (FDA), January 9, 2015; Text under the heading
"Tips to Prevent an Accidental Overdose" is excerpted from "Ten
Tips to Prevent an Accidental Overdose," U.S. Food and Drug
Administration (FDA), June 6, 2016.

Understanding Medication Errors

On May 4, 2011, the U.S. Food and Drug Administration (FDA)
issued a final guidance for industry with the Agency's recommendations for improving dosage delivery devices, such as cups and droppers,
for over-the-counter (OTC) (i.e., non-prescription) orally ingested liquid
drug products. The intent of this guidance is to suggest ways manufacturers can improve their labeling in order to minimize the risk of
accidental overdose.

The following questions and answers provide background on accidental overdose of OTC liquid drug products and describe the steps manufacturers and consumers can take to reduce medication dosing errors.

What Are OTC Orally Ingested Liquid Drug Products?

Over-the-counter (OTC) drugs are those medications sold without a
prescription in drug stores, grocery stores, and other retail establish-
ments. The orally ingested liquid drug products are medications that
are in a liquid form; such as a syrup, solution, suspension, or elixir;
that are intended to be consumed by swallowing (orally ingested).
Examples of these products include the liquid forms of pain relievers, cold medicine, cough syrups, and digestion aids. Liquid oral drug
products are often intended for use in children and require careful
administration by a parent or adult caregiver using an appropriate
dosage delivery device.

What Are OTC Dosage Delivery Devices?

Calibrated cups, spoons, needleless syringes, and droppers are examples of dosage delivery devices used to administer orally ingested liquid drug products. These dosage devices are generally marked in measured increments such as tablespoons (tbsp), teaspoons (tsp), or milliliters (mL). Dosage delivery devices are intended to assist consumers in measuring the appropriate dose of a liquid oral drug product and should be used only with the products they are packaged with.

Why Is FDA Concerned about OTC Dosage Delivery Devices?

FDA is concerned about over-the-counter (OTC) dosage delivery devices because accidental dosing errors can result from markings on the device that are misleading or inconsistent with the dosage directions listed on the product package. For example, FDA identified and monitored the recall of a potentially unsafe nasal decongestant product where the directions stated, "take 2 teaspoonful (tsp) every 4-6 hours." The dosage delivery device packaged with the product did not display a "2 tsp" marking; rather, it displayed a marking for two table spoonful as "2TBS" instead. Misunderstanding or misreading this device marking could potentially lead to a dangerous three-fold increase in the administered dose.

Accidental overdoses can also occur when patients and caregivers cannot read or understand the markings on the dosage delivery device and may improvise and use household utensils such as spoons to measure teaspoon or tablespoon doses. Since household utensils can vary widely in size, patients and caregivers may be administering an inaccurate dose of medicine and may inadvertently under or overdose themselves or the patient.

FDA believes better dosage devices will help minimize these types of accidental dosing errors.

Why Did FDA Issue a Guidance for Industry on OTC Dosage Delivery Devices?

FDA issued a guidance on over-the-counter (OTC) dosage delivery devices because of safety concerns about the serious risk of accidental drug overdoses, especially in children. Accidental overdosing can be caused by dosage delivery devices with unclear markings or markings that are inconsistent with the labeled dosing instructions.

The guidance for industry is aimed at improving the clarity of the markings on dosing devices and the consistency between product labeling and dosing devices by providing recommendations for making liquid dosage delivery devices that are easier for consumers to use and understand.

Better measuring devices for OTC liquid drug products will help patients, parents, and other caregivers use the right amount of these medications—the safest and most effective dose—especially when administering liquid drug products to children.

What Are the Main Points of the Guidance for Industry?

The main points of the guidance for industry are as follows:

- Dosage delivery devices should be included for all orally ingested OTC products that are liquid formulations.

- Dosage devices should be marked with calibrated units of liquid measurement (e.g., teaspoon, tablespoon, or milliliter) that are the same as the units of liquid measure specified in the labeled dosage directions on the product packaging and in any written instructions.

- If units of liquid measure are abbreviated on the dosage delivery device, the abbreviation used on the device should be the same abbreviation used in the labeled dosage directions, outside packaging (carton labeling), bottle, and any accompanying written instructions.

- Any decimals or fractions included on dosage delivery devices should be listed as clearly as possible.

- Dosage delivery devices should not have extraneous measurement markings.

- Manufacturers should try to ensure that the dosage delivery devices are only used to administer the product they are packaged with.

- Dosage delivery devices should not be significantly larger than the largest single dose allowed and should allow accurate delivery of the smallest dose described in the product labeling.

- The liquid measure markings on dosage delivery devices should be clearly visible both before and after a liquid product is added to the device.

How Will FDA Determine If This Guidance Is Effective in Minimizing the Risk of Accidental Overdose of OTC Orally Ingested Liquid Drug Products?

FDA routinely monitors and surveys the over-the-counter (OTC) drug marketplace and will take appropriate measures to address OTC liquid drug products that are packaged with misleading dosage delivery devices and may pose serious safety concerns. FDA expects that widespread industry compliance with this guidance will help consumers better understand how to dispense a correct dose of an OTC medication and thereby help to reduce accidental OTC overdoses.

Tips to Prevent an Accidental Overdose

For a medicine to work for you—and not against you—you've got to take the right dose.

Many over-the-counter liquid medicines—such as pain relievers, cold medicine, cough syrups, and digestion aids—come with spoons, cups, oral droppers, or syringes designed to help consumers measure the proper dose. These "dosage delivery devices" usually have measurement markings on them—such as teaspoons (tsp), tablespoons (tbsp), or milliliters (mL).

But the markings aren't always clear or consistent with the directions on the medicine's package. The U.S. Food and Drug Administration (FDA) has received numerous reports of accidental overdoses—especially in young children—that were attributed, in part, to the use of dosage delivery devices that were unclear or incompatible with the medicine's labeled directions for use.

On May 4, 2011, FDA issued a guidance to firms that manufacture, market, or distribute over-the-counter liquid medicines. The guidance calls for them to provide dosage delivery devices with markings that are easy to use and understand.

Parents and caregivers can do their part, too, to avoid giving too much or too little of an over-the-counter medicine.

Section 38.4

Antibiotics Aren't Always the Answer

This section includes text excerpted from "Antibiotics Aren't Always the Answer," Centers for Disease Control and Prevention (CDC), November 14, 2016.

Dependence on Antibiotics

Antibiotic use is the leading cause of antibiotic resistance. Up to one-third to one-half of antibiotic use in humans is either unnecessary or inappropriate. Each year in the United States, 47 million unnecessary antibiotic prescriptions are written in doctor's offices, emergency rooms, and hospital-based clinics, which makes improving antibiotic prescribing and use a national priority.

To combat antibiotic resistance and avoid adverse drug reactions, we must use antibiotics appropriately. This means using antibiotics only when needed and, if needed, using them correctly.

Antibiotics do not fight infections caused by viruses like colds, flu, most sore throats, and bronchitis. Even many sinus and ear infections can get better without antibiotics. Instead, symptom relief might be the best treatment option for these infections.

What You Can Do

Just because your healthcare professional doesn't give you an antibiotic doesn't mean you aren't sick. Talk with your healthcare professional about the best treatment for your or your child's illness.

To feel better when you or your child has a viral infection:

- Ask your healthcare professional about over-the-counter treatment options that may help reduce symptoms.

- Drink more fluids.

- Get plenty of rest.

- Use a cool-mist vaporizer or saline nasal spray to relieve congestion.

- Soothe your throat with crushed ice, sore throat spray, or lozenges. (Do not give lozenges to young children.)

- Use honey to relieve cough. (Do not give honey to an infant under one year of age.)

- If you are diagnosed with the flu, there are flu antiviral drugs that can be used to treat flu illness. They are prescription drugs.

Taking antibiotics for viral infections, such as colds, flu, most sore throats, and bronchitis:

- Will not cure the infection

- Will not keep other people from getting sick

- Will not help you or your child feel better

- May cause unnecessary and harmful side effects

- May contribute to antibiotic resistance, which is when bacteria are able to resist the effects of an antibiotic and continue to cause harm

Rest, fluids, and over-the-counter products may be your or your child's best treatment options for symptoms associated with viral infections. Remember, there are potential risks when taking any prescription drug. Unneeded antibiotics may lead to harmful side effects and future antibiotic-resistant infections.

What Not to Do

- Do not demand antibiotics when your healthcare professional says they are not needed.

- Do not take an antibiotic for a viral infection.

- Do not take antibiotics prescribed for someone else. The antibiotic may not be right for your illness. Taking the wrong medicine may delay correct treatment and allow bacteria to grow.

If your healthcare professional prescribes an antibiotic for a bacterial infection:

- Do not skip doses.

- Do not stop taking the antibiotics early unless your healthcare professional tells you to do so.

- Do not save any of the antibiotics for the next time you or your child gets sick.

Chapter 39

Adverse Drug Events

What Is Adverse Drug Event (ADE)?

An adverse drug event (ADE) has been defined by the Institute of Medicine as "an injury resulting from medical intervention related to a drug." This broad term encompasses harms that occur during medical care that are directly caused by the drug including but are not limited to medication errors, adverse drug reactions, allergic reactions, and overdoses. A medication error is defined as "inappropriate use of a drug that may or may not result in harm;" such errors may occur during prescribing, transcribing, dispensing, administering, adherence, or monitoring of a drug. In contrast, an adverse drug reaction (ADR) is "harms directly caused by a drug at normal doses."

ADE Prevention Is a Patient Safety Priority

A large majority of ADEs are preventable. In 2006, 82 percent of the United States population reported using at least one prescription medication, over-the-counter medication, or dietary supplement, and 29 percent reported using five or more prescription medications.

This chapter contains text excerpted from the following sources: Text beginning with the heading "What Is Adverse Drug Event (ADE)?" is excerpted from "National Action Plan for the Prevention of Adverse Drug Events," Office of Disease Prevention and Health Promotion (ODPHP), U.S. Department of Health and Human Services (HHS), October 4, 2013. Reviewed January 2017; Text under the heading "Strategies to Prevent ADE" is excerpted from "Sustainment Guide for Adverse Drug Events," U.S. Department of Health and Human Services (HHS), January 24, 2014.

Among older adults (65 years of age or older), 57–59 percent reported taking five to nine medications and 17–19 percent reported taking 10 or more over the course of that year. Given the U.S. population's large and ever-increasing magnitude of medication exposure, the potential for harms from ADEs constitutes a critical patient safety and public health challenge. ADEs can occur in any healthcare setting, including inpatient (e.g., acute care hospitals), outpatient, and institutional and noninstitutional long-term care (LTC) settings (e.g., nursing homes, group homes). The likelihood of ADEs occurring may also increase during transitions of care (e.g., discharge from a hospital to a nursing home or patients' move from one healthcare provider or setting to another), when information may not be adequately transferred between healthcare providers or patients may not completely understand how to manage their medications.

In inpatient settings, research indicates that ADEs are among the largest contributors to hospital-related complications. It has been estimated that ADEs comprise one-third of hospital adverse events, affect approximately 2 million hospital stays annually, and prolong hospital length of stay by approximately 1.7 to 4.6 days. Data regarding how ADEs contribute to postdischarge complications or during other types of care transitions are lacking. One single-center study based in a tertiary care academic medical center identified ADEs as the most common cause of postdischarge complications occurring within 3 weeks of hospital discharge (accounting for two-thirds of postdischarge complications); in this study, 24 percent of postdischarge ADEs were judged to be preventable, and in another, similar study, 27 percent of postdischarge ADEs were judged to be preventable and 33 percent ameliorable. In outpatient settings, nationally representative surveillance data indicate that ADEs account for more than 3.5 million physician office visits, an estimated 1 million emergency department (ED) visits, and approximately 125,000 hospital admissions each year. An analysis of 2011 data indicated that ADEs were three times more likely to be present on admission than during the hospital stay.

The economic impact of ADEs has been inadequately studied. Older data indicate that ADEs impose a large financial burden on healthcare expenditures; one study estimated ADEs incurred $5.6 million (1993 USD) in excess hospital costs. National estimates suggest that ADEs contribute an additional $3.5 billion (2006 USD) to U.S. healthcare costs. Older adults experience the highest population rates of ADEs resulting in ED visits and are seven times more likely than younger persons to have an ADE that requires emergent hospital admission.

Analysis of 2011 data indicated that Medicare beneficiaries are at the highest risk of acquiring an ADE during a hospital stay with Medicare reimbursing 75 percent of inpatient ADEs attributable to the most common medications. These ED visits and hospital admissions from ADEs, a significant number of which are considered preventable, contribute to an enormously overburdened Medicare system.

Focus on High-Impact Targets and Populations

The National Action Plan for Adverse Drug Event Prevention focuses on common, clinically significant, preventable, and measurable ADEs. A key group of ADEs are particularly dangerous and largely preventable, and for these reasons, they are high-priority targets for national and local ADE prevention efforts.

Medication Classes Most Commonly Implicated in ADEs

In a nationally representative sample of hospitalized Medicare beneficiaries, the targets of the ADE Action Plan were identified as three of the most commonly implicated drug classes in ADEs: anticoagulants, opioids, and insulin. Conservative estimates indicate that hospitalized patients experience 380,000 to 450,000 ADEs each year, with a large majority of these attributable to anticoagulants and opioids. A large percentage of these ADEs were judged to be preventable.

In outpatient settings, national public health surveillance data indicate that a small group of key medication classes—those that are characterized by a narrow therapeutic index or require routine laboratory monitoring—cause the most outpatient medication-related harms. In a recent, nationally representative sample of hospital admissions for ADEs among older adults, an estimated twothirds of admissions involved just four medication classes, three of which are preventable targets of the ADE Action Plan: anticoagulants (e.g., warfarin), insulin, and oral diabetes agents (e.g., sulfonylurea)

A significant proportion of ADEs in this sample resulted from unintentional overdoses or supratherapeutic effects (e.g., bleeding due to excessive anticoagulation or hypoglycemia from excessive insulin administration).

Most Vulnerable Populations

It is recognized that several patient populations may be especially vulnerable to ADEs, including the very young (pediatric patients), older adults, individuals with low socioeconomic status (SES) or low health literacy, those with limited access to healthcare services, and certain minority races or ethnic groups.

To date, data commonly implicate age as a principle underlying risk factor for ADEs and suggest that older adults are particularly vulnerable to ADEs, likely owing to altered pharmacokinetics, polypharmacy, or cognitive decline. For example, older adults comprise approximately 35 percent of all inpatient stays but contribute to approximately 53 percent of inpatient stays complicated by ADEs. Analyses of cost data indicate that Medicare-covered patients experience significantly higher rates of ADEs than both privately insured and Medicaid-covered patients. In the outpatient setting, national surveillance data indicate that older adults are two to three times more likely to have an ADE requiring a physician office or ED visit and seven times more likely to have an ADE requiring hospital admission. The aging of the population and the vulnerability of older adults to ADEs will have significant implications for Medicare. In 2050, the number of Americans aged 65 and older is projected to be 88.5 million, more than double its population in 2010 of 40.2 million.

Spending in the United States for prescription drugs in 2010 was $259.1 billion and is expected to double over the next decade. Total expenditures on the Medicare Part D program alone in 2012 were $66.9 billion and are projected to reach $165.1 billion by 2022.

Underserved and Rural Communities

Any steps to reduce the incidence of ADEs should take into consideration the available resources of the healthcare provider, institution, and surrounding community. In underserved and rural communities, limited access to healthcare services, shortages of qualified healthcare personnel, slower adoption of electronic health records (EHRs), higher rates of older adults with chronic conditions, low health literacy, and reduced revenue may affect the successful implementation of approaches outlined in this document.

Limited staff resources and slower adoption of EHRs affect current surveillance efforts, which rely on clinical chart abstractions. In a rural or underserved community, the healthcare provider may be forced to choose between dedicating time to patient care and investing time in reporting rates of ADEs. Even as the Nation moves toward a more seamless system for reporting these errors through the use of EHRs, underserved communities will be at a disadvantage, as EHR adoption rates continue to be higher within facilities with more financial resources, and rural communities continue to lag behind their urban counterparts.

Implementing ADE prevention efforts requires extensive staff training, investment of financial resources, and coordination of providers—all of which may be challenging in communities where staffing is limited, providers are not located within the same geographic community, and financial resources are scarce. In rural communities especially, coordination of medications across healthcare providers may be limited, as only generalists may be available in the community and prescribing specialists may be many miles away. Rural and underserved communities may be less capable of taking advantage of advances in technology, such as the use of clinical decision support (CDS) in EHRs, and are less likely to

have access to e-prescribing systems, which serve as a valuable tool to track inappropriate dosages, drug-drug interactions, and drug-allergy interactions.

The complexity of the care that pharmacists provide patients necessitates that patients should have access to the healthcare provider responsible for their care during all aspects of medication therapy.

Although such local access is not always possible in low-volume, rural settings, leveraging technology to access remotely delivered care can result in both direct intervention and enhanced patient education.

Provider involvement is crucial to supporting consumer engagement in shared decisionmaking regarding medication management. This may be more challenging within underserved and rural communities, as evidence suggests that individuals in rural communities and those with lower SES have lower health literacy.

Rural healthcare providers like critical access hospitals (CAHs) are not subject to some of the same reporting requirements and financial incentive programs as other providers. For example, although the majority of CAHs report quality measure information to the Centers for Medicare and Medicaid Services' (CMS) Hospital Compare Web site, these hospitals are exempt from this requirement, which means that changes in CMS programs and policies may not have the same impact on some rural populations.

Finally, within underserved communities, there is a significant delay in the translation of research into practice. Thus, even proven interventions or new findings related to reducing ADEs may take many years to benefit rural and underserved communities.

Strategies to Prevent ADE

Strategies cited by the Agency for Healthcare Research and Quality (AHRQ) and the General Accounting Office (GAO) to improve the medication delivery system include:

- Improve incident reporting systems (i.e., Patient Safety Reporting System)
- Create a better atmosphere for healthcare providers to report ADEs so that the person
- reporting the error does not fear repercussions or punishment
- Rely more on pharmacists to advise providers in prescribing medications and promote
- education on medications
- Improve nursing medication administration and monitoring systems
- Implement a standardized medication reconciliation form
- Improve communication between providers and patients about risks and benefits of medication
- Dispense drugs from pharmacy in single-unit/single-dose packages
- Install automated dispensing systems
- Barcode hospital medications
- Institute Look-Alike/Sound-Alike alerts
- Include pharmacists in hospital rounds
- Use the FDA's MedWatch program to report serious adverse drug reactions

Chapter 40

Drug Interactions: What You Should Know

There are more opportunities today than ever before to learn about your health and to take better care of yourself. It is also more important than ever to know about the medicines you take. If you take several different medicines, see more than one doctor, or have certain health conditions, you and your doctors need to be aware of all the medicines you take. Doing so will help you to avoid potential problems such as drug interactions.

Drug interactions may make your drug less effective, cause unexpected side effects, or increase the action of a particular drug. Some drug interactions can even be harmful to you. Reading the label every time you use a nonprescription or prescription drug and taking the time to learn about drug interactions may be critical to your health. You can reduce the risk of potentially harmful drug interactions and side effects with a little bit of knowledge and common sense. Drug interactions fall into three broad categories:

- **Drug-drug interactions** occur when two or more drugs react with each other. This drug-drug interaction may cause you to experience an unexpected side effect. For example, mixing a drug you take to help you sleep (a sedative) and a drug you take

This chapter includes text excerpted from "Drug Interactions: What You Should Know," U.S. Food and Drug Administration (FDA), September 25, 2013. Reviewed January 2017.

for allergies (an antihistamine) can slow your reactions and make driving a car or operating machinery dangerous.

- **Drug-food/beverage interactions** result from drugs reacting with foods or beverages. For example, mixing alcohol with some drugs may cause you to feel tired or slow your reactions.

- **Drug-condition interactions** may occur when an existing medical condition makes certain drugs potentially harmful. For example, if you have high blood pressure you could experience an unwanted reaction if you take a nasal decongestant.

Drug Interactions and Over-the-Counter Medicines

Table 40.1. Drug Interaction Information

Category	Drug Interaction Information
Acid Reducers H2 Receptor Antagonists (drugs that prevent or relieve heartburn associated with acid indigestion and sour stomach)	**For products containing cimetidine, ask a doctor or pharmacist before use if you are:** • taking theophylline (oral asthma drug), warfarin (blood thinning drug), or phenytoin (seizure drug)
Antacids (drugs for relief of acid indigestion, heartburn, and/or sour stomach)	**Ask a doctor or pharmacist before use if you are:** • allergic to milk or milk products if the product contains more than 5 grams lactose in a maximum daily dose • taking a prescription drug **Ask a doctor before use if you have:** • kidney disease
Antiemetics (drugs for prevention or treatment of nausea, vomiting, or dizziness associated with motion sickness)	**Ask a doctor or pharmacist before use if you are:** • taking sedatives or tranquilizers **Ask a doctor before use if you have:** • a breathing problem, such as emphysema or chronic bronchitis • glaucoma • difficulty in urination due to an enlarged prostate gland **When using this product:** • avoid alcoholic beverages

Table 40.1. Continued

Category	Drug Interaction Information
Antihistamines (drugs that temporarily relieve runny nose or reduce sneezing, itching of the nose or throat, and itchy watery eyes due to hay fever or other upper respiratory problems)	**Ask a doctor or pharmacist before use if you are taking:** • sedatives or tranquilizers • a prescription drug for high blood pressure or depression **Ask a doctor before use if you have:** • glaucoma or difficulty in urination due to an enlarged prostate gland • breathing problems, such as emphysema, chronic bronchitis, or asthma **When using this product:** • alcohol, sedatives, and tranquilizers may increase drowsiness • avoid alcoholic beverages
Antitussives Cough Medicine (drugs that temporarily reduce cough due to minor throat and bronchial irritation as may occur with a cold)	**Ask a doctor or pharmacist before use if you are:** • taking sedatives or tranquilizers **Ask a doctor before use if you have:** glaucoma or difficulty in urination due to an enlarged prostate gland
Bronchodilators (drugs for the temporary relief of shortness of breath, tightness of chest and wheezing due to bronchial asthma)	**Ask a doctor before use if you:** • have heart disease, high blood pressure, thyroid disease, diabetes, or difficulty in urination due to an enlarged prostate gland • have ever been hospitalized for asthma or are taking a prescription drug for asthma
Laxatives (drugs for the temporary relief of constipation)	**Ask a doctor before use if you have:** • kidney disease and the laxative contains phosphates, potassium, or magnesium • stomach pain, nausea, or vomiting
Nasal Decongestants (drugs for the temporary relief of nasal congestion due to a cold, hay fever, or other upper respiratory allergies)	**Ask a doctor before use if you:** • have heart disease, high blood pressure, thyroid disease, diabetes, or difficulty in urination due to an enlarged prostate gland

Table 40.1. Continued

Category	Drug Interaction Information
Nicotine Replacement Products (drugs that reduce withdrawal symptoms associated with quitting smoking, including nicotine craving)	**Ask a doctor before use if you:** • have high blood pressure not controlled by medication • have heart disease or have had a recent heart attack or irregular heartbeat, since nicotine can increase your heart rate **Ask a doctor or pharmacist before use if you are:** • taking a prescription drug for depression or asthma (your dose may need to be adjusted) • using a prescription non-nicotine stop smoking drug **Do not use:** • if you continue to smoke, chew tobacco, use snuff, or use other nicotine-containing products
Nighttime Sleep Aids (drugs for relief of occasional sleeplessness)	**Ask a doctor or pharmacist before use if you are:** • taking sedatives or tranquilizers **Ask a doctor before use if you have:** • a breathing problem such as emphysema or chronic bronchitis • glaucoma • difficulty in urination due to an enlarged prostate gland **When using this product:** • avoid alcoholic beverages
Pain Relievers (drugs for the temporary relief of minor body aches, pains, and headaches)	**Ask a doctor before taking if you:** • consume three or more alcohol-containing drinks per day (The following ingredients are found in different over-the-counter(OTC) pain relievers: acetaminophen, aspirin, ibuprofen, ketoprofen, magnesium salicylate, and naproxen. It is important to read the label of pain reliever products to learn about different drug interaction warnings for each ingredient.)

Table 40.1. Continued

Category	Drug Interaction Information
Stimulants (drugs that help restore mental alertness or wakefulness during fatigue or drowsines)	**When using this product:** • limit the use of foods, beverages, and other drugs that have caffeine. Too much caffeine can cause nervousness, irritability, sleeplessness, and occasional rapid heart beat • be aware that the recommended dose of this product contains about as much caffeine as a cup of coffee
Topical Acne (drugs for the treatment of acne)	**When using this product:** • increased dryness or irritation of the skin may occur immediately following use of this product or if you are using other topical acne drugs at the same time. If this occurs, only one drug should be used unless directed by your doctor

Learning More about Drug Interactions

Talk to your doctor or pharmacist about the drugs you take. When your doctor prescribes a new drug, discuss all over-the-counter (OTC) and prescription drugs, dietary supplements, vitamins, botanicals, minerals and herbals you take, as well as the foods you eat. Ask your pharmacist for the package insert for each prescription drug you take. The package insert provides more information about potential drug interactions.

Before taking a drug, ask your doctor or pharmacist the following questions:

• Can I take it with other drugs?

• Should I avoid certain foods, beverages or other products?

• What are possible drug interaction signs I should know about?

• How will the drug work in my body?

• Is there more information available about the drug or my condition (on the Internet or in health and medical literature)?

Know how to take drugs safely and responsibly. Remember, the drug label will tell you:

• what the drug is used for

- how to take the drug

- how to reduce the risk of drug interactions and unwanted side effects

If you still have questions after reading the drug product label, ask your doctor or pharmacist for more information

Remember that different OTC drugs may contain the same active ingredient. If you are taking more than one OTC drug, pay attention to the active ingredients used in the products to avoid taking too much of a particular ingredient. Under certain circumstances—such as if you are pregnant or breast-feeding—you should talk to your doctor before you take any medicine. Also, make sure you know what ingredients are contained in the medicines you take. Doing so will help you to avoid possible allergic reactions.

Chapter 41

Preventing Medication Errors: Drug Name Confusion

To minimize confusion between drug names that look or sound alike, the U.S. Food and Drug Administration (FDA) reviews about 300 drug names a year before they are marketed. "About one-third of the names that drug companies propose are rejected," says Phillips. The agency tests drug names with the help of about 120 FDA health professionals who volunteer to simulate real-life drug order situations. "FDA also created a computerized program that assists in detecting similar names and that will help take a more scientific approach to comparing names," Phillips says.

After drugs are approved, the FDA tracks reports of errors due to drug name confusion and spreads the word to health professionals, along with recommendations for avoiding future problems. For example, the FDA has reported errors involving the inadvertent administration of methadone, a drug used to treat opiate dependence, rather than the intended Metadate ER (methylphenidate) for the treatment of attention deficit hyperactivity disorder (ADHD). One report involved the death of an 8-year-old boy after a possible medication error at the dispensing pharmacy. The child, who was being treated for ADHD, was

---

This chapter includes text excerpted from "Strategies to Reduce Medication Errors: Working to Improve Medication Safety," U.S. Food and Drug Administration (FDA), October 23, 2015.

found dead at home. Methadone substitution was the suspected cause of death. Some FDA recommendations regarding drug name confusion have encouraged pharmacists to separate similar drug products on pharmacy shelves and have encouraged physicians to indicate both brand and generic drug names on prescription orders, as well as what the drug is intended to treat.

The last time the FDA changed a drug name after it was approved was in 2004 when the cholesterol-lowering medicine Altocor was being confused with the cholesterol-lowering medicine Advicor. Now Altocor is called Altoprev, and the agency hasn't received reports of errors since the name change. Other examples of drug name confusion reported to the FDA include:

- Serzone (nefazodone) for depression and Seroquel (quetiapine) for schizophrenia

- Lamictal (lamotrigine) for epilepsy, Lamisil (terbinafine) for nail infections, Ludiomil (maprotiline) for depression, and Lomotil (diphenoxylate) for diarrhea

- Taxotere (docetaxel) and Taxol (paclitaxel), both for chemotherapy

- Zantac (ranitidine) for heartburn, Zyrtec (cetirizine) for allergies, and Zyprexa (olanzapine) for mental conditions

- Celebrex (celecoxib) for arthritis and Celexa (citalopram) for depression

What Consumers Can Do

- Know what kind of errors occur. The FDA evaluated reports of fatal medication errors that it received from 1993 to 1998 and found that the most common types of errors involved administering an improper dose (41 percent), giving the wrong drug (16 percent), and using the wrong route of administration (16 percent). The most common causes of the medication errors were performance and knowledge deficits (44 percent) and communication errors (16 percent). Almost half of the fatal medication errors occurred in people over 60. Older people are especially at risk for errors because they often take multiple medications. Children are also a vulnerable population because drugs are often dosed based on their weight, and accurate calculations are critical.

- Find out what drug you're taking and what it's for. Rather than simply letting the doctor write you a prescription and send you on your way, be sure to ask the name of the drug. Cohen says, "I would also ask the doctor to put the purpose of the prescription on the order." This serves as a check in case there is some confusion about the drug name. If you're in the hospital, ask (or have a friend or family member ask) what drugs you are being given and why.

- Find out how to take the drug and make sure you understand the directions. If you are told to take a medicine three times a day, does that mean eight hours apart exactly or at mealtimes? Should the medicine be stored at room temperature or in the refrigerator? Are there any medications, beverages, or foods you should avoid? Also, ask about what medication side effects you might expect and what you should do about them. And read the bottle's label every time you take a drug to avoid mistakes. In the middle of the night, you could mistake ear drops for eye drops, or accidentally give your older child's medication to the baby if you're not careful. Use the measuring device that comes with the medicine, not spoons from the kitchen drawer. If you take multiple medications and have trouble keeping them straight, ask your doctor or pharmacist about compliance aids, such as containers with sections for daily doses. Family members can help by reminding you to take your medicine.

- Keep a list of all medications, including over-the-counter (OTC) drugs, as well as dietary supplements, medicinal herbs, and other substances you take for health reasons, and report it to your healthcare providers. The often-forgotten things that you should tell your doctor about include vitamins, laxatives, sleeping aids, and birth control pills. One National Institutes of Health (NIH) study showed a significant drug interaction between the herbal product St. John's wort and indinavir, a protease inhibitor used to treat human immunodeficiency virus (HIV) infection. Some antibiotics can lower the effectiveness of birth control pills. If you see different doctors, it's important that they all know what you are taking. If possible, get all your prescriptions filled at the same pharmacy so that all of your records are in one place. Also, make sure your doctors and pharmacy know about your medication allergies or other unpleasant drug reactions you may have experienced.

303

- If in doubt, ask, ask, ask. Be on the lookout for clues of a problem, such as if your pills look different than normal or if you notice a different drug name or different directions than what you thought. Krawisz says it's best to be cautious and ask questions if you're unsure about anything. "If you forget, don't hesitate to call your doctor or pharmacist when you get home," he says. "It can't hurt to ask."

Hospital Strategies

Hospitals and other healthcare organizations work to reduce medication errors by using technology, improving processes, zeroing in on errors that cause harm, and building a culture of safety. Here are a couple of examples.

Pharmacy intervention: It was a challenge for healthcare providers, especially surgeons, at Fairview Southdale Hospital in Edina, Minn., to ensure that patients continued taking their regularly prescribed medicines when they entered the hospital, says Steven Meisel, Pharm.D., director of medication safety at Fairview Health Services. "Surgeons are not typically the original prescribers," he says. The solution was to have pharmacy technicians record complete medication histories on a form. In a pilot program, the technicians called most patients on the phone a couple of days before surgery. A pharmacist reviewed the information, and then the surgeon decided which medications should be continued. After three months, the number of order errors per patient dropped by 84 percent, and the pilot program became permanent.

Computerized Physician Order Entry (CPOE): Studies have shown that CPOE is effective in reducing medication errors. It involves entering medication orders directly into a computer system rather than on paper or verbally. The Institute for Safe Medication Practices (ISMP) conducted a survey of 1,500 hospitals in 2001 and found that about 3 percent of hospitals were using CPOE, and the number is rising. Eugene Wiener, M.D., medical director at the Children's Hospital of Pittsburgh, says, "There is no misinterpretation of handwriting, decimal points, or abbreviations. This puts everything in a digital world."

The Pittsburgh hospital unveiled its CPOE system in October 2002. Developed by the hospital and the Cerner Corp. in Kansas City, Mo., Children's Net has replaced most paper forms and prescription pads. Wiener says that, unlike with adults, most drug orders for children are generally based on weight. "The computer won't let you put an order in if the child's weight isn't in the system," he says, "and if the weight changes, the computer notices." The system also provides all kinds of information about potential drug complications that the doctor might not have thought about. "Doctors always have a choice in dealing with the alerts," Wiener says. "They can choose to move past an alert, but the alert makes them stop and think based on the specific patient indications."

Chapter 42

Misused, Counterfeit, and Unapproved Drugs

Chapter Contents

307

Section 42.1

Misuse and Abuse of Prescription Drugs

This section includes text excerpted from "Combating
Misuse and Abuse of Prescription Drugs: Question and
Answer with Michael Klein, Ph.D.," U.S. Food and Drug
Administration (FDA), August 30, 2015.

When a person takes a legal prescription medication for a purpose
other than the reason it was prescribed, or when that person takes
a drug not prescribed to him or her, that is misuse of a drug. Misuse
can include taking a drug in a manner or at a dose that was not recommended by a healthcare professional. This can happen when the
person hopes to get a bigger or faster therapeutic response from medications such as sleeping or weight loss pills. It can also happen when
the person wants to "get high," which is an example of prescription
drug abuse.

What Is the Difference between Misuse and Abuse?

It mostly has to do with the individual's intentions or motivations.
For example, let's say that a person knows that he will get a pleasant
or euphoric feeling by taking the drug, especially at higher doses than
prescribed. That is an example of drug abuse because the person is
specifically looking for that euphoric response.

In contrast, if a person isn't able to fall asleep after taking a single
sleeping pill, they may take another pill an hour later, thinking, "That
will do the job" or a person may offer his headache medication to a
friend who is in pain. Those are examples of drug misuse because, even
though these people did not follow medical instructions, they were not
looking to "get high" from the drugs. They were treating themselves,
but not according to the directions of their healthcare providers.

However, no matter the intention of the person, both misuse and
abuse of prescription drugs can be harmful and even life-threatening
to the individual. This is because taking a drug other than the way
it is prescribed can lead to dangerous outcomes that the person may
not anticipate.

What Are the Dangers Linked to Misuse and Abuse of Prescription Drugs?

It's important to note that all drugs can produce adverse events (side effects), but the risks associated with prescription drugs are managed by a healthcare professional. Thus, the benefits outweigh the risks when the drug is taken as directed.

However, when a person misuses or abuses a prescription drug, there is no medical oversight of the risks. A person can die from respiratory depression from misusing or abusing prescription painkillers; for example, opioids. Prescription sedatives like benzodiazepines can cause withdrawal seizures. Prescription stimulants such as medications for attention deficit hyperactivity disorder (ADHD) can lead to dangerous increases in blood pressure. The risks from these drugs are worse when they are combined with other drugs, or alcohol.

Additionally, when a person misuses a prescription drug, even on a single occasion, that individual might enjoy the experience so much that they begin to seek out the drug more often. Thus, drug abuse and drug dependence are serious risks of misusing prescription drugs.

Why Do People Misuse and Abuse Prescription Drugs?

Prescription drugs are often readily accessible in the home, so it's easy to take more of them than recommended for a therapeutic reason, or to sneak a few from someone else's bottle to see if you can "get high."

One feature of prescription drug abuse is when a person continues to take the drug after it's no longer needed, medically. This is usually because the drug produces euphoric responses. Prescription drugs are often preferred for abuse because of the mistaken belief that the drugs provide a "safe high."All drugs carry risks, and if these risks are not being managed by a healthcare professional, people can get into serious trouble.

How Big Is This Problem?

The prevalence of misuse and abuse of prescription medications is concerning. The Substance Abuse and Mental Health Services Administration (SAMHSA), a federal health agency, reports that in 2008, 52 million persons in the United States age 12 or older had used prescription drugs non-medically at least once in their lifetime, and 6.2 million had used them in the past month. SAMHSA also reported that between 1998 and 2008, there was a 400 percent increase in substance abuse treatment admissions for opioid prescription pain relievers.

A recent Centers for Disease Control and Prevention (CDC) survey found that one in five high school students had taken a prescription drug without a doctor's prescription. According to SAMHSA, the majority of these teenagers are obtaining the drugs from friends or relatives for free. Most concerning, the perception of risk of prescription drug abuse declined 20 percent from 1992 to 2008, based on data from a National Institute on Drug Abuse (NIDA) survey.

What Prescription Drugs Are Being Misused and Abused?

SAMHSA reports that in 2008, nonmedical use of psychotherapeutic prescription drugs fell into four major classes: pain relievers, tranquilizers, stimulants, and sedatives.

Nearly 35 million Americans reported that they had nonmedical use of prescription pain relievers—including opioid-containing drugs such as hydrocodone (Vicodin), oxycodone (OxyContin, Percodan, Percocet), and fentanyl (Duragesic)—at least once during their lifetime.

Approximately 21.5 million Americans have used prescription tranquilizers for nonmedical purposes at least once. These include drugs prescribed for anxiety or insomnia, such as benzodiazepines—including diazepam (Valium), alprazolam (Xanax) and clonazepam (Klonapin)—and non-benzodiazepines such as zolpidem (Ambien), zaleplon (Sonata) and eszopiclone (Lunesta).

Similarly, about 21.2 million Americans have used prescription stimulants non-medically at least once. These include drugs prescribed for ADHD such as amphetamine (Adderall), methylphenidate (Ritalin, Concerta, and Daytrana), and methamphetamine. Notably, almost 13 million people reported they had used prescription methamphetamine at least once during their lifetime.

Finally, nearly 9 million Americans have used prescription sedatives non-medically at least once. These sedatives include barbiturates such as amobarbital (Amytal), pentobarbital (Nembutal), and secobarbital (Seconal).

Who Is Misusing and Abusing These Medications?

Prescription drugs are being misused and abused by a wide variety of people. According to SAMHSA, about 26 million Americans between the ages of 26 and 50 report they have used prescription drugs non-medically at some point in their life. Other age groups have lower lifetime incidents: 13 million who are age 50 or older, 9 million who are age 18 to 25, and 3 million who are 12 to 17 years of age.

There also appears to be regional differences across the United States. For example, SAMHSA reports that the highest past-year rates of nonmedical use of prescription pain relievers occur in Arkansas, Kentucky, Nevada, Oklahoma, Oregon, Tennessee, and Wisconsin.

Should a Person's Healthcare Professional Tell Them about the Risks Associated with a Medication with Abuse Potential?

Yes. The healthcare professional should talk to a patient about all of the warnings and precautions listed in the drug label for the medication being prescribed. In addition, if a medication guide is available, it will explain the risks of the drug in plain language. The pharmacy will provide the medication guide when a person picks up the prescription.

FDA also recommends that patients be vigilant when it comes to matters of their health. Reading information and asking questions are good practices, though they are only the first steps. For instance, individuals may not realize they are developing a drug abuse problem with a prescription drug, especially if they were initially using the drug as directed when they were patients.

Healthcare professionals should encourage patients to be aware of early signs of drug abuse, which can include using the prescription more frequently or at higher doses, but without medical direction to do so. Using the drug compulsively or not being able to carry out normal daily activities because of drug misuse are also signs of abuse.

Finally, healthcare professionals and pharmacists have a responsibility to remind patients not to share their medications with friends or family. Not only is this a dangerous practice health-wise, it is also illegal.

How Does FDA Help Prevent Misuse and Abuse of Prescription Medicines?

FDA works hard to meet the challenges of preventing misuse and abuse of prescription drugs, while making sure that medically appropriate drugs are available for the patients who need them.

The primary way FDA works to prevent misuse and abuse is through educating patients, caregivers, and healthcare professionals.

This often occurs through the information FDA provides to each of these groups, such as in drug labels, medication guides, and alerts.

But long before a patient can obtain a prescription, FDA has already evaluated whether the drug is safe and effective for a particular medical condition. FDA only approves those drug applications that have been shown to be safe and effective for a specific indication, and the data from this review is then used to create informational materials.

FDA is also part of the wider national strategy involving other government agencies, the pharmaceutical industry, medical organizations, and community groups, among other entities. This combined effort addresses improved treatment, prevention, enforcement, and emerging drugs of abuse.

How Is a Prescription Medication Classified as Having Potential for Abuse?

During FDA's drug review process, certain data can give indications that a drug has abuse potential. The chemical structure may be similar to a known drug of abuse. When the drug is given to animals, it may produce behaviors that are like those produced by abusable drugs. In humans, the drug may produce a high rate of euphoria.

FDA considers these and all abuse-related data to make a determination regarding abuse potential, which is a part of the safety evaluation of a drug. If a drug is deemed to have abuse potential, Drug Enforcement Administration (DEA) is informed and they may add the drug to the list of substances covered by the Controlled Substances Act (CSA).

In addition, FDA can become aware that a drug has abuse potential through other means. For example, there may be epidemiological reports of abuse that only became evident after the drug was marketed. Also, DEA informs that there is an increase in law enforcement actions related to a specific drug. In both cases, FDA reviews all available data and makes a scientific and medical assessment of whether the drug has abuse potential. If it does, DEA is informed and may schedule the drug under the CSA.

What Are the Keys to Preventing Abuse of Prescription Medicines?

Be informed about the effects of prescription drugs and be vigilant. Know what medications your loved ones are taking and watch for signs of changes in behavior. For instance, have you noticed negative changes in your child's behavior or grades? Is your spouse evasive about how much medication he or she is taking? Do you have friends that you suspect might be pilfering prescription drugs from your medicine cabinet?

If you are taking medications that have abuse potential, use the drugs only as directed. Don't share them, and store them in a safe, secure place. Count the pills regularly to make sure no one else is using them. If you are having a house party or an open house, make sure the medications are properly secured.

Finally, all drugs should be disposed of properly after they are no longer needed. If no specific disposal directions are given with the medication, discard the drugs by mixing with undesirable substances, sealing them in a container, and placing them in the trash. You can also call your local DEA office for advice on alternative disposal methods.

What Can I Do If I Find That Someone I Know Is Abusing Prescription Drugs, or If I Find Myself Becoming Dependent on Them?

SAMHSA has a website (www.samhsa.gov) and a telephone hotline (800-662-HELP [800-662-4357]) to aid in finding treatment facilities in different areas of the country.

Section 42.2

Counterfeit Drugs

This section includes text excerpted from "Counterfeit Drugs Questions and Answers," U.S. Food and Drug Administration (FDA), April 27, 2016.

What Is the Definition of a Counterfeit Drug?

United States law defines counterfeit drugs as those sold under a product name without proper authorization. Counterfeiting can apply to both brand name and generic products, where the identity of the source is mislabeled in a way that suggests that it is the authentic approved product. Counterfeit products may include products without the active ingredient, with an insufficient or excessive quantity of the active ingredient, with the wrong active ingredient, or with fake packaging.

What Risks Are Involved with Taking Counterfeit Drugs?

An individual who receives a counterfeit drug may be at risk for a number of dangerous health consequences. Patients may experience unexpected side effects, allergic reactions, or a worsening of their medical condition. A number of counterfeit products do not contain any active ingredients, and instead contain inert substances, which do not provide the patient any treatment benefit. Counterfeit drugs may also contain incorrect ingredients, improper dosages of the correct ingredients, or they may contain hazardous ingredients.

What Is the Prevalence of Counterfeit Drugs in the United States?

Drug counterfeiting occurs less frequently in the United States than in other countries due to the strict regulatory framework that governs the production of drug products and the distribution chain, and enforcement against violators. However, the United States has recently experienced three highly publicized examples of counterfeit drugs within the U.S. distribution system:

- Lipitor tablets, a cholesterol-lowering medication,
- Procrit, an injectable drug used to stimulate red blood cell growth,
- Alli, an over-the-counter weight-loss drug.

FDA continues to believe, and works to ensure, that the overall quality of drug products that consumers purchase from U.S. pharmacies remains high. The American public can be confident that these medications are safe and effective.

How Can Pharmacists, Physicians, and Other Healthcare Professionals Identify Counterfeit Medications?

Pharmacists, physicians, and other healthcare professionals should familiarize themselves with those drugs most likely to be counterfeited and how to identify these products. FDA periodically places updated information regarding counterfeiting on its website at www.fda.gov/counterfeit. Healthcare professionals should suspect that a patient may have received a counterfeit drug if the patient has experienced an unexplained worsening of their medical condition or an unexpected side effect. Also, if a patient reports that the drug tastes or looks different, if tablets are chipped or cracked, or if the patient experiences burning at the injection site for an injectable drug, they might have a counterfeit.

Healthcare professionals who believe that a patient has received a counterfeit drug should contact the FDA immediately. In addition, any irregularity in packaging or labeling of a drug product should be reported to the FDA and to the manufacturer immediately.

What Can Consumers Do to Protect Themselves from Counterfeit Drugs?

Consumers can protect themselves from the risks associated with counterfeit drugs by purchasing prescription medications from state-licensed pharmacies in the U.S. Consumers must be vigilant when examining their personal medications, paying attention to the presence of altered or unsealed containers or changes in the packaging of the product. Differences in the physical appearance of the product, taste, and unexpected side effects experienced should alert the patient to contact their physician, pharmacist, or other healthcare professional who is providing treatment.

What Should Consumers Do If They Suspect That They Have a Counterfeit Drug?

If a consumer believes that they may have received a counterfeit drug, they should check with their pharmacist first. The pharmacist will know if the manufacturer recently changed the appearance, flavor, or packaging of a drug product. Also, if a pharmacy changes from one generic manufacturer to another generic manufacturer for dispensing the same drug, the color or shape of the drug product may be different. In this event, your pharmacist can verify that it is not a counterfeit and can explain the change.

Section 42.3

Unapproved Drugs

This section contains text excerpted from the following sources: Text beginning with the heading "Unapproved Use of Approved Drugs "Off Label"" is excerpted from "Understanding Unapproved Use of Approved Drugs "Off Label,"" U.S. Food and Drug Administration (FDA), June 2, 2016; Text under the heading "Unapproved Drugs and Their Availability in the Market" is excerpted from "What Are Unapproved Drugs and Why Are They on the Market?" U.S. Food and Drug Administration (FDA), May 12, 2016; Text under the heading "Unapproved Drugs: FDA's Concern" is excerpted from "FDA's Concerns about Unapproved Drugs," U.S. Food and Drug Administration (FDA), December 7, 2015. Text under the heading "Unapproved Drugs Initiative" is excerpted from "Unapproved Drugs Initiative," U.S. Food and Drug Administration (FDA), December 15, 2014.

Unapproved Use of Approved Drugs "Off Label"

Has your healthcare provider ever talked to you about using an U.S. Food and Drug Administration (FDA)-approved drug for an unapproved use (sometimes called an "off-label" use) to treat your disease or medical condition?

It is important to know that before a drug can be approved, a company must submit clinical data and other information to FDA for review. The company must show that the drug is safe and effective for its intended uses. "Safe" does not mean that the drug has no side effects. Instead, it means the FDA has determined the benefits of using the drug for a particular use outweigh the potential risks.

When you are prescribed a drug for its approved use, you can be sure:

- That FDA has conducted a careful evaluation of its benefits and risks for that use.

- The decision to use the drug is supported by strong scientific data.

- There is approved drug labeling for healthcare providers on how to use the drug safely and effectively for that use.

The approved drug labeling for healthcare providers gives key information about the drug that includes:

- The specific diseases and conditions that the drug is approved to treat.

- How to use the drug to treat those specific diseases and conditions.

- Information about the risks of the drug.

- Information that healthcare providers should discuss with patients before they take a drug.

Some drugs may also have labeling information for patients such as Medication Guides, Patient Package Inserts and Instructions for Use.

Why Might an Approved Drug Be Used for an Unapproved Use?

From the FDA perspective, once the FDA approves a drug, healthcare providers generally may prescribe the drug for an unapproved use when they judge that it is medically appropriate for their patient.

You may be asking yourself why your healthcare provider would want to prescribe a drug to treat a disease or medical condition that the drug is not approved for. One reason is that there might not be an approved drug to treat your disease or medical condition. Another is that you may have tried all approved treatments without seeing any benefits. In situations like these, you and your healthcare provider may talk about using an approved drug for an unapproved use to treat your disease or medical condition.

What Are Examples of Unapproved Uses of Approved Drugs?

Unapproved use of an approved drug is often called "off-label" use. This term can mean that the drug is:

- Used for a disease or medical condition that it is not approved to treat, such as when a chemotherapy is approved to treat one type of cancer, but healthcare providers use it to treat a different type of cancer.

- Given in a different way, such as when a drug is approved as a capsule, but it is given instead in an oral solution.

317

- Given in a different dose, such as when a drug is approved at a dose of one tablet every day, but a patient is told by their healthcare provider to take two tablets every day.

If you and your healthcare provider decide to use an approved drug for an unapproved use to treat your disease or medical condition, remember that FDA has not determined that the drug is safe and effective for the unapproved use.

Unapproved Drugs and Their Availability in the Market

The original Federal Food and Drugs Act of 1906 brought drug regulation under federal law. That Act prohibited the sale of adulterated or misbranded drugs, but did not require that drugs be approved by the U.S. Food and Drug Administration (FDA). In 1938, Congress required that new drugs be approved for safety. In 1962, Congress amended the 1938 law to require manufacturers to show that their drug products were effective, as well as safe. As a result, all drugs approved between 1938 and 1962 had to be reviewed again for effectiveness. To be consistent with current regulations and to ensure that all drugs have been shown to be safe and effective, all new drugs are required to have an approved application for continued marketing.

Many healthcare providers are unaware of the unapproved status of drugs and have continued to unknowingly prescribe them because the drugs' labels do not disclose that they lack FDA approval. In addition, since many unapproved drugs are marketed without brand names and have been available for many years, it is often assumed that these unapproved drugs are generic drugs. This is not correct. Generic drugs have been evaluated and approved by FDA to demonstrate bioequivalence to a brand name reference drug. Healthcare professionals and consumers can be assured that FDA-approved generic drug products have met the same quality, strength, purity and stability as brand name drugs. Additionally, the generic manufacturing, packaging, and testing sites must meet the same quality standards as those of brand name drugs. Unapproved drug products have not been evaluated and approved by FDA. Unapproved drugs are not generic medications, and neither their safety nor their efficacy can be assured.

Unapproved Drugs: FDA's Concern

The agency has serious concerns that drugs marketed without required FDA approval may not meet modern standards for safety, effectiveness, quality, and labeling. The FDA drug approval process provides a review of product-specific information that is critical to ensuring the safety and efficacy of a finished drug product. For instance, the applicant must demonstrate that its manufacturing processes can reliably produce drug products of expected identity, strength, quality, and purity. Furthermore, FDA's review of the applicant's labeling insures that healthcare professionals and patients have the information necessary to understand a drug product's risks and its safe and effective use.

There are prescription and over-the-counter (OTC) drugs marketed illegally without FDA approval. The manufacturers of drug products have not received FDA approval and do not conform to a monograph for making OTC drugs. These manufacturers circumvent the FDA approval process. The lack of evidence demonstrating that these unapproved drugs are safe and effective is a significant public health concern.

Unapproved Drugs Initiative

In June 2006, the FDA announced a new drug safety initiative to remove unapproved drugs from the market, including a final guidance entitled "Marketed Unapproved Drugs—Compliance Policy Guide (CPG)," outlining its enforcement policies aimed at efficiently and rationally bringing all such drugs into the approval process. The FDA uses a risk-based enforcement program in order to concentrate its resources on those products that pose the highest threat to public health and without imposing undue burdens on consumers, or unnecessarily disrupting the market. For all unapproved drugs, the CPG gives highest enforcement priority to the following:

- Drugs with potential safety risks

- Drugs that lack evidence of effectiveness

- Health fraud drugs

- Drugs that present direct challenges to the new drug approval and OTC drug monograph systems

- Unapproved new drugs that are also violative of the Act in other ways

- Drugs that are reformulated to evade an FDA enforcement action

319

Questions You May Want to Consider

If your healthcare provider is thinking about using an approved drug for an unapproved use, you may want to ask your healthcare provider questions like these:

- What is the drug approved for?

- Are there other drugs or therapies that are approved to treat my disease or medical condition?

- What scientific studies are available to support the use of this drug to treat my disease or medical condition?

- Is it likely that this drug will work better to treat my disease or medical condition than using an approved treatment?

- What are the potential benefits and risks of treating my disease or medical condition with this drug?

- Will my health insurance cover treatment of my disease or medical condition with this drug?

- Are there any clinical trials studying the use of this drug for my disease or medical condition that I could enroll in?

Chapter 43

Imported Drugs

Under the Federal Food, Drug, and Cosmetic Act (FD&C Act), the interstate shipment of any prescription drug that lacks required FDA approval is illegal. Interstate shipment includes importation—bringing drugs from a foreign country into the United States.

Drugs sold in the United States also must have proper labeling that conforms with the FDA's requirements, and must be made in accordance with good manufacturing practices. As part of the FDA's high standards, drugs can be manufactured only at plants registered with the agency, whether those facilities are domestic or foreign. If a foreign firm is listed as a manufacturer or supplier of a drug's ingredient on a new drug application, the FDA generally travels to that site to inspect it.

After the FDA approves a drug, manufacturers still are subject to FDA inspections and must continue to comply with good manufacturing practices. "With an unapproved drug, you can't be sure that it has been shipped, handled, and stored under conditions that meet U.S. requirements," McCallion says.

Along with legal requirements on manufacturing, U.S. pharmacists and wholesalers must be licensed or authorized in the states where they operate, and limits on how drugs can be distributed lessen the likelihood that counterfeit or poor-quality drugs will turn up. It's because of such safeguards that the process of getting drugs onto U.S. pharmacy shelves is commonly referred to as a "closed" distribution system.

This chapter includes text excerpted from "Imported Drugs Raise Safety Concerns," U.S. Food and Drug Administration (FDA), May 4, 2016.

Counterfeit drugs—phony replicas of pharmaceuticals—can surface anywhere. Historically, they have been more common in foreign countries than in the United States. And while the Internet has given customers the convenience of buying drugs from the privacy of their own homes, it's also opened up windows for crooks to crawl through.

Limits on Re-Importation

The FD&C Act also states that prescription drugs made in the United States and exported to a foreign country can only be re-imported by the drug's original manufacturer. Even when original manufacturers re-import drugs, the drugs must be real, properly handled, and relabeled for sale in the United States if necessary.

The Medicine Equity and Drug Safety Act (MEDS), enacted in 2000, would have allowed prescription drugs manufactured in the United States and exported to certain foreign countries to be re-imported from those countries for sale to American consumers. Supporters of the bill hoped that lower drug pricing in other countries would be passed along to consumers. But former Health and Human Services (HHS) Secretary Tommy G. Thompson responded by saying that, while he believed strongly in access to affordable drugs, he could not implement the act because it would sacrifice public safety by opening up the closed distribution system in the United States.

Though the law was enacted in 2000, before the bill can take effect, one provision requires that the HHS secretary determine whether adequate safety could be maintained and whether costs could be reduced significantly. Both Thompson and his predecessor, Donna Shalala, concluded that these conditions could not be guaranteed.

"Once an FDA-approved prescription drug is exported for sale in another country, it is no longer subject to U.S. requirements and it can no longer be monitored by U.S. regulators," Thompson wrote in a letter to Sen. James Jeffords, Ind-Vt., one of the bill's sponsors. "In addition, it may not have the U.S.-approved labeling. Instead it may have labeling for the country to which it is exported."

Guidance on Personal Use

Although importing unapproved prescription drugs is illegal, the FDA's guidance on importing prescription drugs for personal use recognizes that there may be circumstances in which the FDA can exercise discretion to not take action against the illegal importation.

The personal use guidance was first adopted in 1954, and it was modified in 1988 in response to concerns that certain acquired immune deficiency syndrome (AIDS) treatments were not available in the United States. The guidance allows individuals with serious conditions, such as a rare form of cancer, to get treatments that are legally available in foreign countries but are not approved in the United States.

The current policy is not a law or a regulation, but serves as guidance for FDA personnel. The importation of certain unapproved prescription medications for personal use may be allowed in some circumstances if all of these factors apply:

- if the intended use is for a serious condition for which effective treatment may not be available domestically

- if the product is not considered to represent an unreasonable risk

- if the individual seeking to import the drug affirms in writing that it is for the patient's own use and provides the name and address of the U.S.-licensed doctor responsible for his or her treatment with the drug or provides evidence that the drug is for continuation of a treatment begun in a foreign country

- if the product is for personal use and is a three-month supply or less and not for resale, since larger amounts would lend themselves to commercialization

- if there is no known commercialization or promotion to U.S. residents by those involved in distribution of the product

That means if you buy your high blood pressure or other medication from a foreign country because it's cheaper—even though a drug with the same name is approved for sale in the United States—generally the drug will be considered unapproved and the FDA's personal use guidance will not apply. The Drug Enforcement Administration (DEA) has additional requirements for controlled drugs.

How the FDA Works with U.S. Customs and Border Protection

The exact amount of imported drugs that come into the United States is hard to track, and the high volume makes it impossible to examine them all. In one pilot program, the Food and Drug Administration

(FDA) and the U.S. Customs and Border Protection (CBP) examined 1,908 packages of drug products from 19 countries that came through a mail facility in Carson, Calif., during a five-week period.

The FDA estimates that a total of 16,500 packages could have been set aside if there had been enough resources to handle them. Of the 1,908 packages, 721 were detained, and the addressees were notified that the products appeared to violate the Federal Food, Drug, and Cosmetic Act.

The FDA's enforcement efforts focus on drugs for commercial use, fraudulent drugs, and products that pose an unreasonable health risk.

- If a bag or package arouses suspicion, customs will set it aside and contact the nearest office of the FDA or the Drug Enforcement Agency (DEA) for advice on whether to release or detain the drug product.

- Even though your bag may not be checked, it is against the law not to properly declare imported medications to customs. Failure to declare products could result in penalties.

- Possession of certain medications without a prescription from a licensed physician may violate federal, state, and local laws.

- Prescription drugs should be stored in their original containers, and you should have a copy of your doctor's prescription or letter of instruction.

- If a drug is detained, the FDA is required by law to send you a written notice asking whether you can show that the product meets legal requirements. If you can't, the drug could be destroyed or returned to the sender.

Potential Health Risks with Imported Drugs

Quality assurance concerns. Medications that have not been approved for sale in the United States may not have been manufactured under quality assurance procedures designed to produce a safe and effective product.

Counterfeit potential. Some imported medications—even those that bear the name of a United States approved product—may, in fact, be counterfeit versions that are unsafe or even completely ineffective.

Presence of untested substances. Imported medications and their ingredients, although legal in foreign countries, may not have been evaluated for safety and effectiveness in the United States. These products may be addictive or contain other dangerous substances.

Risks of unsupervised use. Some medications, whether imported or not, are unsafe when taken without adequate medical supervision. You may need a medical evaluation to ensure that the medication is appropriate for you and your condition. Or, you may require medical checkups to make sure that you are taking the drug properly, it is working for you, and that you are not having unexpected or life-threatening side effects.

Labeling and language issues. The medication's label, including instructions for use and possible side effects, may be in a language you do not understand or may make medical claims and suggest specific uses that have not been adequately evaluated for safety and effectiveness.

Lack of information. An imported medication may lack information that would permit you to be promptly and correctly treated for a dangerous side effect caused by the drug.

Part Five

Managing Chronic Disease

Chapter 44

What's Next after You're Diagnosed with a Chronic Illness

Having a long-term, or chronic, illness can disrupt your life in many ways. You may often be tired and in pain. Your illness might affect your appearance or your physical abilities and independence. You may not be able to work, causing financial problems. For children, chronic illnesses can be frightening, because they may not understand why this is happening to them.

These changes can cause stress, anxiety and anger. If they do, it is important to seek help. A trained counselor can help you develop strategies to regain a feeling of control. Support groups might help, too. You will find that you are not alone, and you may learn some new tips on how to cope.

Next Steps after Your Diagnosis

The below stated describes five basic steps to help you cope with your diagnosis, make decisions, and get on with your life.

This chapter contains text excerpted from the following sources: Text in this chapter begins with excerpts from "Coping with Chronic Illness," MedlinePlus, National Institutes of Health (NIH), July 27, 2016; Text beginning with the heading "Next Steps after Your Diagnosis" is excerpted from "Next Steps after Your Diagnosis," Agency for Healthcare Research and Quality (AHRQ), U.S. Department of Health and Human Services (HHS), June 2016.

Step 1: Take the time you need. Do not rush important decisions about your health. In most cases, you will have time to carefully examine your options and decide what is best for you.

Step 2: Get the support you need. Look for support from family and friends, people who are going through the same thing you are, and those who have "been there." They can help you cope with your situation and make informed decisions.

Step 3: Talk with your doctor. Good communication with your doctor can help you feel more satisfied with the care you receive. Research shows it can even have a positive effect on things such as symptoms and pain. Getting a "second opinion" may help you feel more confident about your care.

Step 4: Seek out information. When learning about your health problem and its treatment, look for information that is based on a careful review of the latest scientific findings published in medical journals.

Step 5: Decide on a treatment plan. Work with your doctor to decide on a treatment plan that best meets your needs.

As you take each step, remember this: Research shows that patients who are more involved in their healthcare tend to get better results and be more satisfied.

Step 1: Take the Time You Need

A Diagnosis Can Change Your Life in an Instant

Like so many other people in your situation, you might be feeling one or more of the following emotions after getting your diagnosis:

- Afraid
- Alone
- Angry
- Anxious
- Ashamed
- Confused
- Depressed
- Helpless
- In denial

- Numb
- Overwhelmed
- Panicky
- Powerless
- Relieved (that you finally know what's wrong)
- Sad
- Shocked.
- Stressed

It is perfectly normal to have these feelings. It is also normal, and very common, to have trouble taking in and understanding information after you receive the news—especially if the diagnosis was a surprise. And it can be even harder to make decisions about treating or managing your disease or condition.

Take Time to Make Your Decisions

No matter how the news of your diagnosis has affected you, do not rush into a decision. In most cases, you do not need to take action right away. Ask your doctor how much time you can safely take.

Taking the time you need to make decisions can help you:

- Feel less anxious and stressed.

- Avoid depression.

- Cope with your condition.

- Feel more in control of your situation.

- Play a key role in decisions about your treatment.

Step 2: Get the Support You Need

You Do Not Have to Go through It Alone

Sometimes the emotional side of illness can be just as hard to deal with as the physical side. You may have fears or concerns. You may feel overwhelmed. No matter what your situation, having other people to turn to will help you know you are not alone. Here are the kinds of support you might want to seek:

- **Family and Friends**. Talking to family and friends you feel close to can help you cope with your illness or condition. Just knowing that someone is there can be a comfort. Sometimes it is hard to ask for help. And sometimes your family and friends want to help, but they do not want to intrude, or they do not know how to ask or what to offer. Think about specific ways people can help you. One idea is to ask someone to come with you to a doctor's appointment to help ask questions, take notes, and talk with you afterward. If you do not have family or friends who can provide support, other people or groups can.

- **Support or Self-Help Groups**. Support groups are made up of people with the same disease or condition who get together to share information and concerns and to help one another. Support groups may or may not be led by experts. Self-help groups are similar to support groups but usually are led by the

331

participants. The names "support group" and "self-help group" sometimes are used to refer to either kind. Research on support groups shows that participants feel less anxious, experience less depression, have a better quality of life, and have more success coping with their disease or condition. Similar findings have been reported for self-help groups.

- **Online Support or Self-Help Groups**. The Internet has support or self-help groups for people whose concerns and situations may be similar to yours. You can also find "message boards," where you can post questions and get answers. These online communities can help you connect with people who can give you support and provide information. But be careful. Not every idea or treatment you come across in these groups will be scientifically proven to be safe and effective. If you read about something interesting and new, check it out with your doctor.

- **Counselor or Therapist**. A good counselor or therapist can help you cope with sadness, depression, and feelings of being overwhelmed. If you think this kind of help might be right for you, ask your doctor or other healthcare professional to recommend someone in your area.

- **People Like You**. You might want to meet and talk with someone in your own situation. Someone who has "been there" can talk about the real-life outcomes of their treatment choices as well as how they have learned to live with their disease or condition. Some advocacy or support groups can help you make this kind of contact.

Step 3: Talk with Your Doctor

Your Doctor Is Your Partner in Healthcare

You probably have many questions about your disease or condition. The first person to ask is your doctor. It is fine to seek more information from other sources; in fact, it is important to do so. But consider your doctor your partner in healthcare—someone who can discuss your situation with you, explain your options, and help you make decisions that are right for you.

It is not always easy to feel comfortable around doctors. But research has shown that good communication with your doctor can actually be good for your health. It can help you to:

- Feel more satisfied with the care you receive.

- Have better outcomes (end results), such as reduced pain and better recovery from symptoms.

Being an active member of your healthcare team also helps to reduce your chances of medical mistakes, and it helps you get high-quality care. Of course, good communication is a two-way street. Here are some ways to help make the most of the time you spend with your doctor:

Prepare for Your Visit

- Think about what you want to get out of your appointment. Write down all your questions and concerns. (Select for a list of suggested questions.)
- Prepare and bring to your doctor visit a list of all the medicines you take.
- Consider bringing along a trusted relative or friend. This person can help ask questions, take notes, and help you remember and understand everything once you leave the doctor's office.

Give Information to Your Doctor

- Do not wait to be asked.
- Tell your doctor everything he or she needs to know about your health—even the things that might make you feel embarrassed or uncomfortable.
- Tell your doctor how you are feeling—both physically and emotionally.
- Tell your doctor if you are feeling depressed or overwhelmed.

Get Information from Your Doctor

- Ask questions about anything that concerns you. Keep asking until you understand the answers. If you do not, your doctor may think you understand everything that is said.
- Ask your doctor to draw pictures if that will help you understand something.
- Take notes.
- Tape record your doctor visit if that will be helpful to you. But first, ask your doctor if this is okay.

- Ask your doctor to recommend resources such as Web sites, booklets, or tapes with more information about your disease or condition.

Do Not Hesitate to Seek a Second Opinion

A second opinion is when another doctor examines your medical records and gives his or her views about your condition and how it should be treated.

You might want a second opinion to:

- Be clear about what you have.

- Know all of your treatment choices.

- Have another doctor look at your choices with you.

It is not pushy or rude to want a second opinion. Most doctors will understand that you need more information before making important decisions about your health. Check to see whether your health plan covers a second opinion. In some cases, health plans require second opinions.

Here are some ways to find a doctor for a second opinion:

- Ask your doctor. Request someone who does not work in the same office, because doctors who work together tend to share similar views.

- Contact your health plan or your local hospital, medical society, or medical school.

Get Information about next Steps

- Get the results of any tests or procedures. Discuss the meaning of these results with your doctor.

- Make sure you understand what will happen if you need surgery.

- Talk with your doctor about which hospital is best for your healthcare needs.

Finally, if you are not satisfied with your doctor, you can do two things:

1. Talk with your doctor and try to work things out.

2. Switch doctors, if you are able to.

It is very important to feel confident about your care.

Ten Important Questions to Ask Your Doctor after a Diagnosis

These ten basic questions can help you understand your disease or condition, how it might be treated, and what you need to know and do before making treatment decisions.

1. What is the technical name of my disease or condition, and what does it mean in plain English?

2. What is my prognosis (outlook for the future)?

3. How soon do I need to make a decision about treatment?

4. Will I need any additional tests, and if so what kind and when?

5. What are my treatment options?

6. What are the pros and cons of my treatment options?

7. Is there a clinical trial (research study) that is right for me?

8. Now that I have this diagnosis, what changes will I need to make in my daily life?

9. What organizations do you recommend for support and information?

10. What resources (booklets, Web sites, audiotapes, videos, DVDs, etc.) do you recommend for further information?

Step 4: Seek out Information

Evidence-Based Information Comes from Research on People Like You

Evidence-based information about treatments generally comes from two major types of scientific studies:

- **Clinical trials** are research studies on human volunteers to test new drugs or other treatments. Participants are randomly assigned to different treatment groups. Some get the research treatment, and others get a standard treatment or may be given a placebo (a medicine that has no effect), or no treatment. The results are compared to learn whether the new treatment is safe and effective.

- **Outcomes research** looks at the impact of treatments and other healthcare on health outcomes (end results) for patients and populations. End results include effects that people care about, such as changes in their quality of life.

Take Advantage of the Evidence-Based Information That Is Available

Health information is everywhere—in books, newspapers, and magazines, and on the Internet, television, and radio. However, not all information is good information. Your best bets for sources of evidence-based information include the Federal Government, national nonprofit organizations, medical specialty groups, medical schools, and university medical centers.

Some resources are listed below, grouped by type of information.

Information

Information about your disease or condition and its treatment is available from many sources. Here are some of the most reliable:

- **healthfinder®:** The healthfinder® site—sponsored by the U.S. Department of Health and Human Services (HHS)—offers carefully selected health information Web sites from government agencies, clearinghouses, nonprofit groups, and universities.

- **Health Information Resource Database:** Sponsored by the National Health Information Center, this database includes 1,400 organizations and government offices that provide health information upon request. Information is also available over the telephone at 800-336-4797.

- **MEDLINEplus®:** MedlinePlus® has extensive information from the National Institutes of Health and other trusted sources on over 650 diseases and conditions. The site includes many additional features.

- **National nonprofit groups** such as the American Heart Association, American Cancer Society, and American Diabetes Association can be valuable sources of reliable information. Many have chapters nationwide. Check your phone book for a local chapter in your community. The Health Information Resource Database can help you find national offices of nonprofit groups.

- **Health or medical libraries** run by government, hospitals, professional groups, and other reliable organizations often welcome consumers. For a list of libraries in your area, use the MedlinePlus® "Find a Library" feature.

Current Medical Research

You can find the latest medical research in medical journals at your local health or medical library, and in some cases, on the Internet. Here are two major online sources of medical articles:

- **MEDLINE®/PubMed®:** PubMed® is the National Library of Medicine's database of references to more than 14 million articles published in 4,800 medical and scientific journals. All of the listings have information to help you find the articles at a health or medical library. Many listings also have short summaries of the article (abstracts), and some have links to the full article. The article might be free, or it might require a fee charged by the publisher.

- **PubMed Central:** PubMed Central is the National Library of Medicine's database of journal articles that are available free of charge to users.

Clinical Trials

Perhaps you wonder whether there is a clinical trial that is right for you. Or you may want to learn about results from previous clinical trials that might be relevant to your situation. Here are two reliable resources:

- **ClinicalTrials.gov:** ClinicalTrials.gov provides regularly updated information about federally and privately supported clinical research on people who volunteer to participate. The site has information about a trial's purpose, who may participate, locations, and phone numbers for more details. The site also describes the clinical trial process and includes news about recent clinical trial results.

- **Cochrane Collaboration:** The Cochrane Collaboration writes summaries ("reviews") about evidence from clinical trials to help people make informed decisions. You can search and read the review abstracts free of charge.

The full Cochrane reviews are available only by subscription. Check with your local medical or health library to see whether you can access the full reviews there.

Outcomes Research

Outcomes research provides research about benefits, risks, and out-comes (end results) of treatments so that patients and their doctors can make better-informed decisions. The U.S. Agency for Healthcare Research and Quality (AHRQ) supports improvements in health outcomes through research, and sponsors products that result from research such as:

- **National Guideline Clearinghouse™:** The National Guide-line Clearinghouse™ is a database of evidence-based clinical practice guidelines and related documents. Clinical practice guidelines are documents designed to help doctors and patients make decisions about appropriate healthcare for specific dis-eases or conditions. The clearinghouse was originally created by AHRQ in partnership with the American Medical Association and America's Health Insurance Plans.

Steer Clear of Deceptive Advertisements and Information

While searching for information either on or off the Internet, beware of "miracle" treatments and cures. They can cost you money and your health, especially if you delay or refuse proper treatment. Here are some tip-offs that a product truly is too good to be true:

- Phrases such as "scientific breakthrough," "miraculous cure," "exclusive product," "secret formula," or "ancient ingredient."
- Claims that the product treats a wide range of ailments.
- Use of impressive-sounding medical terms. These often cover up a lack of good science behind the product.
- Case histories from consumers claiming "amazing" results.
- Claims that the product is available from only one source, and for a limited time only.
- Claims of a "money-back guarantee."
- Claims that others are trying to keep the product off the market.
- Ads that fail to list the company's name, address, or other con-tact information.

Step 5: Decide on a Treatment Plan

At this point, you have learned about your disease or condition and how it can be treated or managed. Your information may have come from the following sources:

- Your doctor.

- Second opinions from one or more other doctors.

- Other people who are or were in the same situation as you.

- Information sources such as Web sites, health or medical libraries, and nonprofit groups.

Work with Your Doctor to Make Decisions

When you are ready to make treatment decisions, you and your doctor can discuss:

- Which treatments have been found to work well, or not work well, for your particular condition.

- The pros and cons of each treatment option.

Make sure that your doctor knows your preferences and feelings about the different treatments—for example, whether you prefer medicine over surgery. Once you and your doctor decide on one or more treatments that are right for you, you can work together to develop a treatment plan. This plan will include everything that will be done to treat or manage your disease or condition—including what you need to do to make the plan work. Remember, being an active member of your healthcare team helps to reduce your chances of medical mistakes, and it helps you get high-quality care.

Take Another Deep Breath

You have taken important steps to cope with your diagnosis, make decisions, and get on with your life. Remember two things:

- Call on others for support as you need it.

- Make use of evidence-based information for any future health decisions.

Chapter 45

Self-Management of Chronic Illness

Chapter Contents

Section 45.1

Take Charge of Your Healthcare

This section includes text excerpted from "Take Charge of
Your Healthcare," Office of Disease Prevention and Health
Promotion (ODPHP), U.S. Department of Health and
Human Services (HHS), April 20, 2016.

When you play an active role in your healthcare, you can improve
the quality of the care you and your family get. Start by speaking up
and asking questions at the doctor's office.

Healthcare is a team effort, and you are the most important member
of the team. Your team also includes doctors, nurses, pharmacists, and
insurance providers.

To take charge of your healthcare:

- Keep track of important health information.
- Know your family health history.
- See a doctor regularly for checkups.
- Be prepared for medical appointments.
- Ask your doctor, nurse, or pharmacist questions.
- Follow up after your appointment

Take Action!

Follow these steps to play an active role in your healthcare.

Keep Track of Important Health Information

Keeping all your health information in one place will make it easier
to manage your healthcare. Take the information with you to every
medical appointment.

To start your own personal health record, write down:

- Your name, birth date, and blood type
- The name and phone number of a friend or relative to call if
  there's an emergency

- Telephone numbers and addresses of places where you get medical care, including your pharmacy

- Dates and results of checkups and screening tests

- All the shots (vaccinations) you've had—and the dates you got them

- Medicines you take, how much you take, and why you take them

- Any health conditions you have, including allergies

If you aren't sure about some of this information, check with your doctor's office.

Know Your Family Health History

Your family's health history is an important part of your personal health record.

See a Doctor Regularly for Checkups

Getting regular checkups with your doctor or nurse can help you stay healthy. Regular checkups can help find problems early, when they may be easier to treat.

What about Cost?

Thanks to the Affordable Care Act (ACA), the health; Public Law Project (PLP) care reform law passed in 2010, insurance plans must cover many preventive services, like screenings and shots. Plans must also cover well-child visits through age 21 and well-woman visits.

Depending on your insurance plan, you may be able to get preventive services at no cost to you. Check with your insurance company for more information.

- Find out which services are covered under the Affordable Care Act.

- Find out which services are covered by Medicare.

If you don't have insurance, check out these resources to help you get healthcare:

- Visit HealthCare.gov to find insurance options for your family.

- For low-cost or free services, find a health center near you and make an appointment.

Write Down Your Questions Ahead of Time

Write down any questions you have about your health and take the list with you to your doctor, nurse, or pharmacist.

Make the Most of Doctor Visits

Take your list of questions and personal health record with you to the appointment. You may also want to ask a family member or friend to go with you to help take notes.

Be sure to talk about any changes since your last visit, like:

- New medicines you are taking, including over-the-counter medicines, herbs or home remedies, and vitamins

- Recent illnesses or surgeries

- Any important changes in your life, like becoming unemployed or a death in the family

- Health concerns or issues

- Health information you've found on the Internet or heard from others

Follow Up after Your Appointment

It can take time and hard work to make the healthy changes you talked about with your doctor or nurse. Remember to:

- Call if you have any questions or side effects from medicine

- Schedule follow-up appointments for tests or lab work, if you need to

Section 45.2

Exercise Can Improve Some Chronic Disease Conditions

This section includes text excerpted from "Physical Activity and Health," Centers for Disease Control and Prevention (CDC), June 4, 2015.

Regular physical activity is one of the most important things you can do for your health. It can help:

- Control your weight

- Reduce your risk of cardiovascular disease

- Reduce your risk for type 2 diabetes and metabolic syndrome

- Reduce your risk of some cancers

- Strengthen your bones and muscles

- Improve your mental health and mood

- Improve your ability to do daily activities and prevent falls, if you're an older adult

- Increase your chances of living longer

If you're not sure about becoming active or boosting your level of physical activity because you're afraid of getting hurt, the good news is that moderate-intensity aerobic activity, like brisk walking, is generally safe for most people.

Start slowly. Cardiac events, such as a heart attack, are rare during physical activity. But the risk does go up when you suddenly become much more active than usual. For example, you can put yourself at risk if you don't usually get much physical activity and then all of a sudden do vigorous-intensity aerobic activity, like shoveling snow. That's why it's important to start slowly and gradually increase your level of activity.

If you have a chronic health condition such as arthritis, diabetes, or heart disease, talk with your doctor to find out if your condition limits, in any way, your ability to be active. Then, work with your doctor to come up with a physical activity plan that matches your abilities. If your condition stops you from meeting the minimum Guidelines, try to do as much as you can. What's important is that you avoid being inactive. Even 60 minutes a week of moderate-intensity aerobic activity is good for you.

The bottom line is-the health benefits of physical activity far outweigh the risks of getting hurt.

If you want to know more about how physical activity improves your health, the section below gives more detail on what research studies have found.

Control Your Weight

Looking to get to or stay at a healthy weight? Both diet and physical activity play a critical role in controlling your weight. You gain weight when the calories you burn, including those burned during physical activity, are less than the calories you eat or drink. When it comes to weight management, people vary greatly in how much physical activity they need. You may need to be more active than others to achieve or maintain a healthy weight.

To maintain your weight. Work your way up to 150 minutes of moderate-intensity aerobic activity, 75 minutes of vigorous-intensity aerobic activity, or an equivalent mix of the two each week. Strong scientific evidence shows that physical activity can help you maintain your weight over time. However, the exact amount of physical activity needed to do this is not clear since it varies greatly from person to person. It's possible that you may need to do more than the equivalent of 150 minutes of moderate-intensity activity a week to maintain your weight.

To lose weight and keep it off. You will need a high amount of physical activity unless you also adjust your diet and reduce the amount of calories you're eating and drinking. Getting to and staying at a healthy weight requires both regular physical activity and a healthy eating plan.

Reduce Your Risk of Cardiovascular Disease

Heart disease and stroke are two of the leading causes of death in the United States. But following the Guidelines and getting at least

150 minutes a week (2 hours and 30 minutes) of moderate-intensity aerobic activity can put you at a lower risk for these diseases. You can reduce your risk even further with more physical activity. Regular physical activity can also lower your blood pressure and improve your cholesterol levels.

Reduce Your Risk of Type 2 Diabetes and Metabolic Syndrome

Regular physical activity can reduce your risk of developing type 2 diabetes and metabolic syndrome. Metabolic syndrome is a condition in which you have some combination of too much fat around the waist, high blood pressure, low High-density lipoproteins (HDL) cholesterol, high triglycerides, or high blood sugar. Research shows that lower rates of these conditions are seen with 120 to 150 minutes (2 hours to 2 hours and 30 minutes) a week of at least moderate-intensity aerobic activity. And the more physical activity you do, the lower your risk will be.

Already have type 2 diabetes? Regular physical activity can help control your blood glucose levels.

Reduce Your Risk of Some Cancers

Being physically active lowers your risk for two types of cancer: colon and breast. Research shows that:

- Physically active people have a lower risk of colon cancer than do people who are not active.

- Physically active women have a lower risk of breast cancer than do people who are not active.

Reduce your risk of endometrial and lung cancer. Although the research is not yet final, some findings suggest that your risk of endometrial cancer and lung cancer may be lower if you get regular physical activity compared to people who are not active.

Improve your quality of life. If you are a cancer survivor, research shows that getting regular physical activity not only helps give you a better quality of life, but also improves your physical fitness.

Strengthen Your Bones and Muscles

As you age, it's important to protect your bones, joints and muscles. Not only do they support your body and help you move, but keeping bones, joints and muscles healthy can help ensure that you're able to do your daily activities and be physically active. Research shows that doing aerobics, muscle-strengthening and bone-strengthening physical activity of at least a moderately-intense level can slow the loss of bone density that comes with age.

Hip fracture is a serious health condition that can have life-changing negative effects, especially if you're an older adult. But research shows that people who do 120 to 300 minutes of at least moderate-intensity aerobic activity each week have a lower risk of hip fracture.

Regular physical activity helps with arthritis and other conditions affecting the joints. If you have arthritis, research shows that doing 130 to 150 (2 hours and 10 minutes to 2 hours and 30 minutes) a week of moderate-intensity, low-impact aerobic activity can not only improve your ability to manage pain and do everyday tasks, but it can also make your quality of life better.

Build strong, healthy muscles. Muscle-strengthening activities can help you increase or maintain your muscle mass and strength. Slowly increasing the amount of weight and number of repetitions you do will give you even more benefits, no matter your age.

Improve Your Mental Health and Mood

Regular physical activity can help keep your thinking, learning, and judgment skills sharp as you age. It can also reduce your risk of depression and may help you sleep better. Research has shown that doing aerobics or a mix of aerobic and muscle-strengthening activities 3 to 5 times a week for 30 to 60 minutes can give you these mental health benefits. Some scientific evidence has also shown that even lower levels of physical activity can be beneficial.

Improve Your Ability to Do Daily Activities and Prevent Falls

A functional limitation is a loss of the ability to do everyday activities such as climbing stairs, grocery shopping, or playing with your grandchildren.

How does this relate to physical activity? If you're a physically active middle-aged or older adult, you have a lower risk of functional limitations than people who are inactive

348

Already have trouble doing some of your everyday activities? Aerobic and muscle-strengthening activities can help improve your ability to do these types of tasks.

Are you an older adult who is at risk for falls? Research shows that doing balance and muscle-strengthening activities each week along with moderate-intensity aerobic activity, like brisk walking, can help reduce your risk of falling.

Increase Your Chances of Living Longer

Science shows that physical activity can reduce your risk of dying early from the leading causes of death, like heart disease and some cancers. This is remarkable in two ways:

1. Only a few lifestyle choices have as large an impact on your health as physical activity. People who are physically active for about 7 hours a week have a 40 percent lower risk of dying early than those who are active for less than 30 minutes a week.

2. You don't have to do high amounts of activity or vigorous-intensity activity to reduce your risk of premature death. You can put yourself at lower risk of dying early by doing at least 150 minutes a week of moderate-intensity aerobic activity.

Everyone can gain the health benefits of physical activity-age, ethnicity, shape or size do not matter.

Section 45.3

Healthy Eating

This section includes text excerpted from "Eat Healthy," Office of Disease Prevention and Health Promotion (ODPHP), U.S. Department of Health and Human Services (HHS), April 18, 2016.

Eating healthy means getting enough vitamins, minerals, and other nutrients—and limiting unhealthy foods and drinks. Eating healthy also means getting the number of calories that's right for you (not eating too much or too little).

To eat healthy, be sure to get plenty of:

- Vegetables, fruits, whole grains, and fat-free or low-fat dairy products

- Seafood, lean meats and poultry, eggs, beans, peas, seeds, and nuts

It's also important to limit:

- Sodium (salt)

- Added sugars–like refined (regular) sugar, brown sugar, corn syrup, high-fructose corn syrup, and honey

- Saturated fats, which come from animal products like cheese, fatty meats, whole milk, and butter, and plant products like palm and coconut oils

- *Trans* fats, which may be in foods including stick margarines, coffee creamers, and some desserts

- Refined grains which are in foods like cookies, white bread, and some snack foods

A Healthy Diet Can Help Keep You Healthy

Eating healthy is good for your overall health. Making smart food choices can also help you manage your weight and lower your risk for certain chronic (long-term) diseases.

When you eat healthy foods–and limit unhealthy foods–you can reduce your risk for:

- Heart disease

- Type 2 diabetes

- High blood pressure

- Some types of cancer

- Osteoporosis (bone loss)

Tips for Shopping

Making small changes to your eating habits can make a big difference for your health over time. Here are some tips and tools you can use to get started.

Keep a Food Diary

Knowing what you eat now will help you figure out what you want to change. Maintain a food diary and write down:

- When you eat
- What and how much you eat
- Where you are and who you are with when you eat
- How you are feeling when you eat

For example, you might write something like:
"Tuesday 3:30 pm, 2 chocolate chip cookies, at work with Mary, feeling stressed."

Shop Smart at the Grocery Store

The next time you go food shopping:

- Make a shopping list ahead of time. Only buy what's on your list.
- Don't shop while you are hungry–eat something before you go to the store.

Use these tips to buy healthy foods:

- Try a variety of vegetables and fruits in different colors.
- Look for low-sodium foods.
- Choose fat-free or low-fat dairy products.
- Replace old favorites with options that have fewer calories and less saturated fat.
- Choose foods with whole grains–like 100 percent whole-wheat or whole-grain bread, cereal, and pasta.
- Buy lean cuts of meat and poultry and other foods with protein–like fish, seafood, and beans.
- Save money by getting fruits and vegetables in season or on sale.

Read the Nutrition Facts Label

Understanding the Nutrition Facts label on food packages can help you make healthy choices.

First, look at the serving size and the number of servings per package–there may be more than 1 serving!

Next, check out the percent Daily Value (% DV) column. The DV lets you know if a food is higher or lower in certain nutrients. Look for foods that are:

- Lower in sodium and saturated fat (5% DV or less)

- Higher in fiber, calcium, potassium, and vitamin D (20% DV or more)

The picture below shows an example of a Nutrition Facts label.

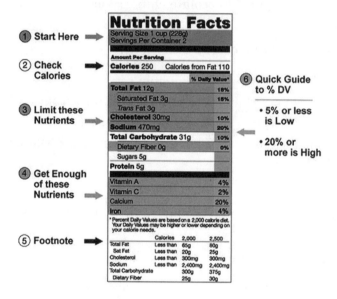

Figure 45.1. *Nutrition Facts*

Read the Ingredients List, Too

To limit added sugars in your food, make sure that added sugars are not listed in the first few ingredients. Names for added sugars include: sugar, corn syrup, high-fructose corn syrup, fruit juice concentrate, maltose, dextrose, sucrose, honey, and maple syrup.

Be a Healthy Family

Parents and caregivers are important role models for healthy eating. You can teach kids how to choose and prepare healthy foods.

- Take your child with you to the store and explain the choices you make.
- Turn cooking into a fun activity for the whole family. Let your young child help with the kitchen tasks.
- Check out these quick tips for making healthy snacks.
- Get more ideas on how to be a healthy role model for your kids.

If you have a family member who has a hard time eating healthy, use these tips to start a conversation about how you can help.

Eat Healthy Away from Home

You can make smart food choices wherever you are–at work, in your favorite restaurant, or out running errands. Try these tips for eating healthy even when you are away from home:

- At lunch, have a sandwich on whole-grain bread instead of white bread.
- Skip the soda–drink water instead.
- In a restaurant, choose dishes that are steamed, broiled, or grilled instead of fried.
- On a long drive or shopping trip, pack healthy snacks like fruit, unsalted nuts, or low-fat string cheese sticks.

If You Are Worried about Your Eating Habits, Talk to a Doctor

If you need help making healthier food choices, your doctor or a registered dietitian can help. A registered dietitian is a health professional who helps people with healthy eating.

If you make an appointment to talk about your eating habits, be sure to take a food diary with you to help start the conversation.

What about Cost?

Thanks to the Affordable Care Act (ACA), the healthcare reform law passed in 2010, health plans must cover diet counseling for people at higher risk for chronic diseases like type 2 diabetes and high blood pressure.

Depending on your insurance, you may be able to get diet counseling at no cost to you. Check with your insurance company to find out what's included in your plan.

For information about other services covered by the Affordable Care Act (ACA), visit HealthCare.gov.

Section 45.4

Tips for Dealing with Pain

This section includes text excerpted from "Pain: You Can Get Help," National Institute on Aging (NIA), National Institutes of Health (NIH), May 2015.

You've probably been in pain at one time or another. Maybe you've had a headache or bruise—pain that doesn't last too long. But, many older people have ongoing pain from health problems like arthritis, cancer, diabetes, or shingles. They may even have many different kinds of pain.

Pain can be your body's way of warning you that something is wrong. Always tell the doctor where you hurt and exactly how it feels.

Acute Pain and Chronic Pain

There are two kinds of pain. Acute pain begins suddenly, lasts for a short time, and goes away as your body heals. You might feel acute pain after surgery or if you have a broken bone, infected tooth, or kidney stone.

Pain that lasts for several months or years is called chronic (or persistent) pain. This pain often affects older people. Examples include rheumatoid arthritis (RA) and sciatica. In some cases, chronic pain follows after acute pain from an injury or other health issue has gone away, like postherpetic neuralgia after shingles.

Living with any type of pain can be very hard. It can cause many other problems. For instance, pain can:

- Get in the way of your daily activities
- Disturb your sleep and eating habits
- Make it difficult to continue working
- Cause depression or anxiety

Describing Pain

Many people have a hard time describing pain. Think about these questions when you explain how the pain feels:

- Where does it hurt?

- When did it start? Does the pain come and go?

- What does it feel like? Is the pain sharp, dull, or burning? Would you use some other word to describe it?

- Do you have other symptoms?

- When do you feel the pain? In the morning? In the evening? After eating?

- Is there anything you do that makes the pain feel better or worse? For example, does using a heating pad or ice pack help? Does changing your position from lying down to sitting up make it better? Have you tried any over-the-counter medications for it?

Your doctor or nurse may ask you to rate your pain on a scale of 0 to 10, with 0 being no pain and 10 being the worst pain you can imagine. Or, your doctor may ask if the pain is mild, moderate, or severe. Some doctors or nurses have pictures of faces that show different expressions of pain. You point to the face that shows how you feel.

Attitudes about Pain

Everyone reacts to pain differently. Many older people have been told not to talk about their aches and pains. Some people feel they should be brave and not complain when they hurt. Other people are quick to report pain and ask for help.

Worrying about pain is a common problem. This worry can make you afraid to stay active, and it can separate you from your friends and family. Working with your doctor, you can find ways to continue to take part in physical and social activities despite being in pain.

Some people put off going to the doctor because they think pain is just part of aging and nothing can help. This is not true! It is important to see a doctor if you have a new pain. Finding a way to manage your pain is often easier if it is addressed early.

Treating Pain

Treating, or managing, chronic pain is important. The good news is that there are ways to care for pain. Some treatments involve medications, and some do not. Your doctor may make a treatment plan that is specific for your needs.

Most treatment plans do not just focus on reducing pain. They also include ways to support daily function while living with pain.

Pain doesn't always go away overnight. Talk with your doctor about how long it may take before you feel better. Often, you have to stick with a treatment plan before you get relief. It's important to stay on a schedule. Sometimes this is called "staying ahead" or "keeping on top" of your pain. As your pain lessens, you can likely become more active and will see your mood lift and sleep improve.

Medicines to Treat Pain

Your doctor may prescribe one or more of the following pain medications:

- **Acetaminophen** may help all types of pain, especially mild to moderate pain. Acetaminophen is found in over-the-counter and prescription medicines. People who drink a lot of alcohol or who have liver disease should not take acetaminophen. Be sure to talk with your doctor about whether it is safe for you to take and what would be the right dose.

- **Nonsteroidal anti-inflammatory drugs (NSAIDs)** include medications like aspirin, naproxen, and ibuprofen. Some types of NSAIDs can cause side effects, like internal bleeding, which make them unsafe for many older adults. For instance, you may not be able to take ibuprofen if you have high blood pressure or had a stroke. Talk to your doctor before taking NSAIDs to see if they are safe for you.

- **Narcotics** (also called opioids) are used for severe pain and require a doctor's prescription. They may be habit-forming. Examples of narcotics are codeine, morphine, and oxycodone.

- **Other medications** are sometimes used to treat pain. These include antidepressants, anticonvulsive medicines, local pain-killers like nerve blocks or patches, and ointments and creams.

As people age, they are at risk for developing more serious side effects from medication. It's important to take exactly the amount of pain medicine your doctor prescribes.

Mixing any pain medication with alcohol or other drugs, such as tranquilizers, can be dangerous. Make sure your doctor knows all the medicines you take, including over-the-counter drugs and herbal supplements, as well as the amount of alcohol you drink.

Remember: If you think the medicine is not working, don't change it on your own. Talk to your doctor or nurse. You might say, "I've been taking the medication as you directed, but it still hurts too much to play with my grandchildren. Is there anything else I can try?"

Pain Specialist

Some doctors receive extra training in pain management. If you find that your regular doctor can't help you, ask him or her for the name of a pain medicine specialist. You also can ask for suggestions from friends and family, a nearby hospital, or your local medical society.

What Other Treatments Help with Pain?

In addition to drugs, there are a variety of complementary and alternative approaches that may provide relief. Talk to your doctor about these treatments. It may take both medicine and other treatments to feel better.

- **Acupuncture** uses hair-thin needles to stimulate specific points on the body to relieve pain.

- **Biofeedback** helps you learn to control your heart rate, blood pressure, and muscle tension. This may help reduce your pain and stress level.

- **Cognitive behavioral therapy** is a form of short-term counseling that may help reduce your reaction to pain.

- **Distraction** can help you cope with pain by learning new skills that may take your mind off your discomfort.

- **Electrical nerve stimulation** uses electrical impulses in order to relieve pain.

- **Guided imagery** uses directed thoughts to create mental pictures that may help you relax, manage anxiety, sleep better, and have less pain.

- **Hypnosis** uses focused attention to help manage pain.

- **Massage therapy** can release tension in tight muscles.

- **Physical therapy** uses a variety of techniques to help manage everyday activities with less pain and teaches you ways to improve flexibility and strength.

Helping Yourself

There are things you can do yourself that might help you feel better. Try to:

- **Keep a healthy weight.** Putting on extra pounds can slow healing and make some pain worse. Keeping a healthy weight might help with knee pain, or pain in the back, hips, or feet.

- **Be active.** Try to keep moving. Pain might make you inactive, which can lead to a cycle of more pain and loss of function. Mild activity can help.

- **Get enough sleep.** It will improve healing and your mood.

- **Avoid tobacco, caffeine, and alcohol.** They can get in the way of your treatment and increase your pain.

- **Join a pain support group.** Sometimes, it can help to talk to other people about how they deal with pain. You can share your ideas and thoughts while learning from others.

- **Participate in activities you enjoy.** Taking part in activities that you find relaxing, like listening to music or doing art, might help take your mind off of some of the pain.

Cancer Pain

Some people with cancer are more afraid of the pain than of the cancer. But, most pain from cancer or cancer treatments can be controlled. As with all pain, it's best to start managing cancer pain early. It might take a while to find the best approach. Talk with your doctor so the pain management plan can be corrected to work for you.

One special concern in managing cancer pain is "breakthrough pain." This is a pain that comes on quickly and can take you by surprise. It can be very upsetting. After one attack, many people worry it will happen again. This is another reason why it is so important to talk with your doctor about having a pain management plan in place.

Alzheimer Disease and Pain

People who have Alzheimer disease may not be able to tell you when they're in pain. When you're caring for someone with Alzheimer disease, watch for clues. A person's face may show signs of being in pain or feeling ill. You may also notice sudden changes in behavior such as increased yelling, striking out, or spending more time in bed.

It's important to find out if there is something wrong. If you're not sure what to do, call the doctor for help.

Pain at the End of Life

Not everyone who is dying is in pain. But if a person has pain at the end of life, there are ways to help. Experts often believe it's best to focus on making the person comfortable, without worrying about possible addiction or drug dependence.

Speak to a palliative care or pain management specialist if you are concerned about pain for yourself or a loved one. These specialists are trained to manage pain and other symptoms for people with serious illnesses.

Caring for Someone in Pain

It's hard to see a loved one hurting. Caring for a person in pain can leave you feeling tired and discouraged. To keep from feeling overwhelmed, you might consider asking other family members and friends for help. Or, some community service organizations might offer short-term, or respite, care. The Eldercare Locator might help you find a local group that offers this service.

Section 45.5

Stress and Your Health

This section includes text excerpted from "Coping with Stress," Centers for Disease Control and Prevention (CDC), October 2, 2015.

Everyone—adults, teens, and even children—experiences stress at times. Stress can be beneficial by helping people develop the skills they need to cope with and adapt to new and potentially threatening situations throughout life. However, the beneficial aspects of stress diminish when it is severe enough to overwhelm a person's ability to take care of themselves and family. Using healthy ways to cope and getting the right care and support can put problems in perspective and help stressful feelings and symptoms subside.

Sometimes after experiencing a traumatic event that is especially frightening—including personal or environmental disasters, or being threatened with an assault—people have a strong and lingering stress reaction to the event. Strong emotions, jitters, sadness, or depression may all be part of this normal and temporary reaction to the stress of an overwhelming event.

What Is Stress?

Stress is a condition that is often characterized by symptoms of physical or emotional tension. It is a reaction to a situation where a person feels threatened or anxious. Stress can be positive (e.g., preparing for a wedding) or negative (e.g., dealing with a natural disaster).

Common reactions to a stressful event can include:

- Disbelief, shock, and numbness
- Feeling sad, frustrated, and helpless
- Fear and anxiety about the future
- Feeling guilty
- Anger, tension, and irritability
- Difficulty concentrating and making decisions
- Crying
- Reduced interest in usual activities
- Wanting to be alone
- Loss of appetite
- Sleeping too much or too little
- Nightmares or bad memories
- Reoccurring thoughts of the event
- Headaches, back pains, and stomach problems
- Increased heart rate, difficulty breathing
- Smoking or use of alcohol or drugs

Healthy Ways to Cope with Stress

Feeling emotional and nervous or having trouble sleeping and eating can all be normal reactions to stress. Engaging in healthy activities and getting the right care and support can put problems in perspective and help stressful feelings subside in a few days or weeks. Some tips for beginning to feel better are:

- Take care of yourself. Talk to others. Share your problems and how you are feeling and coping with a parent, friend, counselor, doctor, or pastor.
    - Eat healthy, well-balanced meals
    - Exercise on a regular basis
    - Get plenty of sleep
    - Give yourself a break if you feel stressed out
- Avoid drugs and alcohol. Drugs and alcohol may seem to help with the stress. In the long run, they create additional problems and increase the stress you are already feeling.
- Take a break. If your stress is caused by a national or local event, take breaks from listening to the news stories, which can increase your stress.

Recognize when you need more help. If problems continue or you are thinking about suicide, talk to a psychologist, social worker, or professional counselor.

If you or someone you know needs immediate help, please contact one of the following crisis hotlines:

- Disaster Distress Helpline: 1-800-985-5990
- National Suicide Prevention Lifeline: 1-800-273-TALK (8255) (1-888-628-9454 for Spanish-speaking callers)
- Youth Mental Health Line: 1-888-568-1112
- Child-Help USA: 1-800-422-4453 (24 hour toll-free) Coping with Stress

Helping Youth Cope with Stress

Because of their level of development, children and adolescents often struggle with how to cope well with stress. Youth can be particularly overwhelmed when their stress is connected to a traumatic event—like a natural disaster (earthquake, tornado, and wildfire), family loss, school shootings, or community violence. Parents and educators can take steps to provide stability and support that help young people feel better.

Tips

Tips for Parents

It is natural for children to worry, especially when scary or stressful events happen in their lives. Talking with children about these stressful events and monitoring what children watch or hear about the events can help put frightening information into a more balanced context. Some suggestions to help children cope are:

- **Maintain a normal routine.** Helping children wake up, go to sleep, and eat meals at regular times provide them a sense of stability. Going to school and participating in typical after-school activities also provide stability and extra support.

- **Talk, listen, and encourage expression.** Create opportunities to have your children talk, but do not force them. Listen to your child's thoughts and feelings and share some of yours. After a traumatic event, it is important for children to feel like they can share their feelings and to know that their fears and worries are understandable. Keep these conversations going by asking them how they feel in a week, then in a month, and so on.

- **Watch and listen.** Be alert for any change in behavior. Are children sleeping more or less? Are they withdrawing from friends or family? Are they behaving in any way out of the ordinary? Any changes in behavior, even small changes, may be signs that the child is having trouble coming to terms with the event.

- **Reassure.** Stressful events can challenge a child's sense of physical and emotional safety and security. Take opportunities to reassure your child about his or her safety and well-being and discuss ways that you, the school, and the community are taking steps to keep them safe.

- **Connect with others.** Make an on-going effort to talk to other parents and your child's teachers about concerns and ways to help your child cope. You do not have to deal with problems alone-it is often helpful for parents, schools, and health professionals to work together to support and ensure the well-being of all children in stressful times.

Tips for Kids and Teens

After a traumatic or violent event, it is normal to feel anxious about your safety and security. Even if you were not directly involved, you may worry about whether this type of event may someday affect you. How can you deal with these fears? Start by looking at the tips below for some ideas.

- **Talk to and stay connected to others.** This connection might be your parent, another relative, a friend, neighbor, teacher, coach, school nurse, counselor, family doctor, or member of your church or temple. Talking with someone can help you make sense out of your experience and figure out ways to feel better. If you are not sure where to turn, call your local crisis intervention center or a national hotline.

- **Get active.** Go for a walk, play sports, write a play or poem, play a musical instrument, or join an after-school program. Volunteer with a community group that promotes nonviolence or another school or community activity that you care about. Trying any of these can be a positive way to handle your feelings and to see that things are going to get better.

- **Take care of yourself.** As much as possible, try to get enough sleep, eat right, exercise, and keep a normal routine. It may be hard to do, but by keeping yourself healthy you will be better able to handle a tough time.

- **Take information breaks.** Pictures and stories about a disaster can increase worry and other stressful feelings. Taking breaks from the news, Internet, and conversations about the disaster can help calm you down.

Tips for School Personals

Kids and teens who experience a stressful event, or see it on television, may react with shock, sadness, anger, fear, and confusion. They may be reluctant to be alone or fearful of leaving secure areas such as the house or classroom. School personnel can help their students restore their sense of safety by talking with the children about their fears. Other tips for school personnel include:

- **Reach out and talk.** Create opportunities to have students talk, but do not force them. Try asking questions like, what do you think about these events, or how do you think these things happen? You can be a model by sharing some of your own thoughts as well as correct misinformation. Children talking about their feelings can help them cope and to know that different feelings are normal.

- **Watch and listen.** Be alert for any change in behavior. Are students talking more or less? Withdrawing from friends? Acting out? Are they behaving in any way out of the ordinary? These changes may be early warning signs that a student is struggling and needs extra support from the school and family.

- **Maintain normal routines.** A regular classroom and school schedule can provide reassurance and promote a sense of stability and safety. Encourage students to keep up with their schoolwork and extracurricular activities but do not push them if they seem overwhelmed.

- **Take care of yourself.** You are better able to support your students if you are healthy, coping well, and taking care of yourself first.

  - Eat healthy, well-balanced meals

  - Exercise on a regular basis

  - Get plenty of sleep

  - Give yourself a break if you feel stressed out

Chapter 46

Preventing Infections

Infection and Types of Infection

When germs, such as bacteria or viruses, invade the body, they attack and multiply. This invasion is called an infection, and the infection is what causes illness. The immune system then has to fight the infection. Once it fights off the infection, the body is left with a supply of cells that help recognize and fight that disease in the future.

Bacterial Infections

Bacteria are living things that have only one cell. Under a microscope, they look like balls, rods, or spirals. They are so small that a line of 1,000 could fit across a pencil eraser. Most bacteria won't hurt you—less than 1 percent of the different types make people sick. Many are helpful. Some bacteria help to digest food, destroy disease-causing cells, and give the body needed vitamins. Bacteria are also used in

This chapter contains text excerpted from the following sources: Text under the heading "Infection and Types of Infection" is excerpted from "Making the Vaccine Decision," Centers for Disease Control and Prevention (CDC), April 15, 2016; Text under the heading "Bacterial Infections" is excerpted from "Bacterial Infections," MedlinePlus, National Institutes of Health (NIH), August 25, 2014; Text under the heading "Viral Infections" is excerpted from "Viral Infections," MedlinePlus, National Institutes of Health (NIH), August 31, 2016; Text beginning with the heading "Wash Your Hands Often" is excerpted from "An Ounce of Prevention Keeps the Germs Away," Centers for Disease Control and Prevention (CDC), May 12, 2006. Reviewed January 2017.

making healthy foods like yogurt and cheese. But infectious bacteria can make you ill. They reproduce quickly in your body. Many give off chemicals called toxins, which can damage tissue and make you sick. Examples of bacteria that cause infections include *Streptococcus*, *Staphylococcus*, and *Escherichia coli*.

Antibiotics are the usual treatment. When you take antibiotics, follow the directions carefully. Each time you take antibiotics, you increase the chances that bacteria in your body will learn to resist them causing antibiotic resistance. Later, you could get or spread an infection that those antibiotics cannot cure.

Viral Infections

Viruses are capsules with genetic material inside. They are very tiny, much smaller than bacteria. Viruses cause familiar infectious diseases such as the common cold, flu and warts. They also cause severe illnesses such as HIV/AIDS, smallpox, and hemorrhagic fevers.

Viruses are like hijackers. They invade living, normal cells and use those cells to multiply and produce other viruses like themselves. This eventually kills the cells, which can make you sick.

Viral infections are hard to treat because viruses live inside your body's cells. They are "protected" from medicines, which usually move through your bloodstream. Antibiotics do not work for viral infections. There are a few antiviral medicines available. Vaccines can help prevent you from getting many viral diseases.

Wash Your Hands Often

Keeping your hands clean is one of the best ways to keep from getting sick and spreading illnesses. Cleaning your hands gets rid of germs you pick up from other people—from the surfaces you touch—and from the animals you come in contact with.

When to Wash

- Before eating.
- Before, during, and after handling or preparing food.
- After contact with blood or body fluids (like vomit, nasal secretions, or saliva).
- After changing a diaper.
- After you use the bathroom.

- After handling animals, their toys, leashes, or waste.
- After touching something that could be contaminated (such as a trash can, cleaning cloth, drain, or soil).
- Before dressing a wound, giving medicine or inserting contact lenses.
- More often when someone in your home is sick.
- Whenever they look dirty.

How to Wash

1. Wet your hands and apply liquid, bar, or powder soap.
2. Rub hands together vigorously to make a lather and scrub all surfaces.
3. Continue for 20 seconds! It takes that long for the soap and scrubbing action to dislodge and remove stubborn germs. Need a timer? Imagine singing "Happy Birthday" all the way through—twice!
4. Rinse hands well under running water.
5. Dry your hands using a paper towel or air dryer.
6. If possible, use your paper towel to turn off the faucet.

If soap and water are not available, use an alcohol-based wipe or hand gel.

Routinely Clean and Disinfect Surfaces

Cleaning and disinfecting are not the same thing. Cleaning removes germs from surfaces—whereas disinfecting actually destroys them. Cleaning with soap and water to remove dirt and most of the germs is usually enough. But sometimes, you may want to disinfect for an extra level of protection from germs.

- While surfaces may look clean, many infectious germs may be lurking around. In some instances, germs can live on surfaces for hours—and even days.
- Disinfectants are specifically registered with the U.S. Environmental Protection Agency (EPA) and contain ingredients that actually destroy bacteria and other germs. Check the product label to make sure it says "Disinfectant" and has an EPA registration number.

Disinfect those areas where there can be large numbers of danger-ous germs—and where there is a possibility that these germs could be spread to others.

In the kitchen:

- Clean and disinfect counters and other surfaces before, during, and after preparing food (especially meat and poultry).

- Follow all directions on the product label, which usually specifies letting the disinfectant stand for a few minutes.

- When cleaning surfaces, don't let germs hang around on clean-ing cloths or towels!

- Use:

  - Paper towels that can be thrown away, or

  - Cloth towels that are later washed in hot water, or

  - Disposable sanitizing wipes that both clean and disinfect.

In the bathroom:

- Routinely clean and disinfect all surfaces. This is especially important if someone in the house has a stomach illness, a cold, or the flu.

Handle and Prepare Food Safely

When it comes to preventing foodborne illness, there are four simple steps to food safety that you can practice every day. These steps are easy—and they'll help protect you and those around you from harmful foodborne bacteria.

Clean Hands and Surfaces Often

Germs that cause foodborne illness can be spread throughout the kitchen and get onto hands from cutting boards, utensils, counter tops, and food. Help stop the spread of these germs! Here's how:

- Clean your hands with warm water and soap for at least 20 sec-onds before and after handling food. If soap and water are not available, use an alcohol-based wipe or hand gel.

- Wash your cutting boards, dishes, utensils, and counter tops with hot soapy water after preparing each food item and before you prepare the next food.

- Consider using paper towels to clean up kitchen surfaces. If you use cloth towels, wash them often using the hot cycle of your washing machine. If using a sponge to clean up, microwave it each evening for 30 seconds or place it in the dishwasher.

- Rinse all fresh fruits and vegetables under running tap water. This includes those with skins and rinds that are not eaten. For firm-skin fruits and vegetables, rub with your hands or scrub with a clean vegetable brush while rinsing.

Don't Cross-Contaminate One Food with Another

Cross-contamination occurs when bacteria spread from a food to a surface—from a surface to another food—or from one food to another. You're helping to prevent cross-contamination when you:

- Separate raw meat, poultry, seafood and eggs from other foods in your grocery cart, grocery bags, and in your refrigerator. Be sure to use the plastic bags available in the meat and produce sections of the supermarket.

- Use one cutting board for fresh produce and a different one for raw meat, poultry, and seafood.

- Never place cooked food on a plate that previously held raw meat, poultry, seafood, or eggs.

- Don't allow juices from meat, seafood, poultry, or eggs to drip on other foods in the refrigerator. Use containers to keep these foods from touching other foods.

- Never re-use marinades that were used on raw food, unless you bring them to a boil first.

Cook Foods to Proper Temperatures

Foods are safely cooked when they are heated for a long-enough time and at a high-enough temperature to kill the harmful bacteria that cause foodborne illness. The target temperature is different for different foods.

The only way to know for sure that meat is cooked to a safe temperature is to use a food thermometer. Make sure it reaches the temperature recommended for each specific food.

369

Refrigerate Foods Promptly

Cold temperatures slow the growth of harmful bacteria. So, refrigerate foods quickly. Do not over-stuff the refrigerator, as cold air must circulate to help keep food safe.

- Keeping a constant refrigerator temperature of 40° F or below is one of the most effective ways to reduce the risk of foodborne illness. Use an appliance thermometer to be sure the temperature is consistently 40° F or below.

- The freezer temperature should be 0° F or below.

- Plan when you shop: Buy perishable foods such as dairy products, fresh meat and hot cooked foods at the end of your shopping trip. Refrigerate foods as soon as possible to extend their storage life. Don't leave perishable foods out for more than two hours.

- If preparing picnic foods, be sure to include an ice pack to keep cold foods cold.

- Store leftovers properly.

Get Immunized

Getting immunizations is easy and low-cost—and most importantly, it saves lives. Make sure you and your children get the shots suggested by your doctor or healthcare provider at the proper time and keep records of all immunizations for the whole family. Also, ask your doctor about special programs that provide free shots for your child.

- Children should get their first immunizations before they are 2 months old. They should have additional doses four or more times before their second birthday.

- Adults need tetanus and diphtheria boosters every 10 years. Shots are also often needed for protection from illnesses when traveling to other countries.

- Get your flu shot. The single best way to prevent the flu is to get vaccinated each fall.

Use Antibiotics Appropriately

Antibiotics are powerful drugs used to treat certain bacterial infections—and they should be taken exactly as prescribed by your healthcare provider.

- Antibiotics don't work against viruses such as colds or the flu. That means children do not need an antibiotic every time they are sick.

- If you do get sick, antibiotics may not always help. If used inappropriately, they can make bacteria resistant to treatment–thus making illnesses harder to get rid of.

When in doubt, check with your healthcare provider—and always follow the antibiotic label instructions carefully.

Be Careful with Pets

Pets provide many benefits to people, including comfort and companionship. However, some animals can also pass diseases to humans. Keep these tips in mind to make sure your pet relationship is a happy and healthy one.

- Pets should be adopted from an animal shelter or purchased from a reputable pet store or breeder.

- All pets should be routinely cared for by a veterinarian. Follow the immunization schedule that the vet recommends.

- Obey local leash laws.

- Clean litter boxes daily. Pregnant women should not clean litter boxes.

- Don't allow children to play where animals go to the bathroom.

- Keep your child's sandbox covered when not in use.

About Children and Pets

Babies and children under 5 are more likely to get diseases from animals—so keep these special guidelines in mind.

- Young children should not be allowed to kiss pets or to put their hands or other objects into their mouths after touching animals.

- Wash your child's hands thoroughly with soap and warm running water after contact with animals.

- Be particularly careful when visiting farms, petting zoos, and fairs

Avoid Contact with Wild Animals

Wild animals can carry diseases that are harmful to you and your pets—but there are simple precautions you can take to avoid contact with a variety of species.

- Keep your house free of wild animals by not leaving any food around and keeping garbage cans sealed.

- Clear brush, grass, and debris from around house foundations to get rid of possible nesting sites for mice and rodents.

- Be sure to seal any entrance holes you discover on the inside or outside of your home.

- Use insect repellent to prevent ticks. Do a routine "tick check" after spending time outdoors. Ticks should be removed immediately with tweezers by applying gentle, steady pressure until they release their bite.

Wild Animals: What are the Risks?

- Mice and other wild animals can carry deadly diseases like Hantavirus and plague.

- Bats, raccoons, skunks, and foxes can transmit rabies.

- Ticks can transmit Rocky Mountain spotted fever and Lyme disease.

Chapter 47

Chronic Illness and Depression

Depression is a real illness. Treatment can help you live to the fullest extent possible, even when you have another illness. It is common to feel sad or discouraged after a heart attack, a cancer diagnosis, or if you are trying to manage a chronic condition like pain. You may be facing new limits on what you can do and feel anxious about treatment outcomes and the future. It may be hard to adapt to a new reality and to cope with the changes and ongoing treatment that come with the diagnosis. Your favorite activities, like hiking or gardening, may be harder to do.

Temporary feelings of sadness are expected, but if these and other symptoms last longer than a couple of weeks, you may have depression. Depression affects your ability to carry on with daily life and to enjoy work, leisure, friends, and family. The health effects of depression go beyond mood—depression is a serious medical illness with many symptoms, including physical ones. Some symptoms of depression are:

- Feeling sad, irritable, or anxious

- Feeling empty, hopeless, guilty, or worthless

- Loss of pleasure in usually-enjoyed hobbies or activities, including sex

This chapter includes text excerpted from "Chronic Illness and Mental Health," National Institute of Mental Health (NIMH), December 18, 2015.

- Fatigue and decreased energy, feeling listless

- Trouble concentrating, remembering details, and making decisions

- Not being able to sleep, or sleeping too much. Waking too early

- Eating too much or not wanting to eat at all, possibly with unplanned weight gain or loss

- Thoughts of death, suicide or suicide attempts

- Aches or pains, headaches, cramps, or digestive problems without a clear physical cause and/or that do not ease even with treatment

People with Other Chronic Medical Conditions Have a Higher Risk of Depression

The same factors that increase risk of depression in otherwise healthy people also raise the risk in people with other medical illnesses. These risk factors include a personal or family history of depression or loss of family members to suicide.

However, there are some risk factors directly related to having another illness. For example, conditions such as Parkinson disease and stroke cause changes in the brain. In some cases, these changes may have a direct role in depression. Illness-related anxiety and stress can also trigger symptoms of depression.

Depression is common among people who have chronic illnesses such as the following:

- Cancer

- Coronary heart disease

- Diabetes

- Epilepsy

- Multiple sclerosis

- Stroke

- Alzheimer disease

- HIV/AIDS

- Parkinson disease

- Systemic lupus erythematosus

- Rheumatoid arthritis

Sometimes, symptoms of depression may follow a recent medical diagnosis but lift as you adjust or as the other condition is treated. In other cases, certain medications used to treat the illness may trigger depression. Depression may persist, even as physical health improves.

Research suggests that people who have depression and another medical illness tend to have more severe symptoms of both illnesses. They may have more difficulty adapting to their co-occurring illness and more medical costs than those who do not also have depression.

It is not yet clear whether treatment of depression when another illness is present can improve physical health. However, it is still important to seek treatment. It can make a difference in day-to-day life if you are coping with a chronic or long-term illness.

People with Depression Are at Higher Risk for Other Medical Conditions

It may have come as no surprise that people with a medical illness or condition are more likely to suffer from depression. The reverse is also true: the risk of developing some physical illnesses is higher in people with depression.

People with depression have an increased risk of cardiovascular disease, diabetes, stroke, and Alzheimer disease, for example. Research also suggests that people with depression are at higher risk for osteoporosis relative to others. The reasons are not yet clear. One factor with some of these illnesses is that many people with depression may have less access to good medical care. They may have a harder time caring for their health, for example, seeking care, taking prescribed medication, eating well, and exercising.

Ongoing research is also exploring whether physiological changes seen in depression may play a role in increasing the risk of physical illness. In people with depression, scientists have found changes in the way several different systems in the body function, all of which can have an impact on physical health:

- Signs of increased inflammation

- Changes in the control of heart rate and blood circulation

- Abnormalities in stress hormones

- Metabolic changes typical of those seen in people at risk for diabetes

Depression Is Treatable Even When Other Illness Is Present

Do not dismiss depression as a normal part of having a chronic illness. Effective treatment for depression is available and can help even if you have another medical illness or condition. If you or a loved one think you have depression, it is important to tell your healthcare provider and explore treatment options.

You should also inform the healthcare provider about all treatments or medications you are already receiving, including treatment for depression (prescribed medications and dietary supplements). Sharing information can help avoid problems with multiple medications interfering with each other. It also helps the provider stay informed about your overall health and treatment issues.

Recovery from depression takes time, but treatment can improve the quality of life even if you have a medical illness. Treatments for depression include:

- **Cognitive behavioral therapy (CBT)**, or talk therapy, that helps people change negative thinking styles and behaviors that may contribute to their depression. Interpersonal and other types of time-limited psychotherapy have also been proven effective, in some cases combined with antidepressant medication.

- **Antidepressant medications,** including, but not limited to, selective serotonin reuptake inhibitors (SSRIs) and serotonin and norepinephrine reuptake inhibitors (SNRIs).

- While **electroconvulsive therapy (ECT)** is generally reserved for the most severe cases of depression, newer brain stimulation approaches, including transcranial magnetic stimulation (TMS), can help some people with depression without the need for general anesthesia and with few side effects.

Chapter 48

Rehabilitative and Assistive Technology

What Is Rehabilitative and Assistive Technology?

Rehabilitative and assistive technology refers to tools, equipment, or products that can help a person with a disability to function successfully at school, home, work, and in the community. Disabilities are disorders, diseases, health conditions, or injuries that affect an individual's physical, intellectual, or mental well-being. Rehabilitative and assistive technologies can help people with disabilities to function more easily in their everyday lives and can also make it easier for a caregiver to care for a disabled person. The term "rehabilitative technology" is sometimes used to refer to aids used to help people recover their functioning after injury or illness. "Assistive technologies" may be as simple as a magnifying glass to improve visual perception or as complex as a computerized communication system.

Some of these technologies are made possible through rehabilitative engineering research, which is the application of engineering and scientific principles to study how people with disabilities function in society. It includes studying barriers to optimal function and designing solutions so that people with disabilities can interact successfully in their environments.

This chapter includes text excerpted from "Rehabilitative and Assistive Technology: Overview," *Eunice Kennedy Shriver* National Institute of Child Health and Human Development (NICHD), December 5, 2012. Reviewed January 2017.

What Are Some Types of Assistive Devices and How Are They Used?

Some examples of assistive technologies are:

- People with physical disabilities that affect movement can use mobility aids, such as wheelchairs, scooters, walkers, canes, crutches, prosthetic devices, and orthotic devices, to enhance their mobility.

- Hearing aids can improve hearing ability in persons with hearing problems.

- Cognitive assistance, including computer or electrical assistive devices, can help people function following brain injury.

- Computer software and hardware, such as voice recognition programs, screen readers, and screen enlargement applications, help people with mobility and sensory impairments use computer technology.

- In the classroom and elsewhere, assistive devices, such as automatic page-turners, book holders, and adapted pencil grips, allow learners with disabilities to participate in educational activities.

- Closed captioning allows people with hearing impairments to enjoy movies and television programs.

- Barriers in community buildings, businesses, and workplaces can be removed or modified to improve accessibility. Such modifications include ramps, automatic door openers, grab bars, and wider doorways.

- Lightweight, high-performance wheelchairs have been designed for organized sports, such as basketball, tennis, and racing.

- Adaptive switches make it possible for a child with limited motor skills to play with toys and games.

- Many types of devices help people with disabilities perform such tasks as cooking, dressing, and grooming. Kitchen implements are available with large, cushioned grips to help people with weakness or arthritis in their hands. Medication dispensers with alarms can help people remember to take their medicine on time. People who use wheelchairs for mobility can use extendable reaching devices to reach items on shelves.

What Are Some Types of Rehabilitative Technologies?

Rehabilitative technologies are any technologies that help people recover function after injury or illness. Just a few examples include the following:

- **Robotics.** Specialized robots help people regain function in arms or legs after a stroke.

- **Virtual reality.** People who are recovering from injury can retrain themselves to perform motions within a virtual environment.

- **Musculoskeletal modeling and simulations.** These computer simulations of the human body can pinpoint the underlying mechanical problems in a person with a movement-related disability. This can help design better assistive aids or physical therapies.

- **Transcranial magnetic stimulation (TMS).** TMS sends magnetic impulses through the skull to stimulate the brain. This system can help people who have had a stroke recover movement and brain function.

- **Transcranial direct current stimulation (tDCS).** In tDCS, a mild electrical current travels through the skull and stimulates the brain of patients recovering from stroke. This can help recover movement.

- **Motion analysis.** Motion analysis captures video of human motion with specialized computer software that analyzes the motion in detail. The technology gives healthcare providers a detailed picture of a person's specific movement challenges to be used as a guide for proper therapy.

For What Conditions Are Assistive Devices Used?

Some disabilities are quite visible, and others are "hidden." Most disabilities can be grouped into four major categories:

- **Cognitive disability:** intellectual and learning disabilities/disorder, distractibility, reading disorders, inability to remember or focus on large amounts of information

- **Hearing disability:** hearing loss or impaired hearing

- **Physical disability:** paralysis, difficulties with walking or other movement, inability to use a computer mouse, slow response time, limited fine or gross motor control

- **Visual disability:** blindness, low vision, color blindness

Mental illness, including anxiety disorders, mood disorders, eating disorders, and psychosis, for example, is also a disability.

Hidden disabilities can include some people with visual impairments and those with dexterity difficulties, such as repetitive strain injury. People who are hard of hearing or have mental health difficulties also may be included in this category.

Some people have disabling medical conditions that may be regarded as hidden disabilities—for example, epilepsy; diabetes; sickle cell conditions; human immunodeficiency virus (HIV)/acquired immune deficiency syndrome (AIDS); cystic fibrosis; cancer; and heart, liver or kidney problems. The conditions may be short term or long term, stable or progressive, constant or unpredictable and fluctuating, controlled by medication or another treatment, or untreatable. Many people with hidden disabilities can benefit from assistive technologies for certain activities or during certain stages of their diseases or conditions.

People who have spinal cord injuries, traumatic brain injury, cerebral palsy, muscular dystrophy, spina bifida, osteogenesis imperfecta, multiple sclerosis, demyelinating diseases, myelopathy, progressive muscular atrophy, amputations, or paralysis often benefit from complex rehabilitative technology. This means that the assistive devices these people use are individually configured to help each person with his or her own unique disability.

How Does Rehabilitative and Assistive Technology Benefit People with Disabilities?

Deciding which type of rehabilitative or assistive technology would be most helpful for a person with a disability is usually made by the disabled person and his or her family and caregivers, along with a team of professionals and consultants. The team is trained to match particular assistive technologies to specific needs to help the person function more independently. The team may include family doctors, regular and special education teachers, speech-language pathologists, rehabilitation engineers, occupational therapists, and other specialists, including representatives from companies that manufacture assistive technology.

Assistive technology enables students with disabilities to compensate for the impairments they experience. This specialized technology promotes independence and decreases the need for other educational support.

Appropriate assistive technology helps people with disabilities overcome or compensate, at least in part, for their limitations. Rehabilitative technology can help restore function in people who have developed a disability due to disease, injury, or aging. Rehabilitative and assistive technology can enable individuals to:

- Care for themselves and their families
- Work
- Learn in schools and other educational institutions
- Access information through computers and reading
- Enjoy music, sports, travel, and the arts
- Participate fully in community life

Assistive technology also benefits employers, teachers, family members, and everyone who interacts with users of the technology. Increasing opportunities for participation benefits everyone.

As assistive technologies are becoming more commonplace, people without disabilities are benefiting from them. For example, people who are poor readers or for whom English is a second language are taking advantage of screen readers. The aging population is making use of screen enlargers and magnifiers.

Chapter 49

Home Modifications for Independence and Safety

Home improvements, modifications, and repairs can help older adults maintain their independence and prevent accidents. Work can range from simple changes, like replacing doorknobs with pull handles, to major structural projects such as installing a wheelchair ramp.

Changes can improve the accessibility, adaptability, and/or universal design of a home. Improving accessibility involves things like widening doorways and lowering countertop and light switch heights for someone who uses a wheelchair. Changes that do not require home redesign, such as installing grab bars in bathrooms, are adaptability features. Universal design is usually built in when a home is constructed. It includes features that are sturdy and reliable, easy for all people to use, and flexible enough to be adapted for special needs.

Evaluating Your Needs

Before any changes are made to the home, evaluate your current and future needs room by room. Once you have explored all areas, make a list of potential problems and solutions.

This chapter includes text excerpted from "Home Improvement Assistance," Eldercare Locator, U.S. Administration on Aging (AOA), June 28, 2016.

Financial Assistance

Minor improvements and repairs can cost between $150 and $2,000. Many home remodeling contractors offer reduced rates or sliding-scale fees based on income and ability to pay. Public and private financing options may also be available. Sources of support include the following.

- Modification and repair funds provided by the Older Americans Act are distributed by Area Agencies on Aging (AAA). To contact your local AAA, contact the Eldercare Locator at 1-800-677-1116 or www.eldercare.gov.

- Rebuilding Together, Inc., a national volunteer organization, is able to assist some low-income seniors through its local affiliates. Visit prebuildingtogether.org to learn more.

- Local energy and social service departments can assist through the U.S. Department of Energy's Low-Income Home Energy Assistance Program (LIHEAP) and Weatherization Assistance Program (WAP). You can also search for state-specific tax credits, rebates, and savings at www.energy.gov/savings.

- Many cities and towns make grant funds available through their local departments of community development.

- Lenders may offer home equity conversion mortgages or reverse mortgages that allow homeowners to utilize home equity to pay for improvements. Learn more by visiting www.ncoa.org/economic-security/home-equity.

- Search for additional resources in your state by visiting www. Homemods.org.

Hiring a Contractor

For some repairs and improvements, you may choose to hire a professional contractor without a public assistance program. In that case, keep these important tips in mind.

- Make sure the contractor is licensed, bonded, and insured for the specific type of work.

- Check with your local Better Business Bureau (BBB) and Chamber of Commerce to see whether any complaints against the contractor are on file.

- Talk with family and friends to get recommendations based on their experiences. Contractors with good reputations can usually be counted on to do a good job again.

- Ask for a written agreement that specifies the exact tasks and timeline.

- Your agreement should outline the total estimated cost and require only a small down payment. The terms should require balance payment when the job is completed.

- Consider asking a trusted friend or family member to help you review the contract and/or monitor work throughout the project.

Chapter 50

Care Coordination and Transition Management

Care Coordination: Overview

Care coordination involves deliberately organizing patient care activities and sharing information among all of the participants concerned with a patient's care to achieve safer and more effective care. This means that the patient's needs and preferences are known ahead of time and communicated at the right time to the right people, and that this information is used to provide safe, appropriate, and effective care to the patient.

Care coordination in the primary care practice involves deliberately organizing patient care activities and sharing information among all of the participants concerned with a patient's care to achieve safer and more effective care.

This chapter contains text excerpted from the following sources: Text beginning with the heading "Care Coordination: Overview" is excerpted from "Care Coordination," Agency for Heathcare Research and Quality (AHRQ), U.S. Department of Health and Human Services (HHS), July 2016; Text under the heading "Transitional Care" is excerpted from "Care Coordination Measures Atlas Update," Agency for Heathcare Research and Quality (AHRQ), U.S. Department of Health and Human Services (HHS), June 2014; Text under the heading "Improving Care Transitions" is excerpted from "Improving Care Transitions," Centers for Medicare and Medicaid Services (CMS), September 9, 2013. Reviewed January 2017.

The main goal of care coordination is to meet patients' needs and preferences in the delivery of high-quality, high-value healthcare. This means that the patient's needs and preferences are known and communicated at the right time to the right people, and that this information is used to guide the delivery of safe, appropriate, and effective care.

There are two ways of achieving coordinated care: using broad approaches that are commonly used to improve healthcare delivery and using specific care coordination activities.

Examples of broad care coordination approaches include:

- Teamwork.

- Care management.

- Medication management.

- Health information technology.

- Patient-centered medical home.

Examples of specific care coordination activities include:

- Establishing accountability and agreeing on responsibility.

- Communicating/sharing knowledge.

- Helping with transitions of care.

- Assessing patient needs and goals.

- Creating a proactive care plan.

- Monitoring and follow-up, including responding to changes in patients' needs.

- Supporting patients' self-management goals.

- Linking to community resources.

- Working to align resources with patient and population needs.

Why Is Care Coordination Important?

Care coordination is identified as a key strategy that has the potential to improve the effectiveness, safety, and efficiency of the American healthcare system. Well-designed, targeted care coordination that is delivered to the right people can improve outcomes for everyone: patients, providers, and payers.

Although the need for care coordination is clear, there are obstacles within the American healthcare system that must be overcome to provide this type of care. Redesigning a healthcare system in order to better coordinate patients' care is important for the following reasons:

- Current healthcare systems are often disjointed, and processes vary among and between primary care sites and specialty sites.

- Patients are often unclear about why they are being referred from primary care to a specialist, how to make appointments, and what to do after seeing a specialist.

- Specialists do not consistently receive clear reasons for the referral or adequate information on tests that have already been done. Primary care physicians do not often receive information about what happened in a referral visit.

- Referral staff deal with many different processes and lost information, which means that care is less efficient.

Transitional Care

Transitions occur when information about or accountability/responsibility for some aspect of a patient's care is transferred between two or more healthcare entities, or is maintained over time by one entity. Often information and responsibility are (or should be) transferred together.

It may be useful to think about two broad categories of transitions:

1. Transitions between entities of healthcare system. Information transfer and/or responsibility shifts:

   - Among members of one care team (receptionist, nurse, physician).

   - Between patient care teams.

   - Between patients/informal caregivers and professional caregivers.

   - Across settings (primary care, specialty care, inpatient, emergency department).

   - Between healthcare organizations.

2. Transitions over time. Information transfer and/or responsibility shifts:

   - Between episodes of care (i.e., initial visit and follow-up visit).

- Across lifespan (e.g., pediatric developmental stages, women's changing reproductive cycle, geriatric care needs).

- Across trajectory of illness and changing levels of coordination need.

Improving Care Transitions

Improving care transitions between care settings is critical to improving individuals' quality of care and quality of life and their outcomes. Effective care transitions:

- Prevent medical errors;

- Identify issues for early intervention;

- Prevent unnecessary hospitalizations and readmissions;

- Support consumers preferences and choices; and

- Avoid duplication of processes and efforts to more effectively utilize resources.

Care transitions include the coordination of medical and long term supports and services (LTSS) when an individual is:

- Admitted to a hospital, emergency room, or other for acute medical care;

- Discharged from a hospital to an institutional long term care (LTC) setting, such as a skilled nursing facility/nursing facility (SNF/NF), inpatient rehabilitation facility (IRF), or intermediate care facility (ICF);

- Discharged to community based LTC; or

- Discharged from an institutional LTC care setting to community LTC or vice versa.

Chapter 51

Palliative Care

What Is Palliative Care?

Dealing with the symptoms of any painful or serious illness is diffi-cult. However, special care is available to make you more comfortable right now. It's called palliative care. You receive palliative care at the same time that you're receiving treatments for your illness. Its primary purpose is to relieve the pain and other symptoms you are experienc-ing and improve your quality of life. Palliative care is a central part of treatment for serious or life threatening illnesses. The information in this chapter will help you understand how you or someone close to you can benefit from this type of care.

Palliative care is comprehensive treatment of the discomfort, symp-toms, and stress of serious illness. It does not replace your primary treatment; palliative care works together with the primary treatment you're receiving. The goal is to prevent and ease suffering and improve your quality of life.

If You Need Palliative Care, Does That Mean You're Dying?

The purpose of palliative care is to address distressing symptoms such as pain, breathing difficulties or nausea, among others. Receiving palliative care does not necessarily mean you're dying.

This chapter includes text excerpted from "Palliative Care," National Institute of Nursing Research (NINR), May 2011. Reviewed January 2017.

Palliative Care Gives You a Chance to Live Your Life More Comfortably

Palliative care provides relief from distressing symptoms including pain, shortness of breath, fatigue, constipation, nausea, loss of appetite, problems with sleep and many other symptoms. It can also help you deal with the side effects of the medical treatments you're receiving. Perhaps, most important, palliative care can help improve your quality of life. Palliative care also provides support for you and your family and can improve communication between you and your healthcare providers.

Palliative care strives to provide you with:

- Expert treatment of pain and other symptoms so you can get the best relief possible.

- Open discussion about treatment choices, including treatment for your disease and management of your symptoms.

- Coordination of your care with all of your healthcare providers.

- Emotional support for you and your family.

Palliative Care Can Be Very Effective

Researchers have studied the positive effects palliative care has on patients. Recent studies show that patients who receive palliative care report improvement in:

- Pain and other distressing symptoms, such as nausea or shortness of breath.

- Communication with their healthcare providers and family members.

- Emotional support.

Other studies also show that palliative care:

- Ensures that care is more in line with patients' wishes.

- Meets the emotional and spiritual needs of patients.

Palliative Care Can Improve Your Quality of Life in a Variety of Ways

Together with your primary healthcare provider, your palliative care team combines vigorous pain and symptom control into every part of your treatment. Team members spend as much time with you and your family as it takes to help you fully understand your condition, care options and other needs. They also make sure you experience a smooth transition between the hospital and other services, such as home care or nursing facilities.

This results in well-planned, complete treatment for all of your symptoms throughout your illness—treatment that takes care of you in your present condition and anticipates your future needs. Palliative care supports you and those who love you by maximizing your comfort. It also helps you set goals for the future that lead to a meaningful, enjoyable life while you get treatment for your illness.

How Do You Know If You Need Palliative Care?

Many adults and children living with illnesses such as cancer, heart disease, lung disease, kidney failure, AIDS and cystic fibrosis, among others, experience physical symptoms and emotional distress related to their diseases. Sometimes these symptoms are related to the medical treatments they are receiving.

You may want to consider palliative care if you or your loved one:

- Suffers from pain or other symptoms due to ANY serious illness.
- Experiences physical or emotional pain that is NOT under control.
- Needs help understanding your situation and coordinating your care.

Start Palliative Care as Soon as You Need It

It's never too early to start palliative care. In fact, palliative care occurs at the same time as all other treatments for your illness and does not depend upon the course of your disease.

There is no reason to wait. Serious illnesses and their treatments can cause exhaustion, anxiety and depression. Palliative care teams understand that pain and other symptoms affect your quality of life and can leave you lacking the energy or motivation to pursue the things you enjoy. They also know that the stress of what you're going through can have a big impact on your family. And they can assist you and your loved ones as you cope with the difficult experience.

Working Together as a Team

Patients who are considering palliative care often wonder how it will affect their relationships with their current healthcare providers. Some of their questions include:

- Will I have to give up my primary healthcare provider?
- What do I say if there is resistance to referring me for palliative care services?
- Will I offend my healthcare provider if I ask questions?

Most important, you do NOT give up your own healthcare provider in order to get palliative care. The palliative care team and your healthcare provider work together.

Most clinicians appreciate the extra time and information the palliative care team provides to their patients. Occasionally a clinician may not refer a patient for palliative care services. If this happens to you, ask for an explanation. Let your healthcare provider know why you think palliative care could help you.

Getting Palliative Care Is as Easy as Asking for It

In most cases, palliative care is provided in the hospital. The process begins when either your healthcare provider refers you to the palliative care team or you ask your healthcare provider for a referral. In the hospital, palliative care is provided by a team of professionals, including medical and nursing specialists, social workers, pharmacists, nutritionists, clergy and others.

Insurance Pays for Palliative Care

Most insurance plans cover all or part of the palliative care treatment you receive in the hospital, just as they would other services. Medicare and Medicaid also typically cover palliative care. If you have concerns about the cost of palliative care treatment, a social worker from the palliative care team can help you.

What Happens When You Leave the Hospital?

When you leave the hospital, your palliative care team will help you make a successful move to your home, hospice or other healthcare setting.

Don't wait to get the help you deserve. Ask for palliative care and start feeling better now.

If you think you need palliative care, ask for it now. Tell your healthcare provider that you'd like to add palliative care specialists to your treatment team and request a consultation. If you want to find a hospital in your area that offers a palliative care program, you can go to the Palliative Care Provider Directory of Hospitals at www.getpalliativecare.org to search by state and city.

Chapter 52

Tips for Caregivers of Individuals with Chronic Disease

The health of caregivers is at risk. Informal or unpaid caregivers (family members or friends) are the backbone of long-term care provided in people's homes. While some aspects of caregiving may be rewarding, caregivers can also be at increased risk for negative health consequences. These may include stress, depression, difficulty in maintaining a healthy lifestyle, and staying up to date on recommended clinical preventive services.

Who Are Caregivers?

Caregivers provide care to people who need some degree of ongoing assistance with everyday tasks on a regular or daily basis. The recipients of care can live either in residential or institutional settings, range from children to older adults, and have chronic illnesses or disabling conditions.

This chapter contains text excerpted from the following sources: Text in this chapter begins with excerpts from "Caregiving," Centers for Disease Control and Prevention (CDC), March 29, 2016; Text under the heading "Caregiver Responsibilities" is excerpted from "Caregivers and Serious Illness," Eldercare Locator, U.S. Administration on Aging (AOA), February 18, 2014; Text under the heading "Help for New Caregivers" is excerpted from "Stepping into Caregiving," Centers for Disease Control and Prevention (CDC), November 2, 2015.

Approximately 25 percent of U.S. adults 18 years of age and older reported providing care or assistance to a person with a long-term illness or disability in the past 30 days, according to 2009 data from Centers for Disease Control and Prevention's (CDC) state-based Behavioral Risk Factor Surveillance System (BRFSS). This is termed "informal or unpaid care" because it is provided by family or friends rather than by paid caregivers. The one year value of this unpaid caregiver activity was estimated as $450 million dollars in 2009.

What Is the Impact of Providing Care for an Older Adult?

Informal or unpaid caregiving has been associated with:

- Elevated levels of depression and anxiety

- Higher use of psychoactive medications

- Worse self-reported physical health

- Compromised immune function

- Increased risk of early death

Over half (53 percent) of caregivers indicate that a decline in their health compromises their ability to provide care. Furthermore, caregivers and their families often experience economic hardships through lost wages and additional medical expenses. In 2009, more than one in four (27 percent) of caregivers of adults reported a moderate to high degree of financial hardship as a result of caregiving.

What Are the Positive Aspects of Caregiving?

For many people, providing care for a family member with a chronic illness or a disabling condition can provide:

- A sense of fulfillment

- Establishment of extended social networks or friendship groups associated with caregiving

- Feeling needed and useful

- Learning something about one's self, others, and the meaning of life

More Caregivers Will Be Needed

As the number of older Americans increases, so will the number of caregivers needed to provide care. The number of people 65 years old and older is expected to double between 2000 and 2030. It is expected that there will be 71 million people aged 65 years old and older when all baby boomers are at least 65 years old in 2030. Currently, there are 7 potential family caregivers per adult. By 2030, there will be only 4 potential family caregivers per adult.

Caregiver Responsibilities

When a family member has a serious illness, you may help with healthcare decision-making, medical procedures and care, and daily activities. You may buy and prepare food; manage finances, legal work, and insurance; provide transportation; do housework; handle your loved one's former responsibilities, such as child care; and provide help with daily activities like bathing and eating.

If your family member has a brain disease like Alzheimer disease or another type of dementia, mental health problems, or a brain injury, you may have even more responsibilities. These can include complex tasks and the most basic human tasks. People with dementia get progressively worse over time so that you may provide more and more help, until the person is totally dependent on you.

As a caregiver, you need clear information and directions about your loved one's condition and healthcare needs. Getting this information from healthcare providers is very important during major changes, like leaving a hospital or nursing home. Having conversations with your loved one about treatment choices and making plans for care is important.

Help for New Caregivers

It is easy to become overwhelmed as a new caregiver. Five tips that can help are:

- **Learn about the person's medical condition or diagnosis.** By learning more you will understand your loved one's disease or condition and can be better able to care for them now and plan for the future. Also, set aside some time to acquaint yourself with their doctors, therapists, prescription drugs, and insurance coverage.

- **Talk about finances and healthcare wishes.** Having these conversations can be difficult but can help you carry out your

399

loved one's wishes and take care of their financial affairs should they no longer be able to do these things themselves.

- **Invite family and close friends to come together and discuss the needed care.** If possible, it's helpful to include the person needing care in this meeting. This meeting gives you a chance to explain what they need, plan for care, and ask others for help.

- **Use community resources.** Services such as Meals on Wheels, adult day programs, and respite care may help relieve your workload and increase your free time. Look for caregiver educational programs that will increase your knowledge and confidence.

- **Take care of yourself.** Don't forget your own mental and physical health by putting your loved one's needs first. Nearly half of caregivers have reported that their health has gotten worse due to caregiving. Of those caregivers who say their health has declined, over half report that declining health has made it harder to support their loved one.

Although caregiving can be a challenge, many people who are caregivers report a tremendous feeling of satisfaction and purpose.

Part Six

Children and Chronic Disease

Chapter 53

Caring for a Seriously Ill Child

Taking care of a chronically ill child is one of the most draining and difficult tasks a parent can face. Beyond handling physical challenges and medical needs, you'll have to deal with your child's emotional needs and the impact that a prolonged illness can have on the entire family.

Luckily, this tough balancing act doesn't have to be done alone: support groups, social workers, and family friends often can lend a helping hand.

Explaining Long-Term Illness to a Child

Honest communication is vital to helping a child adjust to a serious medical condition. It's important for a child to know that he or she is sick and will be getting lots of care. The hospital, tests, and medicine may feel frightening, but they're part of helping your child feel better.

As you explain the illness and its treatment, give clear and honest answers to all questions in a way your child can understand. It's also important to accurately explain and prepare your child for treatments—and any possible discomfort that might go with along with those treatments.

Avoid saying "This won't hurt" if the procedure is likely to be painful. Instead, be honest if a procedure may cause some discomfort, pain, pressure, or stinging. But then reassure your child that it will be temporary and that you'll be there to offer support.

Many hospitals give parents the option to speak to their child about a long-term diagnosis alone, or with the doctor or the entire medical team (doctors, social workers, nurses, etc.) present. Your doctor or other medical professional probably can offer advice on how to talk to your child about the illness.

Tackling Tough Emotions

- Your child will have many feelings about the changes affecting his or her body, and should be encouraged and given opportunities to express those feelings and any concerns and fears. Ask what your child is experiencing and listen to the answers before bringing up your own feelings or explanations.

- This kind of communication doesn't always have to be verbal. Music, drawing, or writing can often help kids express their emotions and escape through a fantasy world of their own design. Kids also may need reminders that they're not responsible for the illness. It's common for them to fear that they brought their sickness on by something they thought, said, or did. Reassure your child that this is not the case, and explain in simple terms what is going on. (You also may want to reassure your other kids that nothing they said or did caused their sibling's illness.)

- For many questions, there won't be easy answers. And you can't always promise that everything is going to be fine. But you can help your child feel better by listening, saying it's OK and completely understandable to have those feelings, and explaining that you and your family will make him or her as comfortable as possible.

- If a child asks "why me?" it's OK to offer an honest "I don't know." Explain that even though no one knows why the illness occurred, the doctors do have treatments for it (if that's the case). If your child says "it's not fair that I'm sick," acknowledge that your child is right. It's important for kids to know it's OK to feel angry about the illness. Your child may ask "am I going to die?" How you answer will depend not only on your child's medical situation, but also your child's age and maturity level. It's important to know, if possible, what specific fears or concerns your child has and to address them specifically. If it is reassuring to your child, you may refer to your religious, spiritual, and cultural beliefs about death. You might want to stay away from euphemisms for death such as "going to sleep." Saying that may cause children to fear going to bed at night.

- Regardless of their age, it's important for kids to know that there are people who love them and will be there for them, and that they'll be kept comfortable.

- Just like any adult, a child will need time to adjust to the diagnosis and the physical changes and is likely to feel sad, depressed, angry, afraid, or even to deny that they are sick. Think about getting professional counseling if you see signs that these feelings are interfering with daily function, or your child seems withdrawn, depressed, and shows radical changes in eating and sleeping habits unrelated to the physical illness.

Behavioral Issues

- Kids with chronic illnesses certainly require extra "tender loving care," but also need the routines of childhood. The foremost— and perhaps trickiest—task for worried parents is to treat a sick child as normally as possible.

- Despite the circumstances, this means setting limits on unacceptable behavior, sticking to normal routines, and avoiding overindulgence. This may seem impossible, but spoiling or coddling can only make it harder for a child to return to daily activities. When your child leaves the hospital for home, normalcy is the goal.

Dealing with Siblings

- Family dynamics can be severely tested when a child is sick. Clinic visits, surgical procedures, and frequent checkups can throw big kinks into everyone's schedules and take an emotional toll on the entire family.

- To ease the pressure, seek help to keep the family routines as close to normal as possible. Friends and family members may be able to help handle errands, carpools, and meals. Siblings should continue to attend school and their usual recreational activities; the family should strive for normalcy and time for everyone to be together.

- Flexibility is key. The "old normal" may have been the entire family around the table for a home-cooked meal at 6:00, while the "new normal" may be takeout pizza on clinic nights. Also, consider talking with your other children's teachers or school counselors and let them know that a sibling in the family is ill. They can keep an eye out for behavioral changes or signs of stress among your kids.

- It's common for siblings of a chronically ill child to become angry, sullen, resentful, fearful, or withdrawn. They may pick fights or fall behind in schoolwork. In all cases, parents should pay close attention, so that their other kids don't feel pushed aside by the demands of their sick brother or sister. It can help if parents reserve some special time for each sibling.

- It can also help them to be included in the treatment process when possible. Depending on their ages and maturity level, visiting the hospital, meeting the nursing and physician staffs, or accompanying their sick sibling to the clinic for treatments can help make the situation less frightening and more under-standable. What they imagine about the illness and hospital visits are often worse than the reality. When they come to the hospital, they can develop a more realistic picture and see that, while unpleasant things may be part of the treatment, there are people who care about their brother or sister and do their best to help.

Lightening Your Load

The stress involved in caring for a child with a long-term illness is considerable, but these tips might ease the strain:

- Break problems into manageable parts. If your child's treatment is expected to be given over an extended time, view it in more manageable time blocks. Planning a week or a month at a time may be less overwhelming.

- Attend to your own needs. Get plenty of rest and, to the extent possible, pay attention to your relationship with your spouse, hobbies, and friendships.

- Depend on friends. Let them carpool siblings to soccer or theater practice. Let others—relatives, friends—share responsibilities of caring for your child. Remember that you can't do it all.

- Ask for help in managing the financial aspects of your child's illness.

- Recognize that everyone handles stress differently. If you and your spouse have distinct coping styles, talk about them and try to accommodate them. Don't pretend that they don't exist.

- Develop working partnerships with healthcare professionals. Realize that you are all part of the team. Ask questions and learn all you can about your child's illness.

- Consult other parents in support groups at your care center or hospital or online. They can offer information and understanding.

- Keep a journal.

- Utilize support staff offered at the treating hospital.

Chapter 54

Palliative Care for Children

What Is Palliative Care?

When a child is seriously ill, each person in the family is affected differently. That is why it is important that you, your child, and your family get the support and care you need during this difficult time. A special type of care called palliative care can help. Palliative care is a key part of care for children living with a serious illness. It is also an important source of support for their families.

How Does Palliative Care Help the Family

Palliative care can ease the symptoms, discomfort, and stress of serious illness for your child and family. Palliative care can help with your child's illness and give support to your family. It can:

- Ease your child's pain and other symptoms of illness.

- Provide emotional and social support that respects your family's cultural values.

- Help your child's healthcare providers, work together and communicate with one another to support your goals.

- Start open discussions with you, your child, and your healthcare team about options for care.

This chapter includes text excerpted from "Palliative Care for Children," National Institute of Nursing Research (NINR), July 2015.

Palliative care provides comfort for your child. Palliative care can help children and teenagers living with many serious illnesses, including genetic disorders, cancer, neurologic disorders, heart and lung conditions, and others. Palliative care is important for children at any age or stage of serious illness. It can begin as soon as you learn about your child's illness. Palliative care can help prevent symptoms and give relief from much more than physical pain. It can also enhance your child's quality of life.

Palliative care gives you and your family an added layer of support. Serious illness in a child affects everyone in the family, including parents and siblings of all ages. Palliative care gives extra support for your whole family. It can ease the stress on all of your children, your spouse, and you during a hard time.

Palliative care surrounds your family with a team of experts who work together to support all of you. It is a partnership between your child, your family, and the healthcare team. This team listens to your preferences and helps you think through the care options for your family. They will work with you and your child to make a care plan for your family. They can also help when your child moves from one care setting (e.g., the hospital) to another (e.g., outpatient care or care at home).

Does Accepting Palliative Care Mean Our Family Is Giving up on Other Treatments?

No. The purpose of palliative care is to ease your child's pain and other symptoms and provide emotional and other support to your entire family. Palliative care can help children, from newborns to young adults, and their families—at any stage of a serious illness. Palliative care works alongside other treatments your child may be receiving. In fact, your child can start getting palliative care as soon as you learn about your child's illness.

Palliative Care Helps Your Child Live a More Comfortable Life

Palliative care can provide direct support for your child by providing relief from distressing symptoms, such as:

- Pain

- Shortness of breath

- Fatigue

- Depression

- Anxiety

- Nausea

- Loss of appetite

- Problems with sleep

Palliative care can help your child deal with side effects from medicines and treatments. Perhaps most important, palliative care can help enhance your child's quality of life. For example, helping to cope with concerns about school and friends might be very valuable to your child.

Palliative care may also include direct support for families such as assistance with:

- Including siblings in conversations.

- Providing respite care for parents to be able to spend time with their other children.

- Locating community resources for services such as counseling and support groups.

Palliative care is effective. Scientists have studied how palliative care can help children living with serious illnesses. Studies show that patients who get palliative care say that it helps with:

- Pain and other distressing symptoms, such as nausea or shortness of breath.

- Communication between healthcare providers and family members.

- Emotional support.

Other studies show that palliative care:

- Helps patients get the kinds of care they want.

- Meets the emotional, developmental, and spiritual needs of patients.

How Do You Know If Your Child or Family Needs Palliative Care?

Children living with a serious illness often experience physical and emotional distress related to their disease. Emotional distress is also common among their parents, siblings, and other family members. If your child has a genetic disorder, cancer, neurologic disorder, heart or lung condition, or another serious illness, palliative care may help reduce pain and enhance quality of life.

Ask your child's healthcare provider about palliative care if your child or any member of your family (including you):

- Suffers from pain or other symptoms due to serious illness.

- Experiences physical pain or emotional distress that is NOT under control.

- Needs help understanding your child's health condition.

- Needs support coordinating your child's care.

Palliative Care Can Start as Soon as Your Child Needs It

It's never too early to start palliative care. In fact, palliative care can take place at the same time as other treatments for your child's illness. It does not depend upon the course or stage of your child's illness. If you feel your child, your family, or you could benefit from palliative care, ask your child's healthcare provider about getting a referral for palliative care services. There is no reason to wait. The sooner you and your child seek palliative care services, the sooner a palliative care team can help your family manage the pain and other symptoms, and emotions that may come with a serious illness.

The Palliative Care Team Works with You, Your Child, and Your Care Team

Together with your child's healthcare providers, palliative care professionals will work with you and your child to make a care plan that is right for your child, your family, and you. The team will help you and your child include pain and other symptom management into every part of your child's care.

Palliative care experts spend as much time with you and your family as it takes to help you fully understand your child's condition, care options, and other needs. They also make sure your child experiences a smooth transition between the hospital and other services, such as getting care at home.

Your team will listen to your preferences and work with you and your child to plan care for all of your child's symptoms throughout the illness. This will include care for your child's current needs and flexibility for future changes.

Your Child's Palliative Care Team Is Unique

Every palliative care team is different. Your child's palliative care team may include:

- Doctors
- Nurses
- Social workers
- Pharmacists
- Chaplains
- Counselors
- Child life specialists
- Nutritionists
- Art and music therapists

How Can Our Family Get Palliative Care?

The palliative care process can begin when your child's healthcare provider refers you to palliative care services. Or, you or your child can ask your provider for a referral if you feel that palliative care would be helpful for your child, your family, or yourself.

If We Start Palliative Care, Can My Child Still See the Same Primary Healthcare Provider?

Yes. Your child does not have to change to a new primary healthcare provider when starting palliative care. The palliative care team and your child's healthcare provider work together to help you and your child decide the best care plan for your child.

What If My Child's Healthcare Provider Is Unsure about Referring Us?

Some parents are afraid they might offend their child's current healthcare providers by asking about palliative care, but this is unlikely. Most healthcare providers appreciate the extra time and information the palliative care team provides to their patients. Occasionally, a clinician may not refer a patient for palliative care services. If this happens, ask for an explanation. Let your child's healthcare provider know why you think palliative care could help your family.

Who Pays for Palliative Care?

Many insurance plans cover palliative care. If you have questions or concerns about costs, you can ask your healthcare team to put you in touch with a social worker, care manager, or financial advisor at your hospital or clinic to look at payment options.

Where Can My Child Get Palliative Care?

Your palliative care team will help you to know what services are available in your community. Your child and family may receive palliative care in a hospital, during clinic visits, or at home. You and your child will likely first meet with your palliative care team in the hospital or at a clinic. After the first visit, some visits may still occur in the clinic or hospital. But many palliative care programs offer services at home and in the community. Home services can occur through telephone calls or home visits.

If palliative care starts in the hospital, your care team can help your child make a successful move to your home or other healthcare setting. Home may feel most comfortable and safe to you and your child. Depending on your child's condition and treatment, the palliative care team may be able to help you find a nursing agency or community care agency to support palliative care for your child at home.

How Can My Child's Pain Be Managed?

The palliative care team can bring your child comfort in many ways. Treating pain often involves medication, but there are also other methods to address a child's discomfort. Your child may feel better with changes like low lighting, comfortable room temperatures, pleasant smells, guided relaxation, and deep breathing techniques. Your child may welcome additional activities like video chats, social media, soothing music, and massage and art therapy that may help decrease pain and anxiety.

If your child has an illness that causes pain that is not relieved by drugs like acetaminophen (Tylenol®) or ibuprofen (Motrin® or Advil®), your child's palliative care team may recommend trying stronger medicines. There is no reason to wait before beginning these medications. Should your child's pain increase, the dose may be safely increased over time to provide relief.

Pain relief can be offered in a hospital, at home, or in other healthcare settings. Your palliative care team will partner with you and your child to learn what is causing discomfort and how best to handle it.

Talk to Your Loved Ones and Healthcare Team about Palliative Care

If your child wants palliative care, or if you think palliative care could be helpful to any member of your family, ask for it now. Talk with your child's healthcare provider about palliative care. To see whether a hospital in your area offers a palliative care program, visit the Palliative Care Provider Directory of Hospitals at www.getpalliativecare.org.

Chapter 55

Questions and Answers about the Pediatric Intensive Care Unit (PICU)

A stay in the hospital can be unnerving for anyone, especially parents with a seriously ill child in the pediatric intensive care unit (PICU). But both adults and children can benefit from a basic understanding of this specialized unit of the hospital. Knowing more about the PICU, what it is designed to do, how it operates, and who works there can help allay some concerns and better prepare parents and kids for a PICU stay.

What Is Pediatric Intensive Care Unit (PICU)?

The PICU is a section of a hospital devoted to providing the highest level of care to critically ill infants, children, and teenagers. With a much higher staff-to-patient ratio than other hospital areas, the PICU is able to ensure that children are monitored very closely and that help will be available immediately if a quick response is required. In addition, the PICU typically has its own dedicated array of medical technology—such as ventilators, dialysis equipment, medication pumps, and computerized monitoring devices—all of which has been designed for the particular needs of young patients.

"Questions and Answers about the Pediatric Intensive Care Unit," © 2017 Omnigraphics. Reviewed January 2017.

What Conditions Require PICU Care?

Children with very serious illnesses or injuries are admitted to the PICU when their conditions cannot be treated in the hospital's emergency room, normal pediatric area, or general medical floors. Examples of such conditions include severe trauma from accidents or injuries, poisoning, pneumonia, childhood cancer, and congenital heart defects. Children are also sent to the PICU following certain surgeries, such as organ transplants, brain and heart surgery, and some reconstructive procedures. Depending on the severity of the condition and the treatment required, PICU stays can range from one day to several months.

Who Takes Care of Children in the PICU?

The PICU is staffed by a multidisciplinary team of medical professionals who are trained in intensive-care procedures and who specialize in treating and working with children. These include:

- **Attending physicians.** These are doctors who undertake a three-year residency after medical school to become a pediatric specialist and then go through several years of additional training in intensive care.

- **Other PICU physicians.** This includes fellows undergoing advanced pediatric training, residents who are who are completing their education in pediatrics, and specialists in various medical areas, such as cardiology, neurology, and oncology.

- **Nurses.** Staff nurses, who have the most interaction with patients and their families, handle the daily care of patients, monitor and record progress, and work with doctors and other team members to plan and implement treatment. There are also charge nurses, nurse managers, and nurse practitioners, all of whom play a role in the daily operation of the PICU.

- **Other team members.** In addition to doctors and nurses, the PICU team may include pharmacists, medical therapists, technicians, social workers, chaplains, and secretaries or receptionists, all of whom contribute to patient care, family support, and the smooth running of the unit.

What Happens in the PICU?

At first, the PICU may seem hectic and scary. Patients don't always know what's going on; they're regularly disturbed by staff monitoring them or treating other patients; lights go on and off at all hours; and there's frequent noise and activity. Learning in advance about some of the PICU's procedures, routines, and equipment can help children and parents be prepared for their stay. These can include:

- **Admission**: Procedures for admission to the PICU vary depending on whether the child is arriving from a scheduled surgery or an emergency situation. In both instances, the patient will be examined by a team of doctors and nurses, and his or her condition will be assessed. In the case of a routine admission, this could be relatively brief, while in an emergency it may be followed by an intense period of treatment and other attention.

- **Morning rounds**: Almost every PICU has regularly scheduled morning rounds, generally beginning around 7:30. Here the medical team visits each patient, discusses progress, and makes plans for the day's activities. Some PICU units also have formal afternoon rounds, and many of these same types of discussions take place during staff shift changes.

- **Daily routine**: Throughout the day, numerous staff members—physicians, nurses, respiratory therapists, dietitians, pharmacists, and social workers—care for the children on the unit. Some medical procedures are performed right in the PICU, and sometimes patients are moved to other parts of the hospital for testing and treatment.

- **Communication**: In addition to discussing patient status and treatment plans among themselves, PICU staff ensure that they give frequent updates to parents. In some hospitals, parents are invited to observe morning rounds and in others there are formal discussions scheduled with members of the medical team. In all cases, parents are encouraged to ask questions and participate as much as possible in their child's care.

- **Monitors and alarms**: All children in the PICU are attached to monitors that keep track of such functions as breathing, heart rate, and blood pressure, and these often make noises that can be unsettling, such as humming and beeping. On occasion, an alarm might sound. Obviously this is to alert the staff that something could be wrong, so it's not unusual for them to come rushing in, ask visitors to leave, and begin examining the patient. Although this can be an indication of a serious medical situation, it's just as likely that the alarm has sounded because a child moved, a sensor wire has come loose, or a technician has made an adjustment to the equipment.

- **Intravenous (IV)**: Most children in the PICU have intravenous (IV) lines inserted into the veins of their hands or arms to administer medication and other fluids. In some cases, a larger tube is needed to deliver greater volumes of fluid. These are called central lines and are inserted into larger blood vessels, such as those in the chest, neck, or groin. There are also arterial lines, which are similar to IVs but are inserted into arteries rather than veins, and may be used to monitor blood pressure and blood oxygen levels.

- **Ventilators.** When kids in the PICU need extra help breathing, they are usually fitted with an oxygen mask on their faces or tubes in their noses. But some patients who need even more help are connected to a ventilator, a machine that actually breathes for them. In these instances, a plastic tube is inserted into the trachea (windpipe) and connected to the ventilator at the other end.

- **Tests.** Since patients in the unit are seriously ill, and treatment must be adjusted frequently, careful monitoring is a vital part of ensuring proper care. Doctors may routinely order tests of the child's blood, urine, and spinal fluid, as well as X-rays, ultrasounds, CT or CAT (computerized tomography) scans, and MRI (magnetic resonance imaging) scans.

- **Medications.** Almost everyone in the PICU is on some kind of medication, and dosages and types might be altered from time to time. Some drugs are given at intervals, such as every few hours, and some are administered continuously through IVs. Because of injury, surgery or medical conditions, children in the PICU may experience pain, so pain medication is frequently given to provide relief. Sedation might also be administered to lessen anxiety and keep the child relaxed.

What Is the Role of Parents in the PICU?

Parents play a critical role in comforting and supporting their children during their stay in the PICU. One important task is to communicate with doctors and nurses and, with older children, explain their condition and prepare them for tests and other procedures. In some hospitals parents may be able to help bathe young children or change infants' diapers. But just as crucial to the patients' well-being is talking to them, touching them, playing their favorite games, coloring, listening to music, reading stories, or watching videos.

It's also important for parents to take care of themselves during the child's stay. Being with a child in the PICU continuously for more than a few days can be both physically and emotionally exhausting, so it's a good idea for parents to leave the unit frequently to visit the cafeteria or watch television or read in a waiting room. Many hospitals provide comfortable sleeping arrangements for parents with children in the PICU, and it's a good idea to take advantage of these facilities to get some much-needed rest.

What Happens When Children Leave the PICU?

Upon leaving the PICU, some patients are sent directly home, but more often they are moved to a regular hospital room where more routine treatment and monitoring will take place for a period of time. Although this is an indication that the child's condition is improving, it can actually be a traumatic experience for some parents who become concerned that their child may not be ready for a reduced level of care. Hospital staff can be a source of support at this time, giving parents detailed updates on progress and providing reassurance. Discharge from the PICU is a significant milestone on the road to recovery, and generally both parents and children are relieved to be in a less intense environment.

References

1. "Pediatric Intensive Care Unit (PICU)," Cincinnati Children's Hospital Medical Center, n.d.

2. "PICU Family Guide," Monroe Carell Jr. Children's Hospital at Vanderbilt, June 1, 2016.

3. "PICU Parents Guide," Pediatric Critical Care Unit, Duke University Medical Center, n.d.

4. Torres, Adalberto, Jr., MD. "When Your Child's in the Pediatric Intensive Care Unit," KidsHealth.org, September 2015.

Chapter 56

Civil Rights of Students with Hidden Disabilities

Section 504 of the Rehabilitation Act of 1973 protects the rights of persons with handicaps in programs and activities that receive Federal financial assistance. Section 504 protects the rights not only of individuals with visible disabilities but also those with disabilities that may not be apparent.

Section 504 provides that: **"No otherwise qualified individual with handicaps in the United States ... shall, solely by reason of her or his handicap, be excluded from the participation in, be denied the benefits of, or be subjected to discrimination under any program or activity receiving Federal financial assistance...."**

The U.S. Department of Education (ED) enforces Section 504 in programs and activities that receive financial assistance from ED. Recipients of this assistance include public school districts, institutions of higher education, and other state and local education agencies. ED maintains an Office for Civil Rights (OCR), with ten regional offices and a headquarters office in Washington, D.C., to enforce Section 504 and other civil rights laws that pertain to recipients of ED funds.

This chapter includes text excerpted from "The Civil Rights of Students with Hidden Disabilities under Section 504 of the Rehabilitation Act of 1973," U.S. Department of Education (ED), October 15, 2015.

Disabilities Covered under Section 504

The ED Section 504 regulation defines an "individual with handicaps" as any person who (i) has a physical or mental impairment which substantially limits one or more major life activities, (ii) has a record of such an impairment, or (iii) is regarded as having such an impairment. The regulation further defines a physical or mental impairment as (A) any physiological disorder or condition, cosmetic disfigurement, or anatomical loss affecting one or more of the following body systems: neurological; musculoskeletal; special sense organs; respiratory, including speech organs; cardiovascular; reproductive; digestive; genitourinary; hemic and lymphatic; skin; and endocrine; or (B) any mental or psychological disorder, such as mental retardation, organic brain syndrome, emotional or mental illness, and specific learning disabilities. The definition does not set forth a list of specific diseases and conditions that constitute physical or mental impairments because of the difficulty of ensuring the comprehensiveness of any such list.

The key factor in determining whether a person is considered an "individual with handicaps" covered by Section 504 is whether the physical or mental impairment results in a substantial limitation of one or more major life activities. Major life activities, as defined in the regulation, include functions such as caring for one's self, performing manual tasks, walking, seeing, hearing, speaking, breathing, learning, and working.

The impairment must have a material effect on one's ability to perform a major life activity. For example, an individual who has a physical or mental impairment would not be considered a person with handicaps if the condition does not in any way limit the individual, or only results in some minor limitation. However, in some cases Section 504 also protects individuals who do not have a handicapping condition but are treated as though they do because they have a history of, or have been misclassified as having, a mental or physical impairment that substantially limits one or more major life activities. For example, if you have a history of a handicapping condition but no longer have the condition, or have been incorrectly classified as having such a condition, you too are protected from discrimination under Section 504. Frequently occurring examples of the first group are persons with histories of mental or emotional illness, heart disease, or cancer; of the second group, persons who have been misclassified as mentally retarded. Persons who are not disabled may be covered by Section 504 also if they are treated as if they are handicapped, for example, if they are infected with the human immunodeficiency virus (HIV).

What Are Hidden Disabilities?

Hidden disabilities are physical or mental impairments that are not readily apparent to others. They include such conditions and diseases as specific learning disabilities, diabetes, epilepsy, and allergy. A disability such as a limp, paralysis, total blindness or deafness is usually obvious to others. But hidden disabilities such as low vision, poor hearing, heart disease, or chronic illness may not be obvious. A chronic illness involves a recurring and long-term disability such as diabetes, heart disease, kidney and liver disease, high blood pressure, or ulcers.

Approximately four million students with disabilities are enrolled in public elementary and secondary schools in the United States. Of these 43 percent are students classified as learning disabled, 8 percent as emotionally disturbed, and 1 percent as other health impaired. These hidden disabilities often cannot be readily known without the administration of appropriate diagnostic tests.

The Responsibilities of ED Recipients in Preschool, Elementary, Secondary, and Adult Education

For coverage under Section 504, an individual with handicaps must be "qualified" for service by the school or institution receiving ED funds. For example, the ED Section 504 regulation defines a "qualified handicapped person" with respect to public preschool, elementary, secondary, or adult education services, as a person with a handicap who is:

- of an age during which persons without handicaps are provided such services;

- of any age during which it is mandatory under state law to provide such services to persons with handicaps; or

- a person for whom a state is required to provide a free appropriate public education under the Individuals with Disabilities Education Act (IDEA).

Under the Section 504 regulation, a recipient that operates a public elementary or secondary education program has a number of responsibilities toward qualified handicapped persons in its jurisdiction. These recipients must:

- Undertake annually to identify and locate all unserved handicapped children;

- Provide a "free appropriate public education" to each student with handicaps, regardless of the nature or severity of the handicap. This means providing regular or special education and related aids and services designed to meet the individual educational needs of handicapped persons as adequately as the needs of non-handicapped persons are met;

- Ensure that each student with handicaps is educated with non-handicapped students to the maximum extent appropriate to the needs of the handicapped person;

- Establish nondiscriminatory evaluation and placement procedures to avoid the inappropriate education that may result from the misclassification or misplacement of students;

- Establish procedural safeguards to enable parents and guardians to participate meaningfully in decisions regarding the evaluation and placement of their children; and

- Afford handicapped children an equal opportunity to participate in nonacademic and extracurricular services and activities.

A recipient that operates a preschool education or day care program, or an adult education program may not exclude qualified handicapped persons and must take into account their needs of qualified handicapped persons in determining the aid, benefits, or services to be provided under those programs and activities.

Students with hidden disabilities frequently are not properly diagnosed. For example, a student with an undiagnosed hearing impairment may be unable to understand much of what a teacher says; a student with a learning disability may be unable to process oral or written information routinely; or a student with an emotional problem may be unable to concentrate in a regular classroom setting. As a result, these students, regardless of their intelligence, will be unable to fully demonstrate their ability or attain educational benefits equal to that of non-handicapped students. They may be perceived by teachers and fellow students as slow, lazy, or as discipline problems.

Whether a child is already in school or not, if his/her parents feel the child needs special education or related services, they should get in touch with the local superintendent of schools. For example, a parent who believes his or her child has a hearing impairment or is having difficulty understanding a teacher, may request to have the child evaluated so that the child may receive appropriate education. A child with behavior problems, or one who is doing poorly academically, may have an undiagnosed hidden disability. A parent has the right to request that the school determine whether the child is handicapped and whether special education or related services are needed to provide the child an appropriate education. Once it is determined that a child needs special education or related services, the recipient school system must arrange to provide appropriate services.

The Responsibilities of ED Recipients in Postsecondary Education

The ED Section 504 regulation defines a qualified individual with handicaps for postsecondary education programs as a person with a handicap who meets the academic and technical standards requisite for admission to, or participation in, the college's education program or activity.

A college has no obligation to identify students with handicaps. In fact, Section 504 prohibits a postsecondary education recipient from making a preadmission inquiry as to whether an applicant for admission is a handicapped person. However, a postsecondary institution is required to inform applicants and other interested parties of the availability of auxiliary aids, services, and academic adjustments, and the name of the person designated to coordinate the college's efforts to carry out the requirements of Section 504. After admission (including the period between admission and enrollment), the college may make confidential inquiries as to whether a person has a handicap for the purpose of determining whether certain academic adjustments or auxiliary aids or services may be needed.

Many students with hidden disabilities, seeking college degrees, were provided with special education services during their elementary and secondary school years. It is especially important for these students to understand that postsecondary institutions also have responsibilities to protect the rights of students with disabilities. In elementary and secondary school, their school district was responsible for identifying, evaluating, and providing individualized special education and related services to meet their needs. At the postsecondary level, however, there are some important differences. The key provisions of Section 504 at the postsecondary level are highlighted below.

At the postsecondary level it is the student's responsibility to make his or her handicapping condition known and to request academic adjustments. This should be done in a timely manner. A student may choose to make his or her needs known to the Section 504 Coordinator, to an appropriate dean, to a faculty advisor, or to each professor on an individual basis.

A student who requests academic adjustments or auxiliary aids because of a handicapping condition may be requested by the institution to provide documentation of the handicap and the need for the services requested. This may be especially important to an institution attempting to understand the nature and extent of a hidden disability.

The requested documentation may include the results of medical, psychological, or emotional diagnostic tests, or other professional evaluations to verify the need for academic adjustments or auxiliary aids.

How Can the Needs of Students with Hidden Disabilities Be Addressed?

The following examples illustrate how schools can address the needs of their students with hidden disabilities:

- A student with a long-term, debilitating medical problem such as cancer, kidney disease, or diabetes may be given special consideration to accommodate the student's needs. For example, a student with cancer may need a class schedule that allows for rest and recuperation following chemotherapy.

- A student with a learning disability that affects the ability to demonstrate knowledge on a standardized test or in certain testing situations may require modified test arrangements, such as oral testing or different testing formats.

- A student with a learning disability or impaired vision that affects the ability to take notes in class may need a note taker or tape recorder.

- A student with a chronic medical problem such as kidney or liver disease may have difficulty in walking distances or climbing stairs. Under Section 504, this student may require special parking space, sufficient time between classes, or other considerations, to conserve the student's energy for academic pursuits.

- A student with diabetes, which adversely affects the body's ability to manufacture insulin, may need a class schedule that will accommodate the student's special needs.

- An emotionally or mentally ill student may need an adjusted class schedule to allow time for regular counseling or therapy.

- A student with epilepsy who has no control over seizures, and whose seizures are stimulated by stress or tension, may need accommodation for such stressful activities as lengthy academic testing or competitive endeavors in physical education.

- A student with arthritis may have persistent pain, tenderness or swelling in one or more joints. A student experiencing arthritic pain may require a modified physical education program.

These are just a few examples of how the needs of students with hidden disabilities may be addressed. If you are a student (or a parent or guardian of a student) with a hidden disability, or represent an institution seeking to address the needs of such students, you may wish to seek further information from OCR.

Chapter 57

Schools and Students with Chronic Illnesses

Healthy Schools

At a Glance 2016

Establishing healthy behaviors during childhood is easier and more effective than trying to change unhealthy behaviors during adulthood. Schools play a critical role in helping children develop lifelong healthy habits. Each day, 132,000 schools provide a setting for 55 million students to learn about health and healthy behaviors. The Centers for Disease Control and Prevention (CDC) is at the forefront of the nation's efforts to promote the health and well-being of children and adolescents in schools.

Public Health Problem

Unhealthy behaviors and chronic diseases are increasingly common in children and adolescents in the United States. The percentage of children aged 6 to 11 years who were obese increased from 7 percent in 1976–1980 to nearly 18 percent in 2011–2014. Similarly, the percentage of adolescents aged 12 to 19 years who were obese increased from 5

This chapter contains text excerpted from the following sources: Text under the heading "Healthy Schools" is excerpted from "Healthy Schools," Centers for Disease Control and Prevention (CDC), June 8, 2016; Text beginning with the heading "Asthma and Schools" is excerpted from "Management of Chronic Conditions," Centers for Disease Control and Prevention (CDC), October 26, 2015.

431

percent to 21 percent during the same period. About 1 in 4 adolescents suffers from a chronic condition, such as diabetes and asthma.

Children with unhealthy behaviors or chronic health conditions may face lower academic achievement, increased disability, fewer job opportunities, and limited community interactions as they enter adulthood. They also may miss more school, which reduces their opportunities and time for learning.

Schools can help children and adolescents improve their dietary and physical activity behaviors and manage their chronic conditions. They can create healthy environments for students by using practices and policies that support healthy eating and regular physical activity and by providing ways for students to learn about and practice these behaviors. Healthier behaviors not only prevent chronic diseases, they are also linked to academic achievement and success.

What Can Schools Do?

Increase the quantity and quality of physical education and physical activity in schools. Regular physical activity in childhood and adolescence improves strength and endurance; helps build healthy bones and muscles; helps control weight; reduces anxiety and stress; increases self-esteem; and may improve academic performance, blood pressure, and cholesterol levels.

Improve the nutritional quality of foods and promote healthy foods and beverages in schools. Healthy eating in childhood and adolescence supports proper growth and development and can prevent health problems like obesity, cavities, iron deficiency, and osteoporosis.

Improve the quantity and quality of health education focused on chronic disease prevention. Preventing chronic diseases is a learning process, and schools are an excellent place to gain skills for understanding and avoiding conditions like obesity, diabetes, and asthma. Students can learn how to make smart food choices; exercise to build strong, fit bodies; and monitor their health.

Improve monitoring and management of chronic conditions. Using proven practices to better manage students with chronic health conditions like diabetes, asthma, and food allergies can help schools improve student health and reduce absenteeism.

Asthma and Schools

Asthma is a leading chronic illness among children and adolescents in the United States. It is also one of the leading causes of school absenteeism. On average, in a classroom of 30 children, about 3 are likely to have asthma. Low-income populations, minorities, and children living in inner cities experience more emergency department visits, hospitalizations, and deaths due to asthma than the general population.

When children and adolescents are exposed to things in the environment—such as dust mites, and tobacco smoke—an asthma attack can occur. These are called asthma triggers.

Asthma-friendly schools are those that make the effort to create safe and supportive learning environments for students with asthma. They have policies and procedures that allow students to successfully manage their asthma. Research and case studies that looked at ways to best manage asthma in schools found that successful school-based asthma programs:

- Establish strong links with asthma care clinicians to ensure appropriate and ongoing medical care

- Target students who are the most affected by asthma at school to identify and intervene with those in greatest need

- Get administrative buy-in and build a team of enthusiastic people, including a full-time school nurse, to support the program

- Use a coordinated, multi-component and collaborative approach that includes school nursing services, asthma education for students and professional development for school staff

- Support evaluation of school-based programs and use adequate and appropriate outcome measures

Diabetes in Schools

Diabetes (type 1 or type 2) is one of the most common chronic diseases in people younger than 20 years affecting about 208,000 (0.25 percent) of all people in this age group in the United States. According to estimates for 2008–2009, about 23,500 persons in this age group were newly diagnosed with diabetes annually.

Ensuring that students with diabetes have the health services they need in school to manage their chronic condition is important in helping them stay healthy and ready to learn. Managing diabetes at school is most effective when there is a partnership among students, parents, school nurse, healthcare providers, teachers, counselors, coaches, transportation, food service employees, and administrators. Support may include helping a student take medications, check blood sugar levels, choose healthy foods in the cafeteria, and be physically active.

Create a diabetes management plan in school:

- Develop a plan to help students care for diabetes and handle any diabetes-related emergencies. Public schools and schools that receive federal funding cannot treat children with diabetes differently by the Americans with Disabilities Act (ADA), the Individuals with Disabilities Education Act (IDEA), and Section 504 of the Rehabilitation Act of 1973

- Work with a child's parents, doctor and school staff to create a Diabetes Medical Management Plan (DMMP). Having a plan helps students and school workers manage diabetes in school and during extracurricular activities such as field trips or sports. Include information on services the school will provide and how to recognize high and low blood sugar levels. A student may need assistance with giving insulin and checking blood sugar levels, and also may need to eat snacks in the classroom.

- Ensure all physician and emergency contacts are updated and provided to school staff.

- Be sure school workers have a glucagon emergency kit and know how to use it if a student experiences a low blood sugar emergency. School staff should be given the *National Diabetes Education Program School Guide* hypoglycemia and hyperglycemia emergency care plans.

Diabetes Self-Management

Help students to manage diabetes at a level right for his or her age.

- If a child is going to monitor his or her blood sugar, ensure that he or she feels comfortable doing so.

- If a trained school employee will do the monitoring, be sure the student knows where and when to go for testing.

- Make sure a child knows who to go to for help with high or low blood sugar episodes. Outline these actions in the Diabetes Medical Management Plan (DMMP).

Encourage students to eat healthy foods.

- Provide and teach the importance of a healthy breakfast, which will help students stay focused and active.

- Encourage students and parents to look at the school menus together to help them make choices for a healthy meal plan. Many schools post their menus online, or you can request this information from school workers.

Be sure students get at least 60 minutes of physical activity every day.

- Having diabetes doesn't mean that a child can't be physically active or participate in physical education classes. In fact, being active can help a child improve his or her blood sugar control.

Help prevent sick days

- Check that students with diabetes have all recommended vaccinations, including the flu shot. If a child with diabetes gets sick, he or she can take longer to recover than children without diabetes. Talk to the student's parents to make sure their child has all the vaccinations they need before starting the school year.

- Encourage students to wash their hands regularly, especially before eating and after using the bathroom.

Diabetes doesn't have to get in the way of a good experience at school. Remember, parents and schools have the same goal: to ensure that students with diabetes are safe and that they're able to learn in a supportive environment.

Epilepsy in Schools

About 0.6 percent of children ages 0–17 have epilepsy in the United States. That is about 460,000 children in 2013. Picture a school with 1,000 students—that means about 6 students would have epilepsy. For many children, epilepsy is easily controlled with medication and they can do what all the other kids can do, and perform as well academically. For others, it can be more challenging.

Compared with students with other health concerns, a Centers for Disease Control and Prevention (CDC) study shows that students aged

6–17 years with epilepsy were more likely to miss 11 or more days of school in the past year. Also, students with epilepsy were more likely to have difficulties in school, use special education services, and have activity limitations such as less participation in sports or clubs compared with students with other medical conditions. CDC also found that a larger percentage of children with epilepsy than those without the disorder lived in very low-income households (below 200 percent of the federal poverty level). This suggests other unmet needs for families of children with epilepsy.

Managing epilepsy while at school may involve:

- Educating the school nurse, teachers, staff, and students about epilepsy and its treatment, seizure first aid, and possible stigma associated with epilepsy.

- Following the seizure action plan and administering first aid (including the use of rescue medications).

- Understanding the importance of medication adherence and supporting students who take daily medications.

- Helping students avoid seizure triggers, such as flashing lights, or other triggers identified in the seizure action plan.

- Monitoring and addressing any related medical conditions, including mental health concerns such as depression.

- Providing case management services for students whose medical condition disrupts their school attendance or academic performance.

- Referring students with uncontrolled seizures to medical services within the community or to the Epilepsy Foundation for more information.

- Understanding the laws related to disability, medical conditions, and special education to ensure that children with epilepsy are able to access the free and appropriate education afforded to them under the law.

- Monitoring student behavior to prevent bullying of students with epilepsy.

Food Allergies in Schools

Food allergies are a growing food safety and public health concern that affect an estimated 4%–6% of children in the United States.

Allergic reactions can be life-threatening and have far-reaching effects on children and their families, as well as on the schools or early care and education (ECE) programs they attend. Staff who work in schools and ECE programs should develop plans for preventing an allergic reaction and responding to a food allergy emergency.

What Is a Food Allergy?

A *food allergy* occurs when the body has a specific and reproducible immune response to certain foods. The body's immune response can be severe and life-threatening, such as anaphylaxis. Although the immune system normally protects people from germs, in people with food allergies, the immune system mistakenly responds to food as if it were harmful.

Eight foods or food groups account for 90 percent of serious allergic reactions in the United States: milk, eggs, fish, crustacean shellfish, wheat, soy, peanuts, and tree nuts.

Symptoms of Food Allergy in Children

- It feels like something is poking my tongue.
- My tongue (or mouth) is tingling (or burning).
- My tongue (or mouth) itches.
- My tongue feels like there is hair on it.
- My mouth feels funny.
- There's a frog in my throat; there's something stuck in my throat.
- My tongue feels full (or heavy).
- My lips feel tight.
- It feels like there are bugs in there (to describe itchy ears).
- It (my throat) feels thick.
- It feels like a bump is on the back of my tongue (throat).

The symptoms and severity of allergic reactions to food can be different between individuals, and can also be different for one person over time. Anaphylaxis is a sudden and severe allergic reaction that may cause death. Not all allergic reactions will develop into anaphylaxis.

Voluntary Guidelines for Managing Food Allergies in Schools and Early Care and Education Programs

In consultation with the U.S. Department of Education (ED) and a number of other federal agencies, CDC developed the Voluntary Guidelines for Managing Food Allergies in Schools and Early Care and Education Centers in fulfillment of the 2011 FDA Food Safety Modernization Act (FSMA) to improve food safety in the United States.

The Voluntary Guidelines for Managing Food Allergies provide practical information and recommendations for each of the five priority areas that should be addressed in each school's or ECE program's Food Allergy and Management Prevention Plan (FAMPP):

1. Ensure the daily management of food allergies in individual children.

2. Prepare for food allergy emergencies.

3. Provide professional development on food allergies for staff members.

4. Educate children and family members about food allergies.

5. Create and maintain a healthy and safe educational environment.

Oral Health in Schools

Tooth decay (cavities) is one of the most common chronic conditions of childhood in the United States. About 1 of 5 (20 percent) children aged 5–11 years have at least one untreated decayed tooth, and about 1 of 7 (13 percent) adolescents aged 12–19 years have at least one untreated decayed tooth. The percentage of children and adolescents aged 5–19 years with untreated tooth decay is twice as high for those from low-income families (25 percent) compared with children from higher-income households (11 percent).

Poor oral health can have a detrimental effect on children's quality of life, their performance at school, and their success later in life. Tooth decay is preventable and ensuring that students have the preventive oral health services they need in school is important in helping them stay healthy and ready to learn.

School-Based and School-Linked Dental Sealant Programs

Sealants prevent tooth decay and also stop cavities from growing. School-based sealant programs provide sealants to children in a school setting, and school-linked programs screen the children in school and refer them to private dental practices or public dental clinics that place the sealants. These programs have been shown to increase the number of children who receive sealants at school, and that dental sealants result in a large reduction in tooth decay among school-aged children 5–16 years of age.

School-based sealant programs are especially important for reaching children from low-income families who are less likely to receive private dental care. When developing, coordinating, and implementing a program, state oral health program strategies should:

- Use evidence-based practices in preventing dental caries through school-based sealant programs.

- Promote policies that allow the use of dental personnel to the top of their licensure when dentists are not required to be on site.

- Develop referral networks with dental practitioners in the community.

- Increase efficiency by collaborating with targeted schools to increase the number of children that can be seen in schools.

Chapter 58

Finding a Camp for a Child with Chronic Health Needs

For many families summer camp has been an annual tradition and a rite of passage for both children and parents. Kids enjoy the chance to gain some independence, experience nature, take part in fun activities, learn new skills, and form new relationships that may last a lifetime. Parents, meanwhile, not only get a bit of a break but also appreciate the lasting positive effect that camp will have on their children.

This holds true for kids with chronic health needs and their families, as well. But of course there are some special considerations in these cases, and both parents and children should be prepared to do considerable research in order to select the most appropriate camp and plan for the child's time away from home. There are more camps for kids with special needs now than ever before, all of which offer a wide array of appropriate physical, mental, social, and therapeutic activities and many that specialize in particular disorders. Learning about the available options and doing a bit of advance preparation can help ensure that camp is a rewarding experience for the entire family.

Types of Camps

There are three primary types of camps that parents of children with chronic health conditions will need to consider: general (or mainstream)

"Finding a Camp for a Child with Chronic Health Needs," © 2017 Omnigraphics. Reviewed January 2017.

camps, those designed for children with a variety of special needs, and those aimed at specific conditions or health requirements.

- **General camps.** Under the Americans with Disabilities Act (ADA), all camps are required to take reasonable steps to accommodate children with special needs. Parents will have to do some research to find out exactly what's available at any given camp, but such accommodations could include wheelchair ramps, medical staff, and special activities. The advantage of this kind of camp is that kids with chronic conditions interact with "mainstream" kids for a potentially more well-rounded experience.

- **Special-needs camps.** These camps welcome children with a wide variety of special needs and conditions. They generally have a broad range of activities designed to accommodate many kinds of disabilities and disorders—physical, behavioral, dietary, allergy, or medical. Another advantage is that they usually have a larger medical team and a better-equipped infirmary than mainstream camps.

- **Camps for specific conditions.** Since the 1970s there has been a dramatic increase in the number of camps aimed at specific chronic disorders. These include cancer, cerebral palsy, epilepsy, diabetes, HIV/AIDS, neurological conditions, and spina bifida, among many others. Not only do these camps tailor activities to the needs and abilities related to that particular condition, but they often include sessions with trained professionals to help kids learn to deal with their disorders successfully. And their medical staff and facilities are prepared to handle these children's special requirements.

Benefits of Camp

Some of the benefits of summer camp are the same for children with chronic health needs as for other kids, and some are unique. These can include:

- **Fun.** An obvious benefit, but one that is certain to be at the top of the child's list. Camp gives kids struggling with chronic conditions a chance to get involved in new activities and enjoy themselves.

- **Independence.** Children with health issues are routinely dependent on parents and medical professionals for care and treatment. Camp provides them with a measure of self-sufficiency that they most likely don't experience on a day-to-day basis.

- **Exercise.** Depending on their condition, kids can get involved in a number of physical activities at camp that can improve coordination, cardiovascular health, and muscle development.

- **Achievement.** Children participating in camp activities gain a sense of accomplishment as they meet goals and learn new skills. This both increases self-confidence and develops abilities that last beyond the duration of camp.

- **Sense of community.** At mainstream camps, kids with chronic issues interact with all sorts of people, become part of a team, and feel less isolated. And at special-needs camps, they not only realize these benefits but also meet others with similar disorders and recognize that they're not alone but are part of a larger community.

- **Learning.** Attending any camp gives children the chance to learn new skills and try new activities, but special-needs camps provide the opportunity to learn more about their particular condition and develop techniques for improving their quality of life.

Searching for a Camp

There are a number of ways to begin looking for a camp for a child with chronic health needs. An Internet search is one way to start. Camps have a lot of useful information on their web sites, such as the special needs they can accommodate, available activities, daily menus, and photos of the staff and facilities. Another good idea is to ask the child's doctor or other medical professional for a recommendation. Hospital departments and associations devoted to specific conditions often run their own camps or, if not, can make some recommendations. Parents or kids in support groups are another good source of ideas.

As the search proceeds, there are a number of questions to consider while trying to sort through the options. These include:

- How far is the camp from home?

- How long has it been in operation?

- Does the physical layout accommodate wheelchairs, crutches, etc.?

- What medical care and facilities are available?

- What provisions are made for emergencies?

- Can special dietary needs be accommodated?

- How many kids are at the camp at any given time?

- What is the age range of the campers?

- What is the camper-to-counselor ratio?

- What training and certification do counselors have?

- Have background checks been conducted on the staff?

- How are the days structured?

- What indoor and outdoor activities are available?

- What kind of educational sessions take place?

- Is transportation available?

- What is the cost, and what's included?

When exploring camp options it's important to involve the child in the research and selection process. Make a list of his or her likes and dislikes, priorities, and questions, and be sure to include these in the search.

A final step is to visit the camp with the child who will be attending. Arrange a tour, inspect the living arrangements, meet the administrators and medical staff, and talk to several counselors. If possible, observe a few of the activities and speak with some of the campers and their parents. It's just as important that both the parents and the child have a good feeling about the camp as it is to ensure that the facilities meet the child's special needs.

References

1. Bachrach, Steven J., MD. "Camps for Kids with Special Needs," KidsHealth.com, January 2014.

2. Grand, Lillieth. "How to Find Just the Right Camp for Special Needs Kids," PDXParent.com, March 10, 2015.

3. McCarthy, Alicia, MSN, CPNP. "Summer Camp for Children and Adolescents with Chronic Conditions," Medscape.com, 2015.

4. Waltari, Mary L., Esq. "Choosing Summer Camp for Kids with Disabilities," Special Needs Alliance, March 3, 2016.

Part Seven

Legal, Financial, and Insurance Issues That Impact Disease Management

Chapter 59

Affordable Care Act (ACA)

The Affordable Care Act enacted in March 2010 has three primary goals.

- Make affordable health insurance available to more people. The law provides consumers with subsidies ("premium tax credits") that lower costs for households with incomes between 100 percent and 400 percent of the federal poverty level.

- Expand the Medicaid program to cover all adults with income below 138 percent of the federal poverty level. (Not all states have expanded their Medicaid programs.)

- Support innovative medical care delivery methods designed to lower the costs of healthcare generally.

About the Law

The Affordable Care Act (ACA) puts consumers back in charge of their healthcare. Under the law, a new "Patient's Bill of Rights" gives the American people the stability and flexibility they need to make informed choices about their health.

This chapter contains text excerpted from the following sources: Text in this chapter begins with excerpts from "Affordable Care Act (ACA)," Centers for Medicare and Medicaid Services (CMS), July 3, 2016; Text beginning with the heading "About the Law" is excerpted from "Health Insurance Marketplace," Centers for Medicare and Medicaid Services (CMS), August 13, 2015.

Coverage

- Ends Pre-Existing Condition Exclusions for Children: Health plans can no longer limit or deny benefits to children under 19 due to a pre-existing condition.

- Keeps Young Adults Covered: If you are under 26, you may be eligible to be covered under your parent's health plan.

- Ends Arbitrary Withdrawals of Insurance Coverage: Insurers can no longer cancel your coverage just because you made an honest mistake.

- Guarantees Your Right to Appeal: You now have the right to ask that your plan reconsider its denial of payment.

Costs

- Ends Lifetime Limits on Coverage: Lifetime limits on most benefits are banned for all new health insurance plans.

- Reviews Premium Increases: Insurance companies must now publicly justify any unreasonable rate hikes.

- Helps You Get the Most from Your Premium Dollars: Your premium dollars must be spent primarily on healthcare–not administrative costs.

Care

- Covers Preventive Care at No Cost to You: You may be eligible for recommended preventive health services. No copayment.

- Protects Your Choice of Doctors: Choose the primary care doctor you want from your plan's network.

- Removes Insurance Company Barriers to Emergency Services: You can seek emergency care at a hospital outside of your health plan's network.

Chapter 60

Americans with Disabilities Act (ADA)

Title I of the Americans with Disabilities Act (ADA) of 1990 prohibits private employers, state and local governments, employment agencies, and labor unions from discriminating against qualified individuals with disabilities in job application procedures, hiring, firing, advancement, compensation, job training, and other terms, conditions, and privileges of employment. The ADA covers employers with 15 or more employees, including state and local governments. It also applies to employment agencies and to labor organizations. The ADA's non-discrimination standards also apply to federal sector employees under section 501 of the Rehabilitation Act, as amended, and its implementing rules.

An individual with a disability is a person who:

- Has a physical or mental impairment that substantially limits one or more major life activities;

- Has a record of such an impairment; or

- Is regarded as having such an impairment.

This chapter contains text excerpted from the following sources: Text in this chapter begins with excerpts from "Facts about the Americans with Disabilities Act," U.S. Equal Employment Opportunity Commission (EEOC), April 9, 2016; Text under the heading "Disability Discrimination" is excerpted from "Disability Discrimination," U.S. Equal Employment Opportunity Commission (EEOC), April 10, 2016.

A qualified employee or applicant with a disability is an individual who, with or without reasonable accommodation, can perform the essential functions of the job in question. Reasonable accommodation may include, but is not limited to:

- Making existing facilities used by employees readily accessible to and usable by persons with disabilities.

- Job restructuring, modifying work schedules, reassignment to a vacant position;

- Acquiring or modifying equipment or devices, adjusting or modifying examinations, training materials, or policies, and providing qualified readers or interpreters.

An employer is required to make a reasonable accommodation to the known disability of a qualified applicant or employee if it would not impose an "undue hardship" on the operation of the employer's business. Reasonable accommodations are adjustments or modifications provided by an employer to enable people with disabilities to enjoy equal employment opportunities. Accommodations vary depending upon the needs of the individual applicant or employee. Not all people with disabilities (or even all people with the same disability) will require the same accommodation. For example:

- A deaf applicant may need a sign language interpreter during the job interview.

- An employee with diabetes may need regularly scheduled breaks during the workday to eat properly and monitor blood sugar and insulin levels.

- A blind employee may need someone to read information posted on a bulletin board.

- An employee with cancer may need leave to have radiation or chemotherapy treatments.

An employer does not have to provide a reasonable accommodation if it imposes an "undue hardship." Undue hardship is defined as an action requiring significant difficulty or expense when considered in light of factors such as an employer's size, financial resources, and the nature and structure of its operation.

An employer is not required to lower quality or production standards to make an accommodation; nor is an employer obligated to provide personal use items such as glasses or hearing aids.

An employer generally does not have to provide a reasonable accommodation unless an individual with a disability has asked for one. If an employer believes that a medical condition is causing a performance or conduct problem, it may ask the employee how to solve the problem and if the employee needs a reasonable accommodation. Once a reasonable accommodation is requested, the employer and the individual should discuss the individual's needs and identify the appropriate reasonable accommodation. Where more than one accommodation would work, the employer may choose the one that is less costly or that is easier to provide.

Title I of the ADA also covers:

Medical examinations and inquiries: Employers may not ask job applicants about the existence, nature, or severity of a disability. Applicants may be asked about their ability to perform specific job functions. A job offer may be conditioned on the results of a medical examination, but only if the examination is required for all entering employees in similar jobs. Medical examinations of employees must be job related and consistent with the employer's business needs.

Medical records are confidential. The basic rule is that with limited exceptions, employers must keep confidential any medical information they learn about an applicant or employee. Information can be confidential even if it contains no medical diagnosis or treatment course and even if it is not generated by a healthcare professional. For example, an employee's request for a reasonable accommodation would be considered medical information subject to the ADA's confidentiality requirements.

Drug and alcohol abuse: Employees and applicants currently engaging in the illegal use of drugs are not covered by the ADA when an employer acts on the basis of such use. Tests for illegal drugs are not subject to the ADA's restrictions on medical examinations. Employers may hold illegal drug users and alcoholics to the same performance standards as other employees.

It is also unlawful to retaliate against an individual for opposing employment practices that discriminate based on disability or for filing a discrimination charge, testifying, or participating in any way in an investigation, proceeding, or litigation under the ADA.

Federal tax incentives to encourage the employment of people with disabilities and to promote the accessibility of public accommodations: The Internal Revenue Code (IRC) includes several provisions aimed at making businesses more accessible to people with disabilities. The following provides general non-legal information about three of the most significant tax incentives. (Employers should check with their accountants or tax advisors to determine eligibility for these incentives or visit the Internal Revenue Service's (IRS) website, www. irs.gov, for more information. Similar state and local tax incentives may be available.)

Small business tax credit (Internal revenue code Section 44: Disabled access credit): Small businesses with either $1,000,000 or less in revenue or 30 or fewer full-time employees may take a tax credit of up to $5,000 annually for the cost of providing reasonable accommodations such as sign language interpreters, readers, materials in alternative format (such as Braille or large print), the purchase of adaptive equipment, the modification of existing equipment, or the removal of architectural barriers.

- **Work opportunity tax credit (Internal revenue code Section 51)**: Employers who hire certain targeted low-income groups, including individuals referred from vocational rehabilitation agencies and individuals receiving Supplemental Security Income (SSI) may be eligible for an annual tax credit of up to $2,400 for each qualifying employee who works at least 400 hours during the tax year. Additionally, a maximum credit of $1,200 may be available for each qualifying summer youth employee.

- **Architectural/Transportation tax deduction (Internal revenue code Section 190 Barrier removal)**: This annual deduction of up to $15,000 is available to businesses of any size for the costs of removing barriers for people with disabilities, including the following: providing accessible parking spaces, ramps, and curb cuts; providing wheelchair-accessible telephones, water fountains, and restrooms; making walkways at least 48 inches wide; and making entrances accessible.

Disability Discrimination

Disability discrimination occurs when an employer or other entity covered by the Americans with Disabilities Act, as amended, or the Rehabilitation Act, as amended, treats a qualified individual with a disability who is an employee or applicant unfavorably because she has a disability.

Disability discrimination also occurs when a covered employer or other entity treats an applicant or employee less favorably because she has a history of a disability (such as cancer that is controlled or in remission) or because she is believed to have a physical or mental impairment that is not transitory (lasting or expected to last six months or less) and minor (even if she does not have such an impairment).

The law requires an employer to provide reasonable accommodation to an employee or job applicant with a disability, unless doing so would cause significant difficulty or expense for the employer ("undue hardship").

The law also protects people from discrimination based on their relationship with a person with a disability (even if they do not themselves have a disability). For example, it is illegal to discriminate against an employee because her husband has a disability.

Federal employees and applicants are covered by the Rehabilitation Act of 1973, instead of the Americans with Disabilities Act. The protections are mostly the same.

Disability Discrimination and Work Situations

The law forbids discrimination when it comes to any aspect of employment, including hiring, firing, pay, job assignments, promotions, layoff, training, fringe benefits, and any other term or condition of employment.

Disability Discrimination and Harassment

It is illegal to harass an applicant or employee because he has a disability, had a disability in the past, or is believed to have a physical or mental impairment that is not transitory (lasting or expected to last six months or less) and minor (even if he does not have such an impairment).

Harassment can include, for example, offensive remarks about a person's disability. Although the law doesn't prohibit simple teasing, offhand comments, or isolated incidents that aren't very serious, harassment is illegal when it is so frequent or severe that it creates a hostile or offensive work environment or when it results in an adverse employment decision (such as the victim being fired or demoted).

The harasser can be the victim's supervisor, a supervisor in another area, a co-worker, or someone who is not an employee of the employer, such as a client or customer.

Chapter 61

Family and Medical Leave Act (FMLA)

The Family and Medical Leave Act (FMLA) entitles eligible employees of covered employers to take unpaid, job-protected leave for specified family and medical reasons. This chapter provides general information about which employers are covered by the FMLA, when employees are eligible and entitled to take FMLA leave, and what rules apply when employees take FMLA leave.

Covered Employers

The FMLA only applies to employers that meet certain criteria. A covered employer is a:

- Private-sector employer, with 50 or more employees in 20 or more workweeks in the current or preceding calendar year, including a joint employer or successor in interest to a covered employer;

- Public agency, including a local, state, or Federal government agency, regardless of the number of employees it employs; or

This chapter contains text excerpted from the following sources: Text in this chapter begins with excerpts from "Wage and Hour Division (WHD)," U.S. Department of Labor (DOL), 2012. Reviewed January 2017; Text under the heading "Final Rule to Amend the Definition of Spouse in the Family and Medical Leave Act Regulations" is excerpted from "Wage and Hour Division (WHD)," U.S. Department of Labor (DOL), February 2015.

- Public or private elementary or secondary school, regardless of the number of employees it employs.

Eligible Employees

Only eligible employees are entitled to take FMLA leave. An eligible employee is one who:

- Works for a *covered employer*;

- Has worked for the employer for at least *12 months*;

- Has at least *1,250 hours of service* for the employer during the 12 month period immediately preceding the leave*; and

- Works at a location where the employer has at least *50 employees within 75 miles*.

* Special hours of service eligibility requirements apply to airline flight crew employees.

The 12 months of employment do not have to be consecutive. That means any time previously worked for the same employer (including seasonal work) could, in most cases, be used to meet the 12-month requirement. If the employee has a break in service that lasted seven years or more, the time worked prior to the break will not count unless the break is due to service covered by the Uniformed Services Employment and Reemployment Rights Act (USERRA), or there is a written agreement, including a collective bargaining agreement, outlining the employer's intention to rehire the employee after the break in service.

Leave Entitlement

Eligible employees may take up to 12 workweeks of leave in a 12-month period for one or more of the following reasons:

- The birth of a son or daughter or placement of a son or daughter with the employee for adoption or foster care;

- To care for a spouse, son, daughter, or parent who has a serious health condition;

- For a serious health condition that makes the employee unable to perform the essential functions of his or her job; or

- For any qualifying exigency arising out of the fact that a spouse, son, daughter, or parent is a military member on covered active duty or call to covered active duty status.

An eligible employee may also take up to 26 workweeks of leave during a "single 12-month period" to care for a covered service member with a serious injury or illness, when the employee is the spouse, son, daughter, parent, or next of kin of the service member. The "single 12-month period" for military caregiver leave is different from the 12-month period used for other FMLA leave reasons.

Under some circumstances, employees may take FMLA leave on an intermittent or reduced schedule basis. That means an employee may take leave in separate blocks of time or by reducing the time he or she works each day or week for a single qualifying reason. When leave is needed for planned medical treatment, the employee must make a reasonable effort to schedule treatment so as not to unduly disrupt the employer's operations. If FMLA leave is for the birth, adoption, or foster placement of a child, use of intermittent or reduced schedule leave requires the employer's approval.

Under certain conditions, employees may choose, or employers may require employees, to "substitute" (run concurrently) accrued paid leave, such as sick or vacation leave, to cover some or all of the FMLA leave period. An employee's ability to substitute accrued paid leave is determined by the terms and conditions of the employer's normal leave policy.

Notice

Employees must comply with their employer's usual and customary requirements for requesting leave and provide enough information for their employer to reasonably determine whether the FMLA may apply to the leave request. Employees generally must request leave 30 days in advance when the need for leave is foreseeable. When the need for leave is foreseeable less than 30 days in advance or is unforeseeable, employees must provide notice as soon as possible and practicable under the circumstances.

When an employee seeks leave for a FMLA-qualifying reason for the first time, the employee need not expressly assert FMLA rights or even mention the FMLA. If an employee later requests additional leave for the same qualifying condition, the employee must specifically reference either the qualifying reason for leave or the need for FMLA leave.

Covered employers must:

1. Post a notice explaining rights and responsibilities under the FMLA (and may be subject to a civil money penalty of up to $110 for willful failure to post);

2. Include information about the FMLA in their employee handbooks or provide information to new employees upon hire;

3. When an employee requests FMLA leave or the employer acquires knowledge that leave may be for a FMLA-qualifying reason, provide the employee with notice concerning his or her eligibility for FMLA leave and his or her rights and responsibilities under the FMLA; and

4. Notify employees whether leave is designated as FMLA leave and the amount of leave that will be deducted from the employee's FMLA entitlement.

Certification

When an employee requests FMLA leave due to his or her own serious health condition or a covered family member's serious health condition, the employer may require certification in support of the leave from a healthcare provider. An employer may also require second or third medical opinions (at the employer's expense) and periodic recertification of a serious health condition.

Job Restoration and Health Benefits

Upon return from FMLA leave, an employee must be restored to his or her original job or to an equivalent job with equivalent pay, benefits, and other terms and conditions of employment. An employee's use of FMLA leave cannot be counted against the employee under a "no-fault" attendance policy. Employers are also required to continue group health insurance coverage for an employee on FMLA leave under the same terms and conditions as if the employee had not taken leave.

Other Provisions

Special rules apply to employees of local education agencies. Generally, these rules apply to intermittent or reduced schedule FMLA leave or the taking of FMLA leave near the end of a school term.

Salaried executive, administrative, and professional employees of covered employers who meet the Fair Labor Standards Act (FLSA) criteria for exemption from minimum wage and overtime under the FLSA regulations, 29 CFR Part 541, do not lose their FLSA-exempt status by using any unpaid FMLA leave. This special exception to the "salary basis" requirements for FLSA's exemption extends only to an eligible employee's use of FMLA leave.

Enforcement

It is unlawful for any employer to interfere with, restrain, or deny the exercise of or the attempt to exercise any right provided by the FMLA. It is also unlawful for an employer to discharge or discriminate against any individual for opposing any practice, or because of involvement in any proceeding, related to the FMLA. The Wage and Hour Division is responsible for administering and enforcing the FMLA for most employees. Most federal and certain congressional employees are also covered by the law but are subject to the jurisdiction of the U.S. Office of Personnel Management or Congress (OPM). If you believe that your rights under the FMLA have been violated, you may file a complaint with the Wage and Hour Division or file a private lawsuit against your employer in court.

Final Rule to Amend the Definition of Spouse in the Family and Medical Leave Act Regulations

In 2013, the Supreme Court in United States v. Windsor struck down section 3 of the Defense of Marriage Act (DOMA) as unconstitutional. In a June 26, 2013, press release responding to the decision, President Obama said: "This ruling is a victory for couples who have long fought for equal treatment under the law, for children whose parents' marriages will now be recognized, rightly, as legitimate; for families that, at long last, will get the respect and protection they deserve; and for friends and supporters who have wanted nothing more than to see their loved ones treated fairly and have worked hard to persuade their nation to change for the better."

The President instructed the Cabinet to review all relevant federal statutes to implement the decision, including its implications for federal benefits and programs. The Department reviewed the application of the President's directive to the Family and Medical Leave Act (FMLA), which entitles eligible employees of covered employers to take unpaid, job-protected leave for specified family and medical reasons.

Immediately following the Windsor decision, the Department announced what the then-current definition of spouse under the FMLA allowed, given the decision: Eligible employees could take leave under the FMLA to care for a same-sex spouse, but only if the employee resided in a state that recognizes same-sex marriage. This ensured that as many families as possible would have the opportunity to deal with serious medical and family situations without fearing the threat of job loss.

In order to provide FMLA rights to all legally married same-sex couples consistent with the Windsor decision and the President's directive, the Department subsequently issued a Final Rule on February 25, 2015, revising the regulatory definition of spouse under the FMLA. The Final Rule amends the regulatory definition of spouse under the FMLA so that eligible employees in legal same-sex marriages will be able to take FMLA leave to care for their spouse or family member, regardless of where they live. This will ensure that the FMLA will give spouses in same-sex marriages the same ability as all spouses to fully exercise their FMLA rights. The Final Rule is effective on March 27, 2015.

Chapter 62

Advance Directives

Advance directives are legal papers that tell your loved ones and doctors what kind of medical care you want if you can't tell them yourself. The papers let you say ahead of time how you want to be treated and to select someone who will make sure your wishes are carried out. It's best to fill these out when you're healthy in case you become ill or unable to make these decisions in the future. Think about taking action now to give someone you trust the right to make medical decisions for you. This is one of the most important things you can do.

Types of Advance Directives

Living Will

This is a document used for people to state whether or not they would like to receive certain types of medical care if they become unable to speak for themselves. The most common types of care addressed by a living will are:

- The use of machines to keep you alive. Examples include dialysis machines and ventilators (also called respirators).

- "Do not resuscitate" (DNR) orders. These instruct the healthcare team not to use cardiopulmonary resuscitation (CPR) if your breathing or heartbeat stops.

This chapter includes text excerpted from "Managing Cancer Care," National Cancer Institute (NCI), March 10, 2015.

- Tube feeding
- Withholding food and fluids
- Organ and tissue donation

Medical Power of Attorney

This is a document that allows people to name another person to make decisions about their medical care if they are unable to make these decisions for themselves. (It is also called a healthcare proxy or durable power of attorney for healthcare.) People often appoint someone they know well and trust to carry out their wishes. This person may be called a healthcare agent, surrogate, or proxy.

Why Advance Directives Are Important

Filling out advance directives gives people control over their healthcare. Choices about end-of-life care can be hard to make even when people are healthy. But if they are already seriously ill, such decisions can seem overwhelming. Some cancer patients want to try every drug or treatment in the hope that something will be effective. Others will choose to stop treatment. Although patients may turn to family and friends for advice, ultimately it is the patient's decision.

It's important to keep in mind that if a day comes where you choose not to receive or to stop treatment to control your disease, medical care to promote your well-being (palliative care) continues. This type of care includes treatment to manage pain and other physical symptoms, as well as support for psychosocial and spiritual needs. You have the right to make your own decisions about treatment. Filling out advance directives gives you a way to be in control.

When to Fill out Advance Directives

Ideally, these documents should be completed when you're healthy. Yet many people connect filling out advance directives to making decisions near the end of life. But you don't need to wait until being diagnosed with a serious illness to think about your wishes for care. In fact, making these choices when you're healthy can reduce the burden on you and your loved ones later on. Talking about these issues ensures that when the time comes, you will face the end of your life with dignity and with treatment that reflects your values.

Talk to your doctor, nurse, or social worker for advice or help with filling out advance directives. Most healthcare facilities have someone who can help. As you prepare your advance directives, you should talk about your decisions with family members and loved ones and explain the reasons behind your choices.

It's hard to talk about these issues. But the benefits of talking to the people close to you about the kind of care you want are:

- Your wishes are known and can be followed.

- It often comforts family members to know what you want.

- It saves family members from having to bring up the subject themselves.

- You may also gain peace of mind. You are making the choices for yourself instead of leaving them to your loved ones.

- It can help you and your loved ones worry less about the future and live each day to the fullest.

If talking with your family and other loved ones is too hard, consider having a family meeting and invite a social worker or member of the faith community to guide the discussion.

Reviewing and Signing Your Advance Directives

Once your advance directives have been completed, the next steps are:

- Review them with a member of your healthcare team or other healthcare professional for accuracy before signing. Most states require a witness to be present at the signing of the documents.

- Provide copies to your doctor, hospital, and family members after you sign them.

- Store copies in a safe, accessible place.

- Consider keeping a card in your wallet with a written statement declaring you have a living will and medical power of attorney and describing where the documents can be found.

Some organizations will store advance directives and make them available on the patient's behalf.

Changing Your Advance Directives

Even after advance directives have been signed, you can change your mind at any time. As a matter of fact, the process of discussing advance directives should be ongoing, rather than taking place just once. This way you can review the documents from time to time and modify them if your situation or wishes change.

To update your document, you should talk to your healthcare providers and loved ones about the new decisions you would like to make. When new advance directives have been signed, the old ones should be destroyed.

Advance Directives and State Laws

Each state has its own laws regarding advance directives. Therefore, special care should be taken to follow the laws of the state where you live or are being treated. A living will or medical power of attorney that is accepted in one state may not be accepted in another state. State-specific advance directives can be downloaded from the National Hospice and Palliative Care Organization (NHPCO).

Chapter 63

Financial Management during Health Crisis

Chapter Contents

Section 63.1

Planning for Reduced Capacity and Illness

This section contains text excerpted from the following sources:
Text in this chapter begins with excerpts from "Preventing Chronic
Disease," Centers for Disease Control and Prevention (CDC),
January 29, 2015; Text beginning with heading "Plan for Diminished
Capacity and Illness" is excerpted from "Planning for Diminished
Capacity and Illness," Consumer Financial Protection
Bureau (CFPB), U.S. Securities and Exchange
Commission (SEC), June 1, 2015.

In the United States the average healthcare spending per person
in 2012 was estimated to be $8,915, with $2.7 trillion total spent on
healthcare. Most of these healthcare expenditures were associated
with care for chronic conditions and associated risk behaviors. In 2012,
118 million (1 in 2) adults lived with at least 1 chronic condition from a
list of 10 selected conditions, and among these adults 60 million lived
with 2 or more chronic conditions.

However, little is known about how combinations of chronic conditions in adults affect total healthcare expenditures. Previous studies
focused on the relationship between total healthcare expenditures and
comorbidity indices or number of chronic conditions or how co-occur-
rence of 2 conditions affected healthcare expenditures. In 2009, average healthcare expenditures were $8,478 for adults with 2 or 3 chronic
conditions and $16,257 for those with 4 or more chronic conditions.

Furthermore, out-of-pocket healthcare spending by individuals and
families also impose an economic burden.

Plan for Diminished Capacity and Illness

Organize Your Important Documents

Organize and store important documents in a safe, easily accessible location. That way, they are readily available in an emergency.
Give copies to trusted loved ones or let them know where to find the
documents. Typically, the following documents will be most relevant
to your finances:

- **Bank and brokerage statements and account information.** Make a list of your accounts with account numbers. Keep a separate list of online bank and brokerage passwords and PINs and keep the lists in a safe place. In addition, make a list of the locations of your safe-deposit boxes, including where the keys to the safe-deposit boxes are located. Also, keep your recent bank and brokerage statements available, as well as information about how to get those statements online if you access them electronically.

- **Mortgage and credit information.** Make a list of your debts and regular payments, with account numbers and names of the financial institutions that issued the loans or credit cards.

- **Insurance policies**

- **Pension and other retirement benefit summaries**

- **Social Security payment information**

- **Contact information for financial and medical professionals,** such as doctors, lawyers, accountants, and securities professionals.

Provide Your Financial Professionals with Trusted Emergency Contacts

If you have a financial professional, such as a broker or investment adviser, provide that person with emergency or alternate contact information in case he or she cannot contact you or suspects something is wrong. You may wish to discuss with your financial professional what you would consider to be an "emergency," and specify when he or she may contact someone on your behalf.

Discuss what information can be shared with your emergency contact. For example, you might provide your financial professional with a simple written instruction, such as: "Please call my son Mark at (222) 555-5555 if:

- you are unable to reach me and there appears to be unusual activity regarding my account;

- you are unable to reach me for two weeks irrespective of any unusual account activity; or

- if you think I am confused or acting strangely."

Providing an emergency contact generally will not enable the person to make investment decisions on your behalf—so be sure to take other steps if you want someone else to manage your accounts if you cannot.

Consider Creating a Durable Financial Power of Attorney

A financial power of attorney gives someone the legal authority to make financial decisions for you if you cannot. That person is called your agent. The document is called "durable" because it remains in effect even if you become incapacitated. You retain the ability to change it or cancel it as long as you are still able to make decisions. A financial power of attorney differs from a healthcare power of attorney, which only covers healthcare decisions. You may want to consult with a lawyer to determine whether a durable financial power of attorney is right for you.

After signing a durable financial power of attorney, you can still manage your money and property as long as you have the ability to make decisions. Also, it is important to remember that you always have the option to change who you choose to act as your appointed representative and the individuals you allow to access your financial information. As you are essentially giving financial decision-making authority to your agent, it is critical that he or she be someone you can trust.

Think about Involving a Trusted Relative, Friend, or Professional

Besides listing them as emergency contacts, you may wish to give a trusted relative, friend, or professional an overview of your finances (even if you don't want to share all the details). For example, you might ask your broker or bank to send duplicate statements to your daughter or accountant. You might also consider asking a trusted friend or relative to join you on periodic visits to your financial professional. This would give someone you trust a sense of your financial situation and with whom you've been doing business. If you choose to involve a relative or friend, it is very important it is someone you are sure you can trust. Consider discussing the selection of the person with a number of other trusted friends or relatives.

Keep Things Up to Date

Be sure that if something changes (for example, you open a new account) you keep your information as current as possible. Also, your trusted contact may change over time. Keep your financial professionals informed of changes regarding who has authority to review your account or whom they should contact in case of an emergency.

Speak Up If Something Goes Wrong

If you ever think someone is taking advantage of you, or that you've been the victim of a fraud, speak up. Sadly, sometimes even financial professionals and people we know commit financial crimes. There's no shame in being a victim, and the sooner you let someone know about it, the better chance there is of putting an end to it.

Helping Others Who May Have Diminished Financial Capacity

You may have a parent or other loved one with diminished financial capacity, or who you worry may face that issue in the future. If so, consider the following steps to help.

Have an open conversation about investments and other financial matters sooner rather than later. Even if it feels awkward, it is important to have an honest conversation about finances. Ask your loved one to consider taking the steps outlined above. Even if he or she does not want to take these steps, ask your relative or friend to consider how he or she wants to maintain control of his or her finances in the future. Explain that advance planning is a way to make sure that a trusted person makes decisions if he or she no longer can.

Help your relative or friend with managing finances. You may also offer to take a more active role in helping your loved one manage his or her financial accounts. Be alert both to mistakes that your loved one may make in managing finances and to any signs of financial abuse. It can be hard to tell whether actions are the result of confusion or of financial exploitation. For example, if you find that a loved one has paid the same bill twice by mistake, you should help him or her fix the error. But beware that multiple or unusual payments could also be a sign of financial exploitation, so don't rule out that possibility without looking into it. Be on guard for any sudden changes in investments that seem out of keeping with the loved one's longstanding goals, values and investment style. These changes may have come about because of confusion or may be a sign of financial exploitation.

If your family member or friend has named you to manage money or property, understand your responsibilities and how you can protect your loved one from financial exploitation. For example, your loved one may have named you as an agent under a power of attorney or a trustee under a revocable living trust. Read the Consumer Financial Protection Bureau's Managing Someone Else's Money guides (consumerfinance.gov/blog/managing-some-one-elses-money). They walk you through your duties, tell you how to watch out for financial exploitation and scams, and tell you where you can go for help. If you've been asked by a loved one or friend to help out with his or her finances, here are some things you can do to help:

Help with ongoing financial responsibilities. You may need to take on immediate tasks, such as helping to pay bills, arranging for benefit claims, preparing tax returns, or helping with investment decisions.

Review their investment portfolio. This might be a good time to help reevaluate the person's portfolio in light of his or her financial and medical situation. Does the person expect a big increase in healthcare, personal care or other costs as a result of his or her illness or disability? If so, will he or she have enough cash or liquid assets on hand to cover those costs? (Liquid investments are assets that the owner can sell readily and without paying a hefty fee to get money when it is needed.) These can be complex questions and you may wish to discuss them with a financial professional. Keep in mind that buying and selling investments on behalf of a loved one requires legal authority, through a power of attorney, a trust or similar arrangement.

Assess the riskiness of their investment portfolio. All investments involve some level of risk. But do the investments present the right level of risk at this stage of the person's life? If not, you may wish to consider contacting a registered investment adviser representative or registered broker-dealer representative for help.

Contact their investment professional. If your loved one has a financial professional and has authorized that person to speak with you, make the professional aware of your loved one's condition. This is critical so that the financial professional can make recommendations appropriate to the client's financial needs and can watch for signs of declining financial skills or potential abuse.

Your financial professional, or that of your loved one, may raise topics discussed in this section. Financial services firms are paying increasing attention to improving communications on this subject. If a financial professional does not raise these topics, however, you should feel free to raise them yourself.

Section 63.2

Managing Multiple Chronic Conditions

This chapter contains text excerpted from the following sources: Text beginning with the heading "The Challenge of Managing Multiple Chronic Conditions" is excerpted from "The Challenge of Managing Multiple Chronic Conditions" Office of the Assistant Secretary for Health (ASH), U.S. Department of Health and Human Services (HHS), December 21, 2010. Reviewed January 2017; Text beginning with the heading "Multiple Chronic Conditions: A Strategic Framework" is excerpted from "How is HHS addressing Multiple Chronic Conditions?" Office of the Assistant Secretary for Health (ASH), U.S. Department of Health and Human Services (HHS), June 30, 2012. Reviewed January 2017.

The Challenge of Managing Multiple Chronic Conditions

Joanne is 78 years old and has six medical conditions that have required long-term treatment—diabetes, high blood pressure, heart failure, emphysema, arthritis and depression. She is discouraged because she doesn't have much energy and often can't do what she'd like. She constantly juggles doctor visits and medications. Joanne feels overwhelmed with all of her medical issues and wishes one of her doctors would coordinate, prioritize and streamline all of her visits, medicines, tests and instructions. She knows she needs more help in preparing nutritious meals, but doesn't really know where to turn for assistance. Her daughter lives too far away to be helpful on a regular basis. Joanne's neighbor looks in on her frequently and is beginning to worry.

Sound familiar? Joanne and those who care about her are grappling with an increasingly common challenge—the management of what many health experts refer to as "multiple chronic conditions." In fact, estimates suggest that about two-thirds of older adults live with two or more chronic conditions. And the aging baby boomer population will only increase the magnitude of this challenge.

Chronic conditions are those that last a year or more and require ongoing medical attention and/or limit activities of daily living. Examples include arthritis, diabetes, heart disease and hypertension. Behavioral health conditions are also increasingly common and include substance use and addiction disorders, as well as mental illnesses, dementia and other cognitive impairments.

The management of multiple chronic conditions has major cost implications. Increased spending on chronic diseases is a key factor driving the overall growth in Medicare spending. And the cost of medications for these conditions can be considerable. There are also non-financial challenges faced by those with multiple chronic conditions, such as learning how to manage fatigue, emotional distress and activity limitations.

And although most individuals have more than one chronic condition, the healthcare system is primarily organized to provide care on a disease-by-disease basis. So when individuals see a number of specialists, the opportunity for confusion escalates. The most common example involves the use of multiple medications: the use of one may contraindicate the use of another. In short, all of this can result in fragmented care. Care coordination is often the missing link. If care is coordinated, then medical and social service providers bring their respective expertise to bear on each individual's health problems in the most effective and coordinated manner.

Multiple Chronic Conditions: A Strategic Framework

The U.S. Department of Health and Human Services (HHS) is focusing on this important issue with the development of a new "Framework on Multiple Chronic Conditions." This framework will be implemented through public-private partnerships and will be bolstered by some of the provisions in the new health reform law.

Recognizing the importance of MCC to patients, caregivers, and the healthcare system, the Assistant Secretary for Health convened an HHS-wide work group on MCC to identify options for improving the health of this population. The work group, in conjunction with other stakeholders, developed Multiple Chronic Conditions: A Strategic Framework. The Framework serves as a national-level roadmap for assisting HHS programs and public and private stakeholders to improve the health of individuals with MCC. It also helps to ensure a more coordinated and comprehensive approach around MCC. Made available in late 2010, the Framework is organized by four major goals:

1. Strengthening the health care and public health systems.

2. Empowering the individual to use self-care management.

3. Equipping health care providers with tools, information, and other interventions.

4. Supporting targeted research about individuals with MCC and effective interventions.

The Framework is directed to clinical practitioners, policy makers, researchers, and others. It is designed to address the needs of all population groups with MCC. Since the Framework's release, HHS agencies and external partners have worked together to align their respective programs, activities, and initiatives in support of the framework's goals, objectives, and strategies. Improving Health for Individuals with Multiple Chronic Conditions: One-Year Achievements Aligned with the HHS Strategic Framework describes HHS achievements during the first year following the release of the Framework.

In early 2012, HHS developed the Implementation of the Strategic Framework, a work plan focusing on several areas of the Framework. Activities in the plan include:

- Examining how the Affordable Care Act supports individuals with MCC.

- Increasing the dissemination of HHS data and patient-centered outcomes research.

- Advancing the quality measures agenda.

- Facilitating self-care management activities.

- Integrating MCC into clinical practice guidelines.

- Including individuals with MCC in clinical trials.

- Promoting MCC curricula for health workforce sectors.

- Educating federal, private, public and international sectors about MCC-related issues.

Inventory of Multiple Chronic Conditions Activities: Database of Programs, Tools, and Research Initiatives to Address the Needs of Individuals with Multiple Chronic Conditions and the Innovative Profiles Report.

In January 2013, HHS expanded its HHS Inventory of Programs, Activities, and Initiatives Focused on Improving the Health of Individuals with Multiple Chronic Conditions (MCC) to include MCC-related programs and activities that take place in the public and private sectors.

This inventory is a database of programs, tools, and initiatives that address individuals with multiple chronic conditions. This new database will benefit researchers, providers, and organizations interested in improving the care of individuals with MCC. The inventory database is organized according to the HHS Strategic Framework on MCC, making it easy to locate programs and activities that address each of the Framework's goals and objectives. OASH also developed a companion piece that provides additional detail on a subset of activities that support the goals of the Framework. The report titled Private Sector Activities Focused on Improving the Health of Individuals with Multiple Chronic Conditions: Innovative Profiles features successful activities that make use of an innovation. The profiles present a new or innovative use of the workforce, a technology, or individuals who themselves have MCC.

Evaluation of the Strategic Framework

HHS evaluated the implementation of the Framework to assess the progress of other federal, public and private organizations in their response to the strategies provided. In support of this effort, a searchable database of MCC-related programs, activities, and initiatives sponsored by other federal, public and private organizations is being developed. Gaps in both inventories were identified to determine which activities further the implementation of the Framework. As a result, the following two stakeholder meetings were held in the summer of 2012:

- Sustaining self-care management

- Identifying the most appropriate interventions for targeted subgroups of individuals with MCC

- The overall aim of the meetings is to continue advancing the HHS goals for MCC.

Multiple Chronic Conditions among Medicare Beneficiaries

The Centers for Medicare and Medicaid (CMS) developed the following data resources which highlight the prevalence of chronic conditions, including MCC, among Medicare beneficiaries:

- Chronic Conditions Chart Book

- Chronic Conditions Dashboard

- State Level Chronic Condition Reports

- MMWR Data Brief

Chapter 64

Medicare, Medicaid, and Hill-Burton Free and Reduced-Cost Healthcare

Chapter Contents

Section 64.1

Medicare and Medicaid

This section contains text excerpted from the following sources: Text under the heading "Medicare" is excerpted from "What's Medicare?" Centers for Medicare and Medicaid Services (CMS), June 2015; Text under the heading "Medicaid" is excerpted from "Medicaid," Centers for Medicare and Medicaid Services (CMS), September 7, 2012. Reviewed January 2017.

Medicare

Medicare is health insurance for:

- People 65 or older
- People under 65 with certain disabilities
- People of any age with End-Stage Renal Disease (ESRD) (permanent kidney failure requiring dialysis or a kidney transplant)

What Are the Different Parts of Medicare?

Part A (Hospital Insurance) helps cover:

- Inpatient care in hospitals
- Skilled nursing facility (SNF) care
- Hospice care
- Home healthcare

Usually, you don't pay a monthly premium for Part A coverage if you or your spouse paid Medicare taxes while working. This is sometimes called premium-free Part A. If you aren't eligible for premium-free Part A, you may be able to buy Part A, and pay a premium.

Part B (Medical Insurance) helps cover:

- Services from doctors and other healthcare providers
- Outpatient care
- Home healthcare

- Durable medical equipment (DME)

- Some preventive services

Most people pay the standard monthly Part B premium. You may want to get coverage that fills gaps in Original Medicare coverage. You can choose to buy a Medicare Supplement Insurance (Medigap) policy from a private company.

Part C (Medicare Advantage):

- Includes all benefits and services covered under Parts A and B

- Usually includes Medicare prescription drug coverage (Part D) as part of the plan

- Run by Medicare-approved private insurance companies

- May include extra benefits and services for an extra cost

Part D (Medicare prescription drug coverage):

- Helps cover the cost of prescription drugs

- Run by Medicare-approved private insurance companies

- May help lower your prescription drug costs and help protect against higher costs in the future

If you have limited income and resources, you may qualify for help paying for your healthcare and prescription drug costs. For more information, visit socialsecurity.gov, call Social Security at 1-800-772-1213, or contact your local State Medical Assistance (Medicaid) office.

Medicaid

Medicaid is a joint federal and state program that helps with medical costs for some people with limited income and resources. Medicaid also offers benefits not normally covered by Medicare, like nursing home care and personal care services.

How to Apply for Medicaid?

Each state has different rules about eligibility and applying for Medicaid. Call your state Medicaid program to see if you qualify and learn how to apply.

Medicaid Spend Down

Even if your income exceeds Medicaid income levels in your state, you may be eligible under Medicaid spend down rules. Under the "spend down" process, some states allow you to become eligible for Medicaid as "medically needy," even if you have too much income to qualify. This process allows you to "spend down," or subtract, your medical expenses from your income to become eligible for Medicaid. To be eligible as "medically needy," your measurable resources also have to be under the resource amount allowed in your state. Call your state Medicaid program to see if you qualify and learn how to apply.

Dual Eligibility

Some people who are eligible for both Medicare and Medicaid are called "dual eligibles." If you have Medicare and full Medicaid coverage, most of your healthcare costs are likely covered.

You can get your Medicare coverage through Original Medicare or a Medicare Advantage Plan (Part C). If you have Medicare and full Medicaid, you'll get your Part D prescription drugs through Medicare. And, you'll automatically qualify for Extra Help paying for your Medicare prescription drug coverage (Part D). Medicaid may still cover some drugs and other care that Medicare doesn't cover.

Who Pays First—Medicaid or Medicare?

Medicaid never pays first for services covered by Medicare. It only pays after Medicare, employer group health plans, and/or Medicare Supplement (Medigap) Insurance have paid.

Section 64.2

Hill-Burton Program

This section includes text excerpted from "Hill-Burton Free and
Reduced-Cost Health Care," Health Resources and Services
Administration (HRSA), March 17, 2016.

In 1946, Congress passed a law that gave hospitals, nursing homes
and other health facilities grants and loans for construction and modernization. In return, they agreed to provide a reasonable volume of
services to persons unable to pay and to make their services available
to all persons residing in the facility's area. The program stopped providing funds in 1997, but about 150 healthcare facilities nationwide
are still obligated to provide free or reduced-cost care.

Since 1980, more than $6 billion in uncompensated services have
been provided to eligible patients through Hill-Burton.

Eligibility and Healthcare Coverages

You are eligible to apply for Hill-Burton free care if your income
is at or below the current U.S. Department of Health and Human
Services (HHS) Poverty Guidelines. You may be eligible for Hill-Burton reduced-cost care if your income is as much as two times (triple
for nursing home care) the HHS Poverty Guidelines. Facilities may
require you to provide documentation that verifies your eligibility,
such as proof of income.

Care at Hill-Burton obligated facilities is not automatically free or
reduced-cost. You must apply at the admissions or business office at an
obligated facility and be found eligible to receive free or reduced-cost
care. You may apply before or after you receive care—you may even
apply after a bill has been sent to a collection agency.

Only facility costs are covered, not your private doctors' bills.

Some facilities may use different eligibility standards and procedures. They are identified on the Hill-Burton list of obligated facilities
as PFCA, CFCA, UACA and 515. Their programs may be called either
a free care, charity care, discounted services, indigent care, etc.

Hill-Burton facilities must post a sign in their admissions and business offices and emergency room that notifies the public that free and reduced-cost care is available. When you apply for Hill-Burton care, the obligated facility must provide you with a written statement that tells you what free or reduced-cost care services you will get or why you have been denied.

Frequently Asked Questions

What services are covered under the Hill-Burton program?

Each facility chooses which services it will provide at no or reduced cost. The covered services are specified in a notice which is published by the facility and also in a notice provided to all persons seeking services in the facility. Services fully covered by a third-party insurance or a government program (e.g., Medicare and Medicaid) are not eligible for Hill-Burton coverage. However, Hill-Burton may cover services not covered by the government programs.

Can I receive Hill-Burton assistance to cover my Medicare deductible and coinsurance amounts or Medicaid co-pay and spenddown amounts?

Medicare deductible and coinsurance amounts are not eligible under the program. However, Medicaid copayment amounts are eligible, except in a long-term care facility. In addition, Medicaid spenddown amounts (the liability a patient must incur before being eligible for Medicaid) are eligible in all Hill-Burton facilities.

Where can I get Hill-Burton free or reduced cost care?

Hill-Burton obligated facilities are obligated to provide a certain amount of free or reduced-cost healthcare each year. Obligated facilities may be hospitals, nursing homes, clinics or other types of healthcare facilities. See the Hill-Burton Obligated Facilities List to find a Hill-Burton obligated facility in your State. You may apply for free or reduced-cost care before or after they are provided at the Admissions Office, Business Office or Patient Accounts Office at the obligated facility.

Who can receive free or reduced cost care through the Hill-Burton program?

Eligibility for Hill-Burton free or reduced cost care is based on a person's family size and income. Income is calculated based on your actual income for the last 12 months or your last 3 month's income times 4, whichever is less. You may qualify if your income falls within the U.S. Department of Health and Human Services poverty guidelines or, at some facilities, if your income is as much as twice (or triple for nursing home services) the poverty guidelines. For complete information on the Hill-Burton program, including the list of facilities obligated to provide it and a link to the poverty guidelines, please see the Hill-Burton Web site.

What does "income" include?

Gross income (before taxes), interest/dividends earned, and child support payments are examples of income. Assets, food stamps, gifts, loans or one-time insurance payments are examples of items not included as income when considering eligibility. For self-employed people, income is determined after deductions for business expenses.

When can I apply for Hill-Burton assistance?

You may apply for Hill-Burton assistance at any time, before or after you receive care. You may even apply after a bill has been sent to a collection agency. If a hospital obtains a court judgment before you applied for Hill-Burton assistance, the solution must be worked out within the judicial system. However, if you applied for Hill-Burton before a judgment was rendered and are found eligible, you will receive Hill-Burton even if a judgment was rendered while you were waiting for a response to your application.

Is United States citizenship required for Hill-Burton eligibility?

No. However, in order for a person to have a Hill-Burton eligibility determination made, one must have lived in the U.S. for at least 3 months.

Can I apply for Hill-Burton assistance on behalf of an uninsured relative or friend?

Yes. You can apply for Hill-Burton assistance on behalf of any patient for whom you can provide the information required to establish eligibility, (i.e., you must be able to provide information regarding the patient's family size and income.)

Do I have to wait until I am sick before I can apply for Hill-Burton assistance?

Hill-Burton is not health insurance. In order to apply for Hill-Burton assistance you must have already received services or know that you will require a specific service in the near future.

What are some reasons I could be denied Hill-Burton care?

The facility may deny your request:

- for non-nursing homes, your income is more than the current poverty guidelines, or more than twice the guidelines if specified in the facility's allocation plan;

- for nursing home services, your income is more than the poverty guidelines, or double or triple the guidelines, if specified in the facility's allocation plan;

- the facility has given out its required amount of free care as specified in its allocation plan; the services you requested or received are not covered in the facility's allocation plan;

- the services you requested or received are to be paid by Medicare/Medicaid, insurance or other financial assistance program;

- the facility asks you to first apply for Medicaid/Medicare or a financial assistance program, and you do not cooperate;

- you do not give the facility requested proof of your income, such as a pay stub.

What can I do if I have a complaint against a Hill-Burton facility?

If you feel you were unfairly denied free care or reduced cost care, a complaint must be filed in writing to the Central Office. You must include:

1. the name and address of the person making the complaint;

2. the name and location of the facility; and

3. a statement of the actions that the complainant considers to violate the requirements of the Hill-Burton program.

Division of Poison Control and Healthcare Facilities,
Parklawn Building,

5600, Fishers Lane,
Room 16C-17,
Rockville, Maryland 20857

What other service obligation does a Hill-Burton facility have?

Under the community service assurance, Hill-Burton facilities are responsible for providing emergency treatment and for treating all persons residing in the service area, regardless of race, color, national origin, creed or Medicare or Medicaid status. This assurance is in effect for the life of the facility. If you feel you were unfairly denied services or discriminated against you should contact the Office for Civil Rights (OCR) at 1-800-368-1019.

How do I apply for free care?

You should contact the Admissions, Business or Patient Accounts Office at a Hill-Burton obligated facility to find out if you qualify for assistance and whether or not a facility provides the specific services needed.

How can I find out which facilities in my area are Hill-Burton facilities?

Check out Hill-Burton Obligated Facilities List for a facility in your State. Be aware that although a facility may be listed, you still need to call the facility to be certain that it still has funds available and that the service you desire would be covered.

Chapter 65

Healthcare Benefit Laws: HIPAA and COBRA

Chapter Contents

Section 65.1

The Health Insurance Portability and Accountability Act (HIPAA)

This section includes text excerpted from "Fact Sheet: The Health Insurance Portability and Accountability Act (HIPAA)," U.S. Department of Labor (DOL), November 2015.

The Health Insurance Portability and Accountability Act (HIPAA) offers protections for millions of America's workers that improve portability and continuity of health insurance coverage.

HIPAA Protects Workers and Their Families By

• Providing additional opportunities to enroll in group health plan coverage when they lose other health coverage, get married or add a new dependent.

• Prohibiting discrimination in enrollment and in premiums charged to employees and their dependents based on any health factors.

• Preserving the states' role in regulating health insurance, including the states' authority to provide greater protections than those available under Federal law.

Special Enrollment Rights

Special enrollment allows individuals who previously declined health coverage to enroll for coverage outside of a plan's open enrollment period. There are two types of special enrollment:

• **Loss of eligibility for other coverage**: Employees and dependents who decline coverage due to other health coverage and then lose eligibility or employer contributions have special enrollment rights. For example, an employee who turns down health benefits for herself and her family because the family already has coverage through her spouse's plan can request special enrollment for her family in her own company's plan.

- **Certain life events**: Employees, spouses, and new dependents are permitted to special enroll because of marriage, birth, adoption, or placement for adoption.

For both types, the employee must request enrollment within 30 days of the loss of coverage or life event triggering the special enrollment.

Nondiscrimination Prohibitions

Employees and their family members cannot be denied eligibility or benefits based on certain "health factors." They also cannot be charged more than similarly situated individuals based on any health factors. "Health factors" include medical conditions, claims experience, and genetic information.

HIPAA and the Affordable Care Act (ACA) also provide protections from impermissible discrimination based on a health factor in wellness programs related to group health plan coverage (such as those that encourage employees to work out, stop smoking or meet certain health standards such as a target cholesterol level).

Preserving the States' Role

If a health plan provides benefits through an insurance company or HMO (an insured plan), HIPAA may be complemented by state laws that offer additional protections. For example, states may increase the number of days parents have to enroll newborns, adopted children, and children placed for adoption or require additional special enrollment circumstances.

Pre-Existing Condition Exclusions

The ACA prohibits plans from imposing preexisting condition exclusions for plan years beginning on or after January 1, 2014. For prior years, HIPAA limited these exclusions and required plans to offset preexisting condition exclusion periods if the individual had prior health coverage.

Section 65.2

Consolidated Omnibus Budget Reconciliation Act (COBRA)

This section contains text excerpted from the following sources:
Text in this section begins with excerpts from "An Employee's
Guide to Health Benefits under COBRA," U.S. Department of Labor
(DOL), September 2015; Text under the heading "FAQs on COBRA
Continuation Health Coverage" is excerpted from "FAQs on COBRA
Continuation Health Coverage," U.S. Department of Labor (DOL),
November 2015.

The Consolidated Omnibus Budget Reconciliation Act (COBRA)
requires most group health plans to provide a temporary continuation
of group health coverage that otherwise might be terminated.

COBRA requires continuation coverage to be offered to covered
employees, their spouses, their former spouses, and their dependent
children when group health coverage would otherwise be lost due to
certain specific events. Those events include the death of a covered
employee, termination or reduction in the hours of a covered employee's employment for reasons other than gross misconduct, divorce
or legal separation from a covered employee, a covered employee's
becoming entitled to Medicare, and a child's loss of dependent status
(and therefore coverage) under the plan.

FAQs on COBRA Continuation Health Coverage

What Is COBRA Continuation Health Coverage?

The Consolidated Omnibus Budget Reconciliation Act (COBRA)
health benefit provisions amend the Employee Retirement Income
Security Act, the Internal Revenue Code and the Public Health Service
Act to require group health plans to provide a temporary continuation
of group health coverage that otherwise might be terminated.

What Does COBRA Do?

COBRA requires continuation coverage to be offered to covered
employees, their spouses, former spouses, and dependent children

when group health coverage would otherwise be lost due to certain specific events. COBRA continuation coverage is often more expensive than the amount that active employees are required to pay for group health coverage, since the employer usually pays part of the cost of employees' coverage and all of that cost can be charged to individuals receiving continuation coverage.

What Group Health Plans Are Subject to COBRA?

The law generally applies to all group health plans maintained by private-sector employers with 20 or more employees, or by state or local governments. The law does not apply to plans sponsored by the Federal Government or by churches and certain church-related organizations. In addition, many states have laws similar to COBRA, including those that apply to health insurers of employers with less than 20 employees (sometimes called mini-COBRA). Check with your state insurance commissioner's office to see if such coverage is available to you.

Who Is Entitled to Continuation Coverage under COBRA?

In order to be entitled to elect COBRA continuation coverage, your group health plan must be covered by COBRA; a qualifying event must occur; and you must be a qualified beneficiary for that event.

Plan Coverage: COBRA covers group health plans sponsored by an employer (private-sector or state/local government) that employed at least 20 employees on more than 50 percent of its typical business days in the previous calendar year. Both full- and part-time employees are counted to determine whether a plan is subject to COBRA. Each part-time employee counts as a fraction of a full-time employee, with the fraction equal to the number of hours that the part-time employee worked divided by the hours an employee must work to be considered full time.

Qualifying Events: Qualifying events are events that cause an individual to lose his or her group health coverage. The type of qualifying event determines who the qualified beneficiaries are for that event and the period of time that a plan must offer continuation coverage. COBRA establishes only the minimum requirements for continuation coverage. A plan may always choose to provide longer periods of continuation coverage.

The following are qualifying events for covered employees if they cause the covered employee to lose coverage:

- Termination of the employee's employment for any reason other than gross misconduct; or

- Reduction in the number of hours of employment.

The following are qualifying events for the spouse and dependent child of a covered employee if they cause the spouse or dependent child to lose coverage:

- Termination of the covered employee's employment for any reason other than gross misconduct;

- Reduction in the hours worked by the covered employee;

- Covered employee becomes entitled to Medicare;

- Divorce or legal separation of the spouse from the covered employee; or

- Death of the covered employee.

In addition to the above, the following is a qualifying event for a dependent child of a covered employee if it causes the child to lose coverage:

- Loss of dependent child status under the plan rules. Under the Patient Protection and Affordable Care Act, plans that offer coverage to children on their parents' plan must make the coverage available until the adult child reaches the age of 26.

Qualified Beneficiaries: A qualified beneficiary is an individual covered by a group health plan on the day before a qualifying event occurred that caused him or her to lose coverage. Only certain individuals can become qualified beneficiaries due to a qualifying event, and the type of qualifying event determines who can become a qualified beneficiary when it happens. A qualified beneficiary must be a covered employee, the employee's spouse or former spouse, or the employee's dependent child. In certain cases involving the bankruptcy of the employer sponsoring the plan, a retired employee, the retired employee's spouse or former spouse, and the retired employee's dependent children may be qualified beneficiaries. In addition, any child born to or placed for adoption with a covered employee during a period of continuation coverage is automatically considered a qualified beneficiary.

An employer's agents, independent contractors, and directors who participate in the group health plan may also be qualified beneficiaries.

How Do I Become Eligible for COBRA Continuation Coverage?

To be eligible for COBRA coverage, you must have been enrolled in your employer's health plan when you worked and the health plan must continue to be in effect for active employees. COBRA continuation coverage is available upon the occurrence of a qualifying event that would, except for the COBRA continuation coverage, cause an individual to lose his or her healthcare coverage.

How Do I Find out about COBRA Coverage?

Group health plans must provide covered employees and their families with certain notices explaining their COBRA rights. Your COBRA rights must be described in the plan's Summary Plan Description (SPD), which you should receive within 90 days after you first become a participant in the plan. In addition, group health plans must give each employee and spouse who becomes covered under the plan a general notice describing COBRA rights, also provided within the first 90 days of coverage.

Before a group health plan must offer continuation coverage, a qualifying event must occur, and the plan must be notified of the qualifying event. Who must give notice of the qualifying event depends on the type of qualifying event.

The employer must notify the plan if the qualifying event is the covered employee's termination or reduction of hours of employment, death, entitlement to Medicare, or bankruptcy of a private-sector employer. The employer must notify the plan within 30 days of the event.

You (the covered employee or one of the qualified beneficiaries) must notify the plan if the qualifying event is divorce, legal separation, or a child's loss of dependent status under the plan. The plan must have procedures 4 for how to give notice of the qualifying event, and the procedures should be described in both the general notice and the plan's SPD. The plan can set a time limit for providing this notice, but it cannot be shorter than 60 days, starting from the latest of:

1. the date on which the qualifying event occurs;

2. the date on which you lose (or would lose) coverage under the plan due to the qualifying event; or

3. the date on which you are informed, through the furnishing of either the SPD or the COBRA general notice, of the responsibility to notify the plan and procedures for doing so.

If your plan does not have reasonable procedures for how to give notice of a qualifying event, you can give notice by contacting the person or unit that handles your employer's employee benefits matters. If your plan is a multiemployer plan, notice can also be given to the joint board of trustees, and, if the plan is administered by an insurance company (or the benefits are provided through insurance), notice can be given to the insurance company.

When the plan receives a notice of a qualifying event, it must give the qualified beneficiaries an election notice which describes their rights to continuation coverage and how to make an election. This notice must be provided within 14 days after the plan receives notice of the qualifying event.

How Long Do I Have to Elect COBRA Coverage?

If you are entitled to elect COBRA coverage, you must be given an election period of at least 60 days (starting on the later of the date you are furnished the election notice or the date you would lose coverage) to choose whether or not to elect continuation coverage.

Each of the qualified beneficiaries for a qualifying event may independently elect COBRA coverage. This means that if both you and your spouse are entitled to elect continuation coverage, you each may decide separately whether to do so. The covered employee or spouse must be allowed to elect on behalf of any dependent children or on behalf of all of the qualified beneficiaries. A parent or legal guardian may elect on behalf of a minor child.

If I Waive COBRA Coverage during the Election Period, Can I Still Get Coverage at a Later Date?

If you waive COBRA coverage during the election period, you must be permitted later to revoke your waiver of coverage and to elect continuation coverage as long as you do so during the election period. Then, the plan need only provide continuation coverage beginning on the date you revoke the waiver.

In addition, certain Trade Adjustment Assistance (TAA) Program participants have a second opportunity to elect COBRA continuation coverage. Individuals who are eligible and receive Trade Readjustment Allowances (TRA), individuals who would be eligible to receive

TRA, but have not yet exhausted their unemployment insurance (UI) benefits, and individuals receiving benefits under Alternative Trade Adjustment Assistance (ATAA) or Reemployment Trade Adjustment Assistance (RTAA), and who did not elect COBRA during the general election period, may get a second election period. This additional, second election period is measured 60 days from the first day of the month in which an individual is determined eligible for the TAA benefits listed above and receives such benefit. For example, if an individual's general election period runs out and he or she is determined eligible for TRA (or would be eligible for TRA but have not exhausted UI benefits) or begin to receive ATAA or RTAA benefits 61 days after separating from employment, at the beginning of the month, he or she would have approximately 60 more days to elect COBRA. However, if this same individual does not meet the eligibility criteria until the end of the month, the 60 days are still measured from the first of the month, in effect giving the individual about 30 days. Additionally, a COBRA election must be made not later than 6 months after the date of the TAA-related loss of coverage. COBRA coverage chosen during the second election period typically begins on the first day of that period.

Under COBRA, What Benefits Must Be Covered?

If you elect continuation coverage, the coverage you are given must be identical to the coverage currently available under the plan to similarly situated active employees and their families (generally, this is the same coverage that you had immediately before the qualifying event). You will also be entitled, while receiving continuation coverage, to the same benefits, choices, and services that a similarly situated participant or beneficiary is currently receiving under the plan, such as the right during open enrollment season to choose among available coverage options. You will also be subject to the same rules and limits that would apply to a similarly situated participant or beneficiary, such as copayment requirements, deductibles, and coverage limits. The plan's rules for filing benefit claims and appealing any claims denials also apply.

Any change made to the plan's terms that apply to similarly situated active employees and their families will also apply to qualified beneficiaries receiving COBRA continuation coverage. If a child is born to or adopted by a covered employee during a period of continuation coverage, the child is automatically considered to be a qualified beneficiary receiving continuation coverage. You should consult your plan for the rules that apply for adding your child to continuation coverage under those circumstances.

How Long Does COBRA Coverage Last?

COBRA requires that continuation coverage extend from the date of the qualifying event for a limited period of 18 or 36 months. The length of time depends on the type of qualifying event that gave rise to the COBRA rights. A plan, however, may provide longer periods of coverage beyond the maximum period required by law.

When the qualifying event is the covered employee's termination of employment or reduction in hours of employment, qualified beneficiaries are entitled to 18 months of continuation coverage.

When the qualifying event is the end of employment or reduction of the employee's hours, and the employee became entitled to Medicare less than 18 months before the qualifying event, COBRA coverage for the employee's spouse and dependents can last until 36 months after the date the employee becomes entitled to Medicare. For example, if a covered employee becomes entitled to Medicare 8 months before the date his/her employment ends (termination of employment is the COBRA qualifying event), COBRA coverage for his/her spouse and children would last 28 months (36 months minus 8 months). For more information on how entitlement to Medicare impacts the length of COBRA coverage, contact the Department of Labor's Employee Benefits Security Administration at askebsa.dol.gov or by calling 1-866-444-3272. For other qualifying events, qualified beneficiaries must be provided 36 months of continuation coverage.

Can Continuation Coverage Be Terminated Early for Any Reason?

A group health plan may terminate coverage earlier than the end of the maximum period for any of the following reasons:

- Premiums are not paid in full on a timely basis;

- The employer ceases to maintain any group health plan;

- A qualified beneficiary begins coverage under another group health plan after electing continuation coverage;

- A qualified beneficiary becomes entitled to Medicare benefits after electing continuation coverage; or

- A qualified beneficiary engages in conduct that would justify the plan in terminating coverage of a similarly situated participant or beneficiary not receiving continuation coverage (such as fraud).

If continuation coverage is terminated early, the plan must provide the qualified beneficiary with an early termination notice. The notice must be given as soon as practicable after the decision is made, and it must describe the date coverage will terminate, the reason for termination, and any rights the qualified beneficiary may have under the plan or applicable law to elect alternative group or individual coverage. If you decide to terminate your COBRA coverage early, you generally won't be able to get a Marketplace plan outside of the open enrollment period.

Can I Extend My COBRA Continuation Coverage?

If you are entitled to an 18 month maximum period of continuation coverage, you may become eligible for an extension of the maximum time period in two circumstances. The first is when a qualified beneficiary is disabled; the second is when a second qualifying event occurs.

Disability: If any one of the qualified beneficiaries in your family is disabled and meets certain requirements, all of the qualified beneficiaries receiving continuation coverage due to a single qualifying event are entitled to an 11-month extension of the maximum period of continuation coverage (for a total maximum period of 29 months of continuation coverage). The plan can charge qualified beneficiaries an increased premium, up to 150 percent of the cost of coverage, during the 11-month disability extension.

The requirements are:

- that the Social Security Administration (SSA) determines that the disabled qualified beneficiary is disabled before the 60th day of continuation coverage; and

- that the disability continues during the rest of the 18-month period of continuation coverage.

The disabled qualified beneficiary or another person on his or her behalf also must notify the plan of the SSA determination. The plan can set a time limit for providing this notice of disability, but the time limit cannot be shorter than 60 days, starting from the latest of:

1. the date on which SSA issues the disability determination;

2. the date on which the qualifying event occurs;

3. the date on which the qualified beneficiary loses (or would lose) coverage under the plan as a result of the qualifying event; or

4. the date on which the qualified beneficiary is informed, through the furnishing of the SPD or the COBRA general notice, of the responsibility to notify the plan and the procedures for doing so.

The right to the disability extension may be terminated if the SSA determines that the disabled qualified beneficiary is no longer disabled. The plan can require qualified beneficiaries receiving the disability extension to notify it if the SSA makes such a determination, although the plan must give the qualified beneficiaries at least 30 days after the SSA determination to do so.

The rules for how to give a disability notice and a notice of no longer being disabled should be described in the plan's SPD (and in the election notice if you are offered an 18-month maximum period of continuation coverage).

Second Qualifying Event: If you are receiving an 18-month maximum period of continuation coverage, you may become entitled to an 18-month extension (giving a total maximum period of 36 months of continuation coverage) if you experience a second qualifying event that is the death of a covered employee, the divorce or legal separation of a covered employee and spouse, a covered employee's becoming entitled to Medicare (in certain circumstances), or a loss of dependent child status under the plan. The second event can be a second qualifying event only if it would have caused you to lose coverage under the plan in the absence of the first qualifying event. If a second qualifying event occurs, you will need to notify the plan.

The rules for how to give notice of a second qualifying event should be described in the plan's SPD (and in the election notice if you are offered an 18-month maximum period of continuation coverage). The plan can set a time limit for providing this notice, but the time limit cannot be shorter than 60 days from the latest of:

1. the date on which the qualifying event occurs;

2. the date on which you lose (or would lose) coverage under the plan as a result of the qualifying event; or

3. the date on which you are informed, through the furnishing of either the SPD or the COBRA general notice, of the responsibility to notify the plan and the procedures for doing so.

How Do I File a COBRA Claim for Benefits?

Health plan rules must explain how to obtain benefits and must include written procedures for processing claims. You should submit a claim for benefits in accordance with these rules. Claims procedures must be described in the Summary Plan Description. Contact the plan administrator for more information on filing a claim for benefits.

Can I Receive COBRA Benefits While on FMLA Leave?

The Family and Medical Leave Act (FMLA) requires an employer to maintain coverage under any group health plan for an employee on FMLA leave under the same conditions coverage would have been provided if the employee had continued working. Coverage provided under the FMLA is not COBRA coverage, and taking FMLA leave is not a qualifying event under COBRA. A COBRA qualifying event may occur, however, when an employer's obligation to maintain health benefits under FMLA ceases, such as when an employee taking FMLA leave decides not to return to work and notifies an employer of his or her intent not to return to work.

I Have Both Medicare and COBRA Coverage, How Do I Know Which Will Pay My Benefits?

Medicare is the Federal health insurance program for people who are 65 or older and certain younger people with disabilities or End-Stage Renal Disease. If you are enrolled in Medicare as well as COBRA continuation coverage, there may be special coordination of benefits rules that determine which coverage is the primary payer of benefits. Check your Summary Plan Description to see if special rules apply or ask your plan administrator.

Am I Eligible for COBRA If My Company Closed or Went Bankrupt and There Is No Health Plan?

If there is no longer a health plan, there is no COBRA coverage available. If, however, there is another plan offered by the company, you may be covered under that plan. Union members who are covered by a collective bargaining agreement that provides for a medical plan also may be entitled to continued coverage.

Where Can I Go If I Have Questions or Want More Information on COBRA?

COBRA continuation coverage laws are administered by several agencies. The Departments of Labor and Treasury have jurisdiction over private-sector group health plans. The Department of Health and Human Services administers the continuation coverage law as it applies to state and local governmental health plans.

The Labor Department's interpretive responsibility for COBRA is limited to the disclosure and notification requirements of COBRA. If you need further information on your rights under a private-sector plan, or about ERISA generally, contact the Employee Benefits Security Administration (EBSA) electronically at askebsa.dol.gov or call toll free 1-866-444-3272.

The Internal Revenue Service, Department of the Treasury, has issued regulations on COBRA provisions relating to eligibility, coverage and payment. Both the Departments of Labor and Treasury share jurisdiction for enforcement of these provisions.

Chapter 66

Eligibility for Medicare Coverage of Home Healthcare

What Is Medicare?

Medicare is the federal health insurance program for people who are 65 or older, certain younger people with disabilities, and people with End-Stage Renal Disease (permanent kidney failure requiring dialysis or a transplant, sometimes called ESRD).

How Often Is It Covered?

Medicare Part A (Hospital Insurance) and/or Medicare Part B (Medical Insurance) covers eligible home health services like these:

- Intermittent skilled nursing care

- Physical therapy

- Speech-language pathology services

This chapter contains text excerpted from the following sources: Text under the heading "What Is Medicare?" is excerpted from "What's Medicare?" Centers for Medicare and Medicaid Services (CMS), August 17, 2012. Reviewed January 2017. Text beginning with the heading "How Often Is It Covered?" is excerpted from "Home Health Services," Centers for Medicare and Medicaid Services (CMS), September 30, 2012. Reviewed January 2017.

- Continued occupational services, and more
- Usually, a home healthcare agency coordinates the services your doctor orders for you.

Medicare doesn't pay for:

- 24-hour-a-day care at home
- Meals delivered to your home
- Homemaker services
- Personal care

Who Is Eligible?

All people with Part A and/or Part B who meet all of these conditions are covered:

- You must be under the care of a doctor, and you must be getting services under a plan of care established and reviewed regularly by a doctor.
- You must need, and a doctor must certify that you need, one or more of these:
  - Intermittent skilled nursing care (other than just drawing blood)
  - Physical therapy, speech-language pathology, or continued occupational therapy services. These services are covered only when the services are specific, safe and an effective treatment for your condition. The amount, frequency and time period of the services needs to be reasonable, and they need to be complex or only qualified therapists can do them safely and effectively. To be eligible, either:
    1. your condition must be expected to improve in a reasonable and generally-predictable period of time, or
    2. you need a skilled therapist to safely and effectively make a maintenance program for your condition, or
    3. you need a skilled therapist to safely and effectively do maintenance therapy for your condition.
- The home health agency caring for you must be Medicare-certified.

- Your must be homebound, and a doctor must certify that you're homebound.

You're not eligible for the home health benefit if you need more than part-time or "intermittent" skilled nursing care.

You may leave home for medical treatment or short, infrequent absences for non-medical reasons, like attending religious services. You can still get home healthcare if you attend adult day care.

Home health services may also include medical social services, part-time or intermittent home health aide services, medical supplies for use at home, durable medical equipment, or injectable osteoporosis drugs.

Your Costs in Original Medicare

Before you start getting your home healthcare, the home health agency should tell you how much Medicare will pay. The agency should also tell you if any items or services they give you aren't covered by Medicare, and how much you'll have to pay for them. This should be explained by both talking with you and in writing. The home health agency should give you a notice called the "Home Health Advance Beneficiary Notice" (HHABN) before giving you services and supplies that Medicare doesn't cover.

To find out how much your specific test, item, or service will cost, talk to your doctor or other healthcare provider. The specific amount you'll owe may depend on several things, like other insurance you may have, how much your doctor charges, whether your doctor accepts assignment, the type of facility, and the location where you get your test, item, or service.

Your doctor or other healthcare provider may recommend you get services more often than Medicare covers. Or, they may recommend services that Medicare doesn't cover. If this happens, you may have to pay some or all of the costs. It's important to ask questions so you understand why your doctor is recommending certain services and whether Medicare will pay for them.

Chapter 67

Purchasing Health Insurance as an Individual

Personal health insurance helps you pay for medical services and sometimes prescription drugs. Once you purchase insurance coverage, you and your health insurer each agree to pay a part of your medical expenses—usually a certain dollar amount or percentage of the expenses.

How to Get Health Coverage

You can get healthcare coverage through:

- A group coverage plan at your job or your spouse or partner's job

- Your parents' insurance plan, if you are under 26 years old

- A plan you purchase on your own directly from a health insurance company or through the health insurance marketplace

- Government programs such as Medicare, Medicaid, or Children's Health Insurance Program (CHIP)

- The Veterans Administration or TRICARE for military personnel

- Your state, if it provides a health insurance plan

This chapter includes text excerpted from "Personal Insurance," USA.gov, U.S. General Services Administration (GSA), September 7, 2016.

- Continuing employer coverage from your former employer, on a temporary basis under the Consolidated Omnibus Budget Reconciliation Act (COBRA)

Types of Health Insurance Plans

When purchasing health insurance, your choices typically fall into one of three categories:

- Traditional fee-for-service health insurance plans are usually the most expensive choice, but they offer you the most flexibility in choosing healthcare providers.

- Health maintenance organizations (HMOs) offer lower copayments and cover the costs of more preventive care, but your choice of healthcare providers is limited to those who are part of the plan.

- Preferred provider organizations (PPOs) offer lower co-payments like HMOs but give you more flexibility in selecting a provider.

Important Questions to Ask When Choosing a Health Insurance Plan

Read the fine print when choosing among different healthcare plans. Also ask a lot of questions, such as:

- Do I have the right to go to any doctor, hospital, clinic, or pharmacy I choose?

- Are specialists, such as eye doctors and dentists, covered?

- Does the plan cover special conditions or treatments such as pregnancy, psychiatric care, and physical therapy?

- Does the plan cover home care or nursing home care?

- Will the plan cover all medications my physician may prescribe?

- What are the deductibles? Are there any copayments? Deductibles are the amount you must pay before your insurance company will pay a claim. These differ from copayments, which are the amount of money you pay when you receive medical services or a prescription.

- What is the most I will have to pay out of my own pocket to cover expenses?

- If there is a dispute about a bill or service, how is it handled?

Chapter 68

High Deductible Health Insurance

A High Deductible Health Plan (HDHP) is a health plan product that combines a Health Savings Account (HSA) or a Health Reimbursement Arrangement (HRA) with traditional medical coverage. It provides insurance coverage and a tax-advantaged way to help save for future medical expenses. The HDHP/HSA or HRA gives you greater flexibility and discretion over how you use your healthcare dollars.

HDHPs have higher annual deductibles and out-of-pocket maximum limits than other types of Federal Employees Health Benefits (FEHB) Program plans. With an HDHP, the annual deductible must be met before plan benefits are paid for services other than in-network preventive care services, which are covered 100 percent.

HDHPs also protect you against catastrophic out-of-pocket expenses for covered services. Once your annual out-of-pocket expenses for covered services from in-network providers, including deductibles, copayments and coinsurance, reaches the pre-determined catastrophic limit, the plan pays 100 percent of the allowable amount for the remainder of the calendar year.

Health Savings Accounts

A Health Savings Account allows individuals to pay for current health expenses and save for future qualified medical expenses on a

This chapter includes text excerpted from "FastFacts—High Deductible Health Plans," U.S. Office of Personnel Management (OPM), March 4, 2014.

pre-tax basis. Funds deposited into an HSA are not taxed, the balance in the HSA grows tax free, and that amount is available on a tax free basis to pay medical costs. When you enroll in an HDHP, the health plan determines whether you are eligible for a Health Savings Account (HSA) or a Health Reimbursement Arrangement (HRA) based on the information you provide.

Who Is Eligible for an HSA?

You are eligible for an HSA if you are:

- Enrolled in an HDHP and not covered by another health plan (including a spouse's health plan, but not including specific injury insurance and accident, disability, dental care, vision care, or long-term care coverage)

- Not enrolled in Medicare

- Not in receipt of U.S. Department of Veterans Affairs (VA) or Indian Health Service (IHS) benefits within the last three months

- Not covered by your own or your spouse's flexible spending account (FSA), and are not claimed as a dependent on someone else's tax return

How Does an HDHP with an HSA Work?

- You enroll in an HDHP under the FEHB Program.

- Your plan establishes an HSA with a fiduciary (each HDHP has more information on how this step works in their brochure).

- Your plan contributes money into your HSA (the premium pass through).

- You can make additional tax-deductible contributions into your HSA, up to an allowable amount determined by IRS rules. Your HSA dollars earn tax-free interest.

- When you need preventive care, your plan will provide it without cost to you, subject to any limits outlined in the plan's brochure.

- When you need non-preventive healthcare, you pay the full cost of that care with funds from your HSA or out of pocket, up to your plan's high deductible.

- If you reach the catastrophic limit, your HDHP will provide needed care with no charge to you (assuming you use in-network providers).

Other Key Features

- Distributions from your HSA are tax-free for qualified medical expenses for you, your spouse and your dependents, even if they are not covered by an HDHP.

- You may withdraw money from your HSA for items other than qualified medical expenses, but it will be subject to income tax and, if you are under 65 years old, an additional 20 percent penalty tax on the amount withdrawn.

- You may allow the contributions in your HSA to grow over time, like a savings account. The HSA is portable—you may take the HSA with you if you leave the Federal government or switch to another plan.

Health Reimbursement Arrangements

An HRA is an employer-funded tax-sheltered account to reimburse allowable medical expenses. HDHP members who do not qualify for an HSA, will be provided an HRA. There is no additional paperwork needed for enrollment into the HRA.

Features of an HRA

- Tax-free withdrawals for qualified medical expenses

- Carryover of unused credits, without limit, from year to year

- Your HRA is administered by the health plan

How Does an HDHP with an HRA Work?

- You enroll in an HDHP under the FEHB Program

- Your plan establishes an HRA for you (each HDHP has more information on how this step works)

- Your plan will credit a portion of the health plan premium to your account at the beginning of each calendar year. Note: The amount for either a Self Only enrollment or a Self and Family enrollment will be the same as the amounts that will be deposited in HSAs in the same plan

- When you need preventive care, your plan will provide it without cost to you, subject to any limits outlined in the plan's brochure

- When you need non-preventive healthcare, you can use funds in your account to help pay your health plan deductible. You also can use the account to pay Medicare premiums.

- If you reach the catastrophic limit, your HDHP will provide needed care with no charge to you (assuming you use in-network providers)

Differences between an HRA and an HSA

- An HRA does not earn interest

- An HRA is not portable—Credits in an HRA are forfeited if you switch health plans, or if you leave federal employment (other than to retire, as long as you stay enrolled in the same health plan)

- You cannot make additional contributions to an HRA

Chapter 69

Children's Health Insurance Program (CHIP)

If your children need health coverage, they may be eligible for the Children's Health Insurance Program (CHIP). If they qualify, you won't have to buy an insurance plan to cover them. CHIP provides low-cost health coverage to children in families that earn too much money to qualify for Medicaid. In some states, CHIP covers pregnant women. Each state offers CHIP coverage, and works closely with its state Medicaid program.

Apply for CHIP

Each state program has its own rules about who qualifies for CHIP. You can apply right now, any time of year, and find out if you qualify. If you apply for Medicaid coverage to your state agency, you'll also find out if your children qualify for CHIP.

Two ways to apply for CHIP:

- Call 1-800-318-2596 (TTY: 1-855-889-4325).

- Fill out an application through the Health Insurance Marketplace. If it looks like anyone in your household qualifies for

---

This chapter contains text excerpted from the following sources: Text in this chapter begins with excerpts from "The Children's Health Insurance Program (CHIP)," Centers for Medicare and Medicaid Services (CMS), August 15, 2014; Text under the heading "Benefits" is excerpted from "Benefits," Centers for Medicare and Medicaid Services (CMS), December 13, 2014.

Medicaid or CHIP, we'll send your information to your state agency. They'll contact you about enrollment. When you submit your Marketplace application, you'll also find out if you qualify for an individual insurance plan with savings based on your income instead.

What CHIP Covers

CHIP benefits are different in each state. But all states provide comprehensive coverage, including:

- Routine check-ups
- Immunizations
- Doctor visits
- Prescriptions
- Dental and vision care
- Inpatient and outpatient hospital care
- Laboratory and X-ray services
- Emergency services

States may provide more CHIP benefits. Check with your state for information about covered services.

What CHIP Costs

Routine "well child" doctor and dental visits are free under CHIP. But there may be copayments for other services. Some states charge a monthly premium for CHIP coverage. The costs are different in each state, but you won't have to pay more than 5 percent of your family's income for the year.

Benefits

The Children's Health Insurance Program (CHIP) provides comprehensive benefits to children. Since states have flexibility to design their own program within Federal guidelines, benefits vary by state and by the type of CHIP program.

Medicaid Expansion Benefits

Medicaid Expansion CHIP programs provide the standard Medicaid benefit package, including Early and Periodic Screening, Diagnostic, and Treatment (EPSDT) services, which includes all medically necessary services like mental health and dental services.

Separate CHIP Benefits Options

States can choose to provide benchmark coverage, benchmark-equivalent coverage, or Secretary-approved coverage:

- Benchmark coverage based on one of the following:
- The standard Blue Cross/Blue Shield preferred provider option service benefit plan offered to Federal employees
- State employee's coverage plan
- HMO plan that has the largest commercial, non-Medicaid enrollment within the state
- Benchmark-Equivalent coverage must be actuarially equivalent and include:
- Inpatient and outpatient hospital services
- Physician's services
- Surgical and medical services
- Laboratory and X-ray services
- Well-baby and well-child care, including immunizations
- Secretary-approved coverage: Any other health coverage deemed appropriate and acceptable by the Secretary of the U.S. Department of Health and Human Services (HHS).

Separate CHIP Dental Benefits

States that provide CHIP coverage to children through a Medicaid expansion program are required to provide the EPSDT benefit. Dental coverage in separate CHIP programs is required to include coverage for dental services "necessary to prevent disease and promote oral health, restore oral structures to health and function, and treat emergency conditions." For more information see CHIP Dental Care Goals and related Federal Policy Guidance.

States with a separate CHIP program may choose from two options for providing dental coverage: a package of dental benefits that meets the CHIP requirements, or a benchmark dental benefit package. The benchmark dental package must be substantially equal to the (1) the most popular federal employee dental plan for dependents, (2) the most popular plan selected for dependants in the state's employee dental plan, or (3) dental coverage offered through the most popular commercial insurer in the state.

States are also required to post a listing of all participating Medicaid and CHIP dental providers and benefit packages on www.insurekidsnow.gov.

Vaccines

Coverage for age-appropriate immunizations is required in CHIP. States with a separate CHIP program (including the separate portion of a combination program) must purchase vaccines to be administered to enrolled children using only CHIP federal and state matching funds. Vaccines for federally vaccine-eligible children (through the Vaccines For Children program) should not be used by children enrolled in separate CHIP programs, and funds available under section 317 of the Public Health Service Act are designated for the purchase of vaccines for the uninsured and may not be used to purchase vaccines for children who have separate CHIP coverage.

States have two options for purchasing vaccines for children enrolled in separate CHIP programs:

1. purchase vaccines using the CDC contract and distribution mechanism, or

2. purchase vaccines through the private sector.

Chapter 70

Health Insurance Fraud

Chapter Contents

Section 70.1

Medical Discount Plans – Service or a Scam?

This section includes text excerpted from "Discount Plan or Health Insurance?" Federal Trade Commission (FTC), November 2014.

Looking for health insurance? Make sure that's what you're buying, or you could find yourself on the hook for big medical bills with no way to pay them. Dishonest marketers make it sound like they're selling affordable health insurance, when really, it's a medical discount plan instead. Medical discount plans can be a way for some people to save money on their healthcare costs, but discount plans aren't health insurance, and aren't a substitute for it.

Health Insurance versus Discount Plans

If you buy a health insurance plan, it generally covers a broad range of services, and pays you or your healthcare provider for a portion of your medical bills. With a medical discount plan, you generally pay a monthly fee to get discounts on specific services or products from a list of participating providers. Medical discount plans don't pay your healthcare costs.

Medical Discount Scams

While there are medical discount plans that provide legitimate discounts, others take people's money and offer very little in return. Dishonest marketers sometimes make it sound like they're selling you health insurance, or lie about what their plans really offer. Here are some ways to ensure you don't get caught up in a discount scam:

Beware of "Up to" Discounts

"Discounts of up to 70%!"—but how often will you save that much? Savings with discount plans typically are a lot less. When you consider a discount plan's monthly premiums and enrollment fees, there may be no "discount" at all. What's more, if you have major health problems or an emergency, you will have to cover most, or all, of the bills if you don't have health insurance.

Confirm the Details

Medical discount plans aren't a substitute for health insurance. Nevertheless, if you are interested in a discount plan, check whether the doctors you use participate. Call your providers, as well as others on the plan's list, before you enroll or pay any fees. Some dishonest plan promoters may tell you that particular local doctors participate when they don't, or they might send you outdated lists. Check out every claim, and get the details of the discount plan in writing before you sign up.

Don't Sign Up on the Spot

Legitimate plans should be willing to point you to written information and give you the chance to check out their claims before you enroll. Pressure to sign up quickly or miss out on a "special deal" is your cue to say, "no thanks."

Some Pitches Are after Your Information

Unfortunately, identity thieves also use pitches for medical discount plans and insurance to get your personal information. Don't give out your financial information to someone who calls you out of the blue, or whose reputation you haven't checked out. You can do that with your state insurance department, your state Attorney General, your local Better Business Bureau (BBB), and even by entering the company's name and the word "complaints" or "scam" in an online search engine to see what others have to say.

Checking out Plans

The idea behind medical discount plans—also known as discount healthcare programs—is that you will save money on products and services your insurance may not cover like dental, vision, hearing, or chiropractic services. Some people automatically get discount programs through their health insurance company.

Many states require medical discount programs to be licensed or registered. Your state insurance commissioner's office can tell you whether a medical discount program—or a health insurance plan—is licensed in your state, and may be able to alert you to a scam. Find your contact at naic.org.

Report Scams

If you've been targeted by a medical discount scam, report it to the Federal Trade Commission (FTC) at ftc.gov/complaint.
Federal Trade Commission (FTC)
600 Pennsylvania Ave. N.W.
Washington, DC 20580
Toll-Free: 877-FTC-HELP (877-382-4357)
Phone: 202-326-2222
Website: www.ftc.gov

Section 70.2

Marketplace Fraud

This section contains text excerpted from the following sources: Text under the heading "Health Insurance Marketplace" is excerpted from "Health Insurance Marketplace," Centers for Medicare and Medicaid Services (CMS), July 20, 2016; Text under the heading "Protect Yourself from Marketplace Fraud" is excerpted from "Protect Yourself from Marketplace Fraud," Centers for Medicare and Medicaid Services (CMS), January 19, 2014.

Health Insurance Marketplace

The Health Insurance Marketplace is a service that helps people shop for and enroll in affordable health insurance. The federal government operates the Marketplace, available at HealthCare.gov, for most states. Some states run their own Marketplaces.

The Health Insurance Marketplace (also known as the "Marketplace" or "exchange") provides health plan shopping and enrollment services through websites, call centers, and in-person help.

Small businesses can use the Small Business Health Options Program (SHOP) Marketplace to provide health insurance for their employees.

When you apply for individual and family coverage through the Marketplace, you'll provide income and household information. You'll find out if you qualify for:

- Premium tax credits and other savings that make insurance more affordable

- Coverage through the Medicaid and Children's Health Insurance Program (CHIP) in your state

Protect Yourself from Marketplace Fraud

When you apply for health coverage through the Health Insurance Marketplace, you can protect yourself from fraud by following a few simple guidelines. After you complete an application, you may get a phone call from the Marketplace to verify or ask for more information.

Be Informed about Your Healthcare Choices

- Spend some time with HealthCare.gov to learn the basics about getting health coverage. It's the official Marketplace website.

- Compare insurance plans carefully before making your decision. If you have questions, contact the Health Insurance Marketplace call center at 1-800-318-2596. TTY users should call 1-855-889-4325.

- Look for official government seals, logos, or web addresses (which end in ".gov") on materials you see in print or online.

- Know the Marketplace Open Enrollment dates. No one can enroll you in a health plan in the Marketplace until Open Enrollment begins or after it ends unless you have special circumstances.

Protect Your Private Healthcare and Financial Information

- Never give your financial information, like your banking, credit card, or account numbers, to someone who calls or comes to your home uninvited, even if they say they are from the Marketplace.

- Never give your personal health information, like your medical history or specific treatments you've received, to anyone who asks you for it. (If you apply for certain Marketplace exemptions, you may be asked for medical documentation.)

Ask Questions and Verify the Answers You Get

- The Marketplace has trained assisters in every state to help you at no cost. You should never be asked to pay for services or help to apply for Marketplace coverage.

- Ask questions if any information is unclear

- Write down and keep a record of the name of a salesperson or anyone who may assist you, who he or she works for, telephone number, street address, mailing address, email address, and website.

- Double check any information that is confusing or sounds fishy. Check out HealthCare.gov to verify things or call the Marketplace at 1-800-318-2596 (TTY: 1-855-889-4325).

If You Get a Call from the Marketplace

After you apply you may get a phone call from the Marketplace asking you to verify or provide more information.

Follow these tips to help prevent fraud:

If your phone has caller ID, check the number. The display may show one of these:

Health Insurance MP

InsMarketplace

701-264-3124

844-477-7500

The customer service representative will say they are calling from the Marketplace and provide a first name and agent ID number. Write them down.

A Marketplace representative may leave a message on your answering machine. If this happens, you won't be able to call back. If the Marketplace can't reach you after 3 tries, you'll get a letter in the mail telling you what to do next.

The Marketplace representative may ask you the following:

- To verify your identity, using information you provided on your application, including your full name and address.

- To provide or verify your Social Security number, application ID, policy ID, user ID, date of birth, or phone number.

- To verify or provide income, household, and employment information, but NOT personal financial information, like a bank name and account number. They will also not ask about any personal health information, like your medical history or conditions.

(If you're applying for certain Marketplace exemptions, you may be asked to provide medical documentation.)

If you don't want to answer over the phone, ask the representative to mail you a letter with instructions for completing your application.

In certain cases, the Marketplace may request additional documentation. If you need to mail any information to the:

Health Insurance Marketplace
465 Industrial Blvd.
London, KY 40750-0001

Don't mail any information to a different address. The ZIP code may end with 4 extra numbers the representative provides.

When to Report Suspected Fraud

It's time to take action if:

- Someone other than the insurance company you've chosen contacts you about health insurance and asks you to pay – or asks for your financial or personal health information

- Someone you don't know contacts you about getting health insurance and asks you to pay – or asks you for your personal financial or health information

- Someone contacts you and claims to be from the government or Medicare – and asks you to pay for a new "Obamacare" insurance card

- You give your personal health, bank account, or credit card information to someone who calls you and says they're from the government

How to Report Suspected Fraud

You can report suspected fraud one of two ways:

- If you suspect identity theft, or feel like you gave your personal information to someone you shouldn't have, use the Federal Trade Commission's online Complaint Assistant. You should also contact your local police department. Visit www.ftc.gov/idtheft to learn more about identity theft.

- Call the Health Insurance Marketplace call center at 1-800-318-2596 (TTY: 1-855-889-4325). Explain what happened and your information will be handled appropriately.

Chapter 71

The Pre-Existing Condition Insurance Plan

Pre-Existing Conditions

Under the Affordable Care Act (ACA), health insurance companies can't refuse to cover you or charge you more just because you have a "pre-existing condition"—that is, a health problem you had before the date that new health coverage starts. They also can't charge women more than men.

These rules went into effect for plan years beginning on or after January 1, 2014.

What This Means for You

Health insurers can no longer charge more or deny coverage to you or your child because of a pre-existing health condition like asthma, diabetes, or cancer. They cannot limit benefits for that condition either.

This chapter contains text excerpted from the following sources: Text beginning with the heading "Pre-Existing Conditions" is excerpted from "Pre-Existing Conditions," U.S. Department of Health and Human Services (HHS), November 18, 2014; Text beginning with the heading "Coverage for Pre-Existing Conditions" is excerpted from "Health Benefits and Coverage," Centers for Medicare and Medicaid Services (CMS), October 9, 2015; Text beginning with the heading "Pre-Existing Condition Insurance Plan (PCIP)" is excerpted from "The Center for Consumer Information and Insurance Oversight," Centers for Medicare and Medicaid Services (CMS), March 2, 2011. Reviewed January 2017.

Once you have insurance, they can't refuse to cover treatment for your pre-existing condition.

One Exception: Grandfathered Plans

The pre-existing coverage rule does not apply to "grandfathered" individual health insurance policies. A grandfathered individual health insurance policy is a policy that you bought for yourself or your family on or before March 23, 2010 that has not been changed in certain specific ways that reduce benefits or increase costs to consumers.

Pre-Existing Condition Insurance Plan (PCIP) Coverage

The Pre-existing Condition Insurance Plan (PCIP) ended on April 30, 2014. The PCIP program provided health coverage options to individuals who were uninsured for at least six months, had a pre-existing condition, and had been denied coverage (or offered insurance without coverage of the pre-existing condition) by a private insurance company. Now, thanks to the Affordable Care Act, health insurance plans can no longer deny anyone coverage for their pre-existing condition, and so PCIP enrollees can transition to a new plan outside of the PCIP program.

Coverage for Pre-Existing Conditions

All marketplace plans must cover treatment for pre-existing medical conditions.

- No insurance plan can reject you, charge you more, or refuse to pay for essential health benefits for any condition you had before your coverage started.

- Once you're enrolled, the plan can't deny you coverage or raise your rates based only on your health.

- Medicaid and the Children's Health Insurance Program (CHIP) also can't refuse to cover you or charge you more because of your pre-existing condition.

Pregnancy Is Covered from the Day Your Plan Starts

- If you're pregnant when you apply, an insurance plan can't reject you or charge you more because of your pregnancy.

- Once you're enrolled, your pregnancy and childbirth are covered from the day your plan starts.

- **If you have a 2017 health plan and give birth or adopt after you enrolled:**

  - If you give birth or adopt before January 31, 2017, you can report the update on your application by logging in to report the change.

  - If you give birth or adopt after January 31, your child's birth or adoption will qualify you for a Special Enrollment Period. This means you can enroll in or change plans outside the annual Open Enrollment Period. Your coverage can start from the date of birth or adoption, even if you enroll up to 60 days afterward.

- **If you have a 2016 health plan and give birth or adopt in the final months of 2016:** Having a baby or adopting a child qualifies you for a Special Enrollment Period so you can enroll in or change plans for the rest of 2016. Your coverage can start the day of the event—even if you enroll in the plan up to 60 days afterward.

Exception: Grandfathered Plans Don't Have to Cover Pre-Existing Conditions

Grandfathered plans don't have to cover pre-existing conditions or preventive care. If you have a grandfathered plan and want pre-existing conditions covered, you have 2 options:

- You can switch to a Marketplace plan that will cover them during Open Enrollment.

- You can buy a Marketplace plan outside Open Enrollment when your grandfathered plan year ends, and you'll qualify for a Special Enrollment Period.

Pre-Existing Condition Insurance Plan (PCIP)

The Affordable Care Act created the Pre-Existing Condition Insurance Plan to make health insurance available to those that have been denied coverage by private insurance companies because of a pre-existing condition.

PCIP provides health coverage options for people who:

- Have been uninsured for at least six months

- Have a pre-existing condition or have been denied health coverage because of a health condition

- Are a U.S. citizen or are residing here legally

PCIP Program Basics:

- PCIP covers a broad range of health benefits, including primary and specialty care, hospital care, and prescription drugs.

- The program will not charge you a higher premium just because of your medical condition.

- PCIP does not base eligibility on income.

State Programs

Previously, many states have run "high-risk pools" or other programs that offer insurance to people with pre-existing conditions. Now, PCIP is available in every state, but the program may vary between states.

The U.S. Department of Health and Human Services (HHS), the Office of Personnel Management (OPM), and United States Department of Agriculture's (USDA) National Finance Center (NFC), are running PCIP in some states. The federal government is contracting with a national insurance plan to administer benefits in those states. States have the option to build on their current programs, choose to run the new program, or elect to rely on HHS to provide coverage.

To learn more about PCIP, including eligibility, how to apply, and benefits, please call 1-866-717-5826.

Chapter 72

Filing a Claim for Your Health or Disability Benefits

If you participate in a health plan or a plan that provides disability benefits, you will want to know how to file a claim for your benefits. The steps outlined below describe some of your plan's obligations and briefly explain the procedures and timelines for filing a health or disability benefits claim.

Before you file, however, be aware of the Employee Retirement Income Security Act of 1974 (ERISA), a federal law that protects your health and disability benefits and sets standards for those who administer your plan. Among other things, the law and rules issued by the U.S. Department of Labor (DOL) include requirements for the processing of benefit claims, the timeline for a decision when you file a claim, and your rights when a claim is denied.

The Affordable Care Act (also called "Obamacare") includes additional requirements for claims processing for group health plans that are "non-grandfathered." A non-grandfathered health plan is a plan that was established, or that has made certain significant changes, after March 23, 2010.

You should know that ERISA does not cover some employee benefit plans (such as those sponsored by government entities and most churches). If, however, you are one of the millions of participants and

---

This chapter includes text excerpted from "Filing a Claim for Your Health or Disability Benefits," U.S. Department of Labor (DOL), March 10, 2007. Reviewed January 2017.

beneficiaries who depend on health or disability benefits from a private-sector employment-based plan, take a few minutes and read on to learn more.

Reviewing Information from Your Plan

A key document related to your plan is the summary plan description (SPD). The SPD is the brochure you receive when you first are covered by your employer's plan. It provides a detailed overview of the plan—how it works, what benefits it provides, and how to file a claim for benefits. It also describes your rights as well as your responsibilities under ERISA and your plan. You also can find answers to many of your questions in the Summary of Benefits and Coverage (SBC), a short, easy-to-understand summary of the benefits available under your plan and detailed information on the out-of-pocket costs for coverage. For some single-employer collectively bargained plans, you should also check the collective bargaining agreement's claim filing, grievance, and appeal procedures as they may apply to claims for health and disability benefits.

Before you apply for health or disability benefits, review the SPD to make sure you meet the plan's requirements and understand the procedures for filing a claim. Sometimes claims procedures are contained in a separate booklet that is handed out with your SPD. If you do not have a copy of your plan's SPD or claims procedures, make a written request for one or both to your plan's administrator. Your plan administrator is required to provide you with a copy.

Filing a Claim

An important first step is to check your SPD and your SBC to make sure you meet your plan's requirements to receive benefits. Your plan might say, for example, that a waiting period must pass before you can enroll and receive benefits or that a dependent is not covered after a certain age. Also, be aware of what your plan requires to file a claim. The SPD or claims procedure booklet must including information on where to file, what to file, and whom to contact if you have questions about your plan, such as the process for providing a required pre-approval for health benefits. Plans generally cannot charge any filing fees or costs for filing claims and appeals.

If, for any reason, that information is not in the SPD or claims procedure booklet, write your plan administrator, your employer's human resource department (or the office that normally handles claims), or your employer to notify them that you have a claim. Keep a copy of the letter for your records. You may also want to send the letter by certified mail, return receipt requested, so you will have a record that the letter was received and by whom.

If it is not you, but an authorized representative who is filing the claim, that person should refer to the SPD and follow your plan's claims procedure. Your plan may require you to complete a form to name the representative. If it is an emergency situation, the treating physician can automatically become your authorized representative without you having to complete a form.

When a claim is filed, be sure to keep a copy for your records.

Types of Claims

All health and disability benefit claims must be decided within a specific time limit, depending on the type of claim filed.

Group health claims are divided into three types: urgent care, pre-service and post-service claims, with the type of claim determining how quickly a decision must be made. The plan must decide what type of claim it is except when a physician determines that the urgent care is needed.

Urgent care claims are a special kind of pre-service claim that requires a quicker decision because your health would be threatened if the plan took the normal time permitted to decide a pre-service claim. If a physician with knowledge of your medical condition tells the plan that a pre-service claim is urgent, the plan must treat it as an urgent care claim.

Pre-service claims are requests for approval that the plan requires you to obtain before you get medical care, such as preauthorization or a decision on whether a treatment or procedure is medically necessary.

Post-service claims are all other claims for benefits under your group health plan, including claims after medical services have been provided, such as requests for reimbursement or payment of the costs of the services provided. Most claims for group health benefits are post-service claims.

Disability claims are requests for benefits where the plan must make a determination of disability to decide the claim.

Waiting For a Decision on Your Claim

As noted, ERISA sets specific periods of time for plans to evaluate your claim and inform you of the decision. The time limits are counted in calendar days, so weekends and holidays are included. These limits do not govern when the benefits must be paid or provided. If you are entitled to benefits, check your SPD for how and when benefits are paid. Plans are required to pay or provide benefits within a reasonable time after a claim is approved.

Urgent care claims must be decided as soon as possible, taking into account the medical needs of the patient, but no later than 72 hours after the plan receives the claim. The plan must tell you within 24 hours if more information is needed; you will have no less than 48 hours to respond. Then the plan must decide the claim within 48 hours after the missing information is supplied or the time to supply it has elapsed. The plan cannot extend the time to make the initial decision without your consent. The plan must give you notice that your claim has been granted or denied before the end of the time allotted for the decision. The plan can notify you orally of the benefit determination so long as a written notification is furnished to you no later than three days after the oral notification.

Pre-service claims must be decided within a reasonable period of time appropriate to the medical circumstances, but no later than 15 days after the plan has received the claim. The plan may extend the time period up to an additional 15 days if, for reasons beyond the plan's control, the decision cannot be made within the first 15 days. The plan administrator must notify you prior to the expiration of the first 15-day period, explaining the reason for the delay, requesting any additional information, and advising you when the plan expects to make the decision. If more information is requested, you have at least 45 days to supply it. The plan then must decide the claim no later than 15 days after you supply the additional information or after the period of time allowed to supply it ends, whichever comes first. If the plan wants more time, the plan needs your consent. The plan must give you written notice that your claim has been granted or denied before the end of the time allotted for the decision.

Post-service health claims must be decided within a reasonable period of time, but not later than 30 days after the plan has received the claim. If, because of reasons beyond the plan's control, more time is needed to review your request, the plan may extend the time period up to an additional 15 days. However, the plan administrator has to let you know before the end of the first 30-day period, explaining the reason for the delay, requesting any additional information needed, and advising you when a final decision is expected. If more information is requested, you have at least 45 days to supply it. The claim then must be decided no later than 15 days after you supply the additional information or the period of time given by the plan to do so ends, whichever comes first. The plan needs your consent if it wants more time after its first extension. The plan must give you notice that your claim has been denied in whole or in part (paying less than 100 percent of the claim) before the end of the time allotted for the decision.

Disability claims must be decided within a reasonable period of time, but not later than 45 days after the plan has received the claim. If, because of reasons beyond the plan's control, more time is needed to review your request, the plan can extend the timeframe up to 30 days. The plan must tell you prior to the end of the first 45-day period that additional time is needed, explaining why, any unresolved issues and additional information needed, and when the plan expects to render a final decision. If more information is requested during either extension period, you will have at least 45 days to supply it. The claim then must be decided no later than 30 days after you supply the additional information or the period of time given by the plan to do so ends, whichever comes first. The plan administrator may extend the time period for up to another 30 days as long as it notifies you before the first extension expires. For any additional extensions, the plan needs your consent. The plan must give you notice whether your claim has been denied before the end of the time allotted for the decision.

If your claim is denied, the plan administrator must send you a notice, either in writing or electronically, with a detailed explanation of why your claim was denied and a description of the appeal process. In addition, the plan must include the plan rules, guidelines, or exclusions (such as medical necessity or experimental treatment exclusions) used in the decision or provide you with instructions on how you can request a copy of these documents from the plan. The notice may also include a specific request for you to provide the plan with additional information in case you wish to appeal your denial.

Appealing a Denied Claim

Claims are denied for various reasons. Perhaps you are not eligible for benefits. Perhaps the services you received are not covered by your plan. Or, perhaps the plan simply needs more information about your claim. Whatever the reason, you have at least 180 days to file an appeal (check your SPD or claims procedure to see if your plan provides a longer period).

Use the information in your claim denial notice in preparing your appeal. You should also be aware that the plan must provide claimants, on request and free of charge, copies of documents, records, and other information relevant to the claim for benefits. The plan also must identify, at your request, any medical or vocational expert whose advice was obtained by the plan. Be sure to include in your appeal all information related to your claim, particularly any additional information or evidence that you want the plan to consider, and get it to the person specified in the denial notice before the end of the 180-day period.

Reviewing an Appeal

On appeal, your claim must be reviewed by someone new who looks at all of the information submitted and consults with qualified medical professionals if a medical judgment is involved. This reviewer cannot be the same person or a subordinate of the person who made the initial decision and the reviewer must give no consideration to that decision.

Plans have specific periods of time within which to review your appeal, depending on the type of claim.

Urgent care claims must be reviewed as soon as possible, taking into account the medical needs of the patient, but not later than 72 hours after the plan receives your request to review a denied claim.

Pre-service claims must be reviewed within a reasonable period of time appropriate to the medical circumstances, but not later than 30 days after the plan receives your request to review a denied claim.

Post-service claims must be reviewed within a reasonable period of time, but not later than 60 days after the plan receives your request to review a denied claim.

If a group health plan needs more time, the plan must get your consent. If you do not agree to more time, the plan must complete the review within the permitted time limit.

Disability claims must be reviewed within a reasonable period of time, but not later than 45 days after the plan receives your request to review a denied claim. If the plan determines special circumstances exist and an extension is needed, the plan may take up to an additional

45 days to decide the appeal. However, before taking the extension, the plan must notify you in writing during the first 45-day period explaining the special circumstances, and the date by which the plan expects to make the decision.

There are two exceptions to these time limits. In general, single-employer collectively bargained plans may use a collectively bargained grievance process for their claims appeal procedure if it has provisions on filing, determination, and review of benefit claims. Multi-employer collectively bargained plans are given special timeframes to allow them to schedule reviews on appeal of post-service claims and disability claims for the regular quarterly meetings of their boards of trustees. If you are a participant in one of those plans and you have questions about your plan's procedures, you can consult your plan's SPD and collective bargaining agreement or contact the Department of Labor's Employee Benefits Security Administration (EBSA).

Plans can require you to go through two levels of review of a denied health or disability claim to finish the plan's claims process. If two levels of review are required, the maximum time for each review generally is half of the time limit permitted for one review. For example, in the case of a group health plan with one appeal level, as noted above, the review of a pre-service claim must be completed within a reasonable period of time appropriate to the medical circumstances but no later than 30 days after the plan gets your appeal. If the plan requires two appeals, each review must be completed within 15 days for pre-service claims. If your claim on appeal is still denied after the first review, the plan has to allow you a reasonable period of time (but not a full 180 days) to file for the second review.

Once the final decision on your claim is made, the plan must send you a written explanation of the decision. The notice must be in plain language that can be understood by participants in the plan. It must include all the specific reasons for the denial of your claim on appeal, refer you to the plan provisions on which the decision is based, tell you if the plan has any additional voluntary levels of appeal, explain your right to receive documents that are relevant to your benefit claim free of charge, and describe your rights to seek judicial review of the plan's decision.

If Your Appeal Is Denied

If the plan's final decision denies your claim, you may want to seek legal advice regarding your rights to bring an action in court to challenge the denial. Normally, you must complete your plan's claim process before filing an action in court to challenge the denial of a claim for benefits. However, if you believe your plan failed to establish or follow a claims procedure consistent with the Department's rules described in this booklet, you may want to seek legal advice regarding your right to ask a court to review your benefit claim without waiting for a decision from the plan. You also may want to contact the nearest EBSA office about your rights if you believe the plan failed to follow any of ERISA's requirements in handling your benefit claim.

If your appeal is denied and you are in a non-grandfathered health plan, you also have the right to external review of the decision, as discussed below. To find out if your plan is not grandfathered, check the documents from your plan describing the plan's benefits. If your plan is grandfathered, it must be disclosed. If there is no disclosure in your plan's documents, your plan likely is not grandfathered.

Additional Protections If Your Plan Is Not Grandfathered under the Affordable Care Act

Non-grandfathered health plans, or insurers to those plans, must provide additional internal claims and appeal rights and a process for external review of benefit claim denials. Internal claims and appeals are your health claims or appeals of denials reviewed by your plan. These rights also apply to rescissions (retroactive cancellations) of coverage.

The additional internal claims and appeal protections include:

- Providing you with new or additional evidence or rationale, and the opportunity to respond to it, before the final decision is made on the claim;

- Ensuring that claims and appeals are adjudicated in an independent and impartial manner;

- Providing detail on the claim involved, the reason for denial (including the denial code and meaning), the internal and external appeals processes that are available, and information on consumer assistance, in all claims denial notices;

- Providing, on request, diagnosis and treatment codes (and their meanings) for any denied claim;

- Providing notices in a culturally and linguistically appropriate manner;

- Allowing you to begin the external review process if the plan fails to follow the internal claims requirements (unless the plan's violation is minimal); and

- Allowing you to resubmit an internal claim if a request for immediate external review is rejected.

Non-grandfathered plans also must provide a process for an external review of claims denials by an independent party. The external review process used depends on whether the plan is self-funded or provides benefits through an insurance company. The notice of the denial of your claim from your plan will describe the external review process and your rights. To request an external review of your claim denial, follow the steps provided in your denial notice.

Chapter 73

Rights to Appeal Health Plan Decisions

Under the Affordable Care Act (ACA), you have the right to appeal a health insurance company's decision to deny payment for a claim or to terminate your health coverage. The following rules for appeals apply to health plans created after March 23, 2010, and to older plans that have been changed in certain ways since that date.

You can appeal your insurance company's decision through an "internal appeal," in which you ask your insurance company to do a full and fair review of its decision. If your insurance company still denies payment or coverage, the law permits you to have an independent third party decide to uphold or overturn the plan's decision. This final process is often referred to as an "external review."

Your state may have a Consumer Assistance Program that can help you file an appeal or request a review of your health insurance company's decision if you are not sure what steps to take. Your insurance company should have provided you with information about how to file an appeal and the appeals process when you were enrolled in coverage, and there may be information about the process on the plan's website.

Internal Appeals

Your internal appeals rights took effect when your plan starts a new plan year or policy year on or after September 23, 2010.

This chapter includes text excerpted from "Appealing Health Plan Decisions, " U.S. Department of Health and Human Services (HHS), September 16, 2014.

External Review

If after an internal appeal the plan still denies your request for payment or services, you can ask for an independent external review. For plan years or policy years that begin on or after July 1, 2011, your plan must include information on your denial notice about how to request this review. If your state has a Consumer Assistance Program, that program can help you with this request. If the external reviewer reverses your insurance company's denial, your insurance company must give you the payments or services you requested in your claim.

What This Means for You

If your insurance company denies payment for a claim or terminates your health coverage, you can request an appeal. When your insurance company receives your request, it is required to review and explain its decision. The insurance company must also let you know how you can disagree with its decision. It is required to start and complete the process in a timely manner.

If you don't speak English, you may be entitled to receive appeals information in the language you speak upon request (Spanish and some other languages are available). This right applies to plan years or policy years that started on or after January 1, 2012.

Some Important Details

- Health plans that started on or before March 23, 2010 may be "grandfathered health plans." The appeals and review rights don't apply to them.

- Appeal rights depend on the state you live in and the type of health plan you have. Some group plans may require more than one level of internal appeal before you can request an external review.

Part Eight

Additional Help and Information

Chapter 74

Glossary of Terms Related to Disease Management

activities of daily living (ADL): The tasks of everyday life. These activities include eating, dressing, getting into or out of a bed or chair, taking a bath or shower, and using the shopping, doing housework, and using a telephone.

advance directive: A legal document that states the treatment or care a person wishes to receive or not receive if he or she becomes unable to make medical decisions (for example, due to being unconscious or in a coma).

anesthesiology: A medical specialty concerned with purposeful depression of nerve function, characterized by loss of feeling or sensation, usually the result of pharmacologic action by anesthetics, and induced to allow performance of surgery or other painful procedures.

antibiotic: A drug used to treat infections caused by bacteria and other microorganisms.

anxiety: Feelings of fear, dread, and uneasiness that may occur as a reaction to stress. A person with anxiety may sweat, feel restless and tense, and have a rapid heart beat.

assessment: In healthcare, a process used to learn about a patient's condition.

This glossary contains terms excerpted from documents produced by several sources deemed reliable.

assistive device: A tool that helps a person with a disability to do a certain task. Examples are a cane, wheelchair, scooter, walker, hearing aid, or special bed.

assistive technology: Any device or technology that helps a disabled person. Examples are special grips for holding utensils, computer screen monitors to help a person with low vision read more easily.

blood transfusion: The administration of blood or blood products into a blood vessel.

blood: A tissue with red blood cells, white blood cells, platelets, and other substances suspended in fluid called plasma. Blood takes oxygen and nutrients to the tissues, and carries away wastes.

cancer: A term for diseases in which abnormal cells divide without control. Cancer cells can invade nearby tissues and can spread to other parts of the body through the blood and lymph systems.

cardiology: A medical subspecialty concerned with the study of the heart, its physiology, and its functions.

cardiopulmonary: Having to do with the heart and lungs.

cell: The individual unit that makes up the tissues of the body. All living things are made up of one or more cells.

chaplain: A member of the clergy in charge of a chapel or who works with the military or with an institution, such as a hospital.

chemotherapy: Treatment with drugs that kill cancer cells.

clinical trial: A type of research study that tests how well new medical approaches work in people. These studies test new methods of screening, prevention, diagnosis, or treatment of a disease; also called a clinical study.

COBRA: An abbreviation for the Consolidated Omnibus Budget Reconciliation Act of 1986, a law that provides for a temporary extension of health plan coverage from a prior group health plan.

counseling: The process by which a professional counselor helps a person cope with mental or emotional distress, and understand and solve personal problems.

cure: To heal or restore health; a treatment to restore health.

depression: A mental condition marked by ongoing feelings of sadness, despair, loss of energy, and difficulty dealing with normal daily life. Other symptoms of depression include feelings of worthlessness and hopelessness, loss of pleasure in activities, changes in eating or sleeping habits, and thoughts of death or suicide.

diagnosis: The process of identifying a disease by the signs and symptoms.

dietitian: A health professional with special training in nutrition who can help with dietary choices, also called a nutritionist.

drug: Any substance, other than food, that is used to prevent, diagnose, treat, or relieve symptoms of a disease or abnormal condition.

durable power of attorney (DPA): A type of power of attorney. A power of attorney is a legal document that gives one person (such as a relative, lawyer, or friend) the authority to make legal, medical, or financial decisions for another person.

enrollment date: The first day of health insurance coverage or the first day of the waiting period (if applicable).

family practice: A medical specialty concerned with the provision of continuing, comprehensive primary healthcare for the entire family.

geriatrics: The subspecialty of medicine concerned with the physiological and pathological aspects of the aged, including, but not limited to, the clinical problems of senescence and senility.

hospice: A program that provides special care for people who are near the end of life and for their families, either at home, in freestanding facilities, or within hospitals.

infection: Invasion and multiplication of germs in the body. Infections can occur in any part of the body and can spread throughout the body. The germs may be bacteria, viruses, yeast, or fungi. They can cause a fever and other problems, depending on where the infection occurs.

insured plan: A plan which provides benefits through an insurance company or HMO. Check your summary plan description (SPD) to see if your plan is insured.

late enrollee: An individual who enrolls in the plan at some time other than when first eligible or a special enrollment opportunity.

living will: A type of legal advance directive in which a person describes specific treatment guidelines that are to be followed by healthcare providers if he or she becomes terminally ill and cannot communicate.

lung: One of a pair of organs in the chest that supplies the body with oxygen and removes carbon dioxide from the body.

mental health: A person's overall psychological and emotional condition. Good mental health is a state of well-being in which a person is able to cope with everyday events, think clearly, be responsible, meet challenges, and have good relationships with others.

nephrology: A subspecialty of internal medicine concerned with the anatomy, physiology, and pathology of the kidney.

neurology: A medical specialty concerned with the study of the structures, functions, and diseases of the nervous system.

nuclear medicine: A subspecialty field of radiology concerned with diagnostic, therapeutic, and investigative use of radioactive compounds in pharmaceutical form.

nurse: A health professional trained to care for people who are ill or disabled.

nursing home: A place that gives care to people who have physical or mental disabilities and need help with activities of daily living (such as taking a bath, getting dressed, and going to the bathroom) but do not need to be in the hospital.

nursing: The profession concerned with the provision of care and services essential to the promotion, maintenance, and restoration of health by attending to a patient's needs.

nutrition: The clinical practice concerned with nutrients and other substances contained in food and their action, interaction, and balance in relation to health and disease.

obstetrics and gynecology: The medical-surgical specialty concerned with management and care of women during pregnancy, parturition, and puerperium; the physiology and disorders primarily of the female genital tract; and female endocrinology and reproductive physiology.

occupational therapist: A health professional trained to help people who are ill or disabled learn to manage their daily activities.

oncology: A subspecialty of internal medicine concerned with the study of neoplasms.

outpatient: A patient who visits a healthcare facility for diagnosis or treatment without spending the night, sometimes called a day patient.

palliative care: Care given to improve the quality of life of patients who have a serious or life-threatening disease. The goal of palliative care is to prevent or treat as early as possible the symptoms of the disease, side effects caused by treatment of the disease, and psychological, social, and spiritual problems related to the disease or its treatment, also called comfort care, supportive care, and symptom management.

pediatrics: A medical specialty concerned with the physical, emotional, and social health of children from birth to young adulthood.

pharmacology: A clinical specialty concerned with the effectiveness and safety of drugs in humans.

physical examination: An exam of the body to check for general signs of disease.

physical medicine and rehabilitation: A medical specialty concerned with the use of physical agents, mechanical apparatuses, and manipulation in rehabilitating patients who are physically diseased, injured, or recovering from elective surgery (e.g., hip replacement) to the maximum degree possible. Physicians practicing this specialty are Physiatrists.

physical therapist: A health professional who teaches exercises and physical activities that help condition muscles and restore strength and movement.

podiatry: A profession concerned with the diagnosis and treatment of disorders, injuries and anatomic defects of the foot.

preexisting condition exclusion period: The amount of time that you are excluded from health insurance coverage of benefits for a preexisting condition (the maximum is 12 months, or 18 months for late enrollees).

psychological: Having to do with how the mind works and how thoughts and feelings affect behavior.

psychologist: A specialist who can talk with patients and their families about emotional and personal matters and can help them make decisions.

psychology: A clinical profession concerned with recognizing and treating behavior disorders.

pump: A device that is used to give a controlled amount of a liquid at a specific rate. For example, pumps are used to give drugs (such as chemotherapy or pain medicine) or nutrients.

quality of life: The overall enjoyment of life.

radiology: The specialty concerned with the use of X-ray and other forms of radiant energy in the diagnosis and treatment of disease.

rehabilitation: In medicine, a process to restore mental or physical abilities lost to injury or disease, in order to function in a normal or near-normal way.

remission: A decrease in or disappearance of signs and symptoms of illness such as cancer.

respirator: In medicine, a machine used to help a patient breathe, also called ventilator.

rheumatology: A subspecialty of internal medicine concerned with the study of inflammatory or degenerative processes and metabolic derangement of connective tissue structures that pertain to a variety of musculoskeletal disorders (e.g., arthritis).

screening: Checking for disease when there are no symptoms.

side effect: A problem that occurs when treatment affects healthy tissues or organs. Some common side effects of cancer treatment are fatigue, pain, nausea, vomiting, decreased blood cell counts, hair loss, and mouth sores.

similarly situated individuals: Permitted distinctions health insurance plans may make among individuals, such as groups of employees, if based on bona fide employment-based classifications consistent with the employer's usual business practice.

social service: A community resource that helps people in need. Services may include help getting to and from medical appointments, home delivery of medication and meals, in-home nursing care, help paying medical costs not covered by insurance, loaning medical equipment, and housekeeping help.

social worker: A professional trained to talk with people and their families about emotional or physical needs and to find them support services.

special enrollment: An opportunity for certain individuals to enroll in a group health plan, regardless of the plan's regular enrollment dates.

speech-language pathology: A clinical profession concerned with the study of speech/language and swallowing disorders and their diagnosis and correction. special enrollment: An opportunity for certain individuals to enroll in a group health plan, regardless of the plan's regular enrollment dates. These opportunities occur when you lose eligibility for other coverage or experience certain life events (marriage, birth, adoption, or placement for adoption).

stage: The extent of a cancer in the body. Staging is usually based on the size of the tumor, whether lymph nodes contain cancer, and whether the cancer has spread from the original site to other parts of the body.

summary plan description (SPD): A document outlining your plan, usually provided when you enroll in the plan.

support group: A group of people with similar disease who meet to discuss how better to cope with their disease and treatment.

supportive care: Care given to improve the quality of life of patients who have a serious or life-threatening disease.

surgery: A medical specialty concerned with manual or operative procedures used in the diagnosis and treatment of diseases, injuries, or deformities.

symptom: An indication that a person has a condition or disease. Some examples of symptoms are headache, fever, fatigue, nausea, vomiting, and pain.

tube feeding: A type of enteral nutrition (nutrition that is delivered into the digestive system in a liquid form). For tube feeding, a small tube may be placed through the nose into the stomach or the small intestine.

waiting period: The time that must pass before coverage can become effective under the terms of a group health plan.

Chapter 75

Directory of Organizations That Provide Information about Disease Management

Government Agencies That Provide Information about Disease Management

Administration on Aging (AoA)
National Aging Information Center
330 C St. S.W.
Washington, DC 20201
Toll-Free: 800-677-1116
(Eldercare Locator)
Phone: 202-619-7501
Website: www.aoa.acl.gov
E-mail: aclinfo@acl.hhs.gov

Agency for Healthcare Research and Quality (AHRQ)
U.S. Department of Health and Human Services (HHS)
5600 Fishers Ln.
Rockville, MD 20857
Toll-Free: 800-358-9295
Phone: 301-427-1364
Website: www.ahrq.gov
E-mail: info@ahrq.gov

Resources in this chapter were compiled from several sources deemed reliable; all contact information was verified and updated in January 2017.

Centers for Medicare and Medicaid Services (CMS)
7500 Security Blvd.
Baltimore, MD 21244
Toll-Free: 800-MEDICARE
(800-633-4227)
Phone: 410-786-3000
Toll-Free TTY: 866-226-1819
TTY: 410-786-0727
Website: www.cms.gov

Centers for Disease Control and Prevention (CDC)
1600 Clifton Rd.
Atlanta, GA 30329-4027
Toll-Free: 800-CDC-INFO
(800-232-4636)
Phone: 404-639-3534
TTY: 888-232-6348
Website: www.cdc.gov
E-mail: cdcinfo@cdc.gov

Equal Employment Opportunity Commission (EEOC)
1801 L St. N.W.
Washington, DC 20507
Toll-Free: 800-669-4000
Phone: 202-663-4500
Toll-Free TDD: 800-669-6820
Fax: 202-653-6034
Website: www.eeoc.gov
E-mail: info@eeoc.gov

Eunice Kennedy Shriver National Institute of Child Health and Human Development (NICHD)
Information Resource Center
P.O. Box 3006
Rockville, MD 20847
Phone: 800-370-2943
TTY: 888-320-6942
Fax: 866-760-5947
Website: www.nichd.nih.gov
E-mail: NICHDInformation
ResourceCenter@mail.nih.gov

Federal Trade Commission (FTC)
600 Pennsylvania Ave. N.W.
Washington, DC 20580
Toll-Free: 877-FTC-HELP
(877-382-4357)
Phone: 202-326-2222
TTY: 866-653-4261
Website: www.ftc.gov

Health Resources and Services Administration (HRSA)
Information Center
P.O. Box 2910
Merrifield, VA 22116
Toll-Free: 888-275-4772
Toll-Free TTY: 877-489-4772
Fax: 703-821-2098
Website: www.hrsa.gov
E-mail: ask@hrsa.gov

Healthfinder®
National Health Information
Center (NHIC)
1101 Wootton Pkwy
Rockville, MD 20852
Fax: 301-984-4256
Website: www.healthfinder.gov
E-mail: healthfinder@hhs.gov

*National Cancer Institute
(NCI)*
Public Inquiries Office
9609 Medical Center Dr.
Bethesda, MD 20892-9760
Toll-Free: 800-4-CANCER
(800-422-6237)
Toll-Free TTY: 800-332-8615
Website: www.cancer.gov
E-mail: cancergovstaff@mail.nih.
gov

*National Diabetes
Information Clearinghouse
(NDIC)*
1 Information Way
Bethesda, MD 20892-3560
Toll-Free: 800-860-8747
TTY: 866–569–1162
Fax: 703-738-4929
Website: www.diabetes.niddk.
nih.gov
E-mail: ndic@info.niddk.nih.gov

*National Center for
Chronic Disease Prevention
and Health Promotion
(NCCDPHP)*
4770 Buford Hwy. N.E.
Atlanta, GA 30341
Toll-Free: 800-311-3435
Phone: 404-639-3534
Website: www.cdc.gov/nccdphp
E-mail: ccdinfo@cdc.gov

*National Center for
Complementary and
Integrative Health (NCCIH)*
9000 Rockville Pike
Bethesda, MD 20892
Toll-Free: 888-644-6226
Phone: 301-519-3153
Toll-Free TTY: 866-464-3615
TTY: 866-464-3615
Fax: 866-464-3616
Website: www.nccih.nih.gov
E-mail: info@nccih.nih.gov

*National Health Information
Center*
P.O. Box 1133
Washington, DC 20013-1133
Toll-Free: 800-336-4797
Phone: 301-565-4167
Fax: 301-984-4256
Website: www.health.gov/NHIC
E-mail: nhicinfo@health.org

National Heart, Lung, and Blood Institute (NHLBI)
P.O. Box 30105
Bethesda, MD 20824-0105
Phone: 301-592-8573
TTY: 240-629-3255
Fax: 301-592-8563
Website: www.nhlbi.nih.gov
E-mail: nhlbiinfo@nhlbi.nih.gov

National Human Genome Research Institute (NHGRI)
National Institutes of Health (NIH)
31 Center Dr. MSC 2152
Bethesda, MD 20892-2152
Phone: 301-402-0911
Fax: 301-402-2218
Website: www.genome.gov

National Institute of Arthritis and Musculoskeletal and Skin Diseases (NIAMS)
1 AMS Circle
Bethesda, MD 20892-3675
Toll-Free: 877-22-NIAMS
(877-226-4267)
Phone: 301-496-8190
TTY: 301-565-2966
Fax: 301-480-2814
Website: www.niams.nih.gov
E-mail: NIAMSinfo@mail.nih. gov.

National Institute of Diabetes and Digestive and Kidney Diseases (NIDDK)
Office of Communications and Public Liaison (OCPL)
31 Center Dr.
Bethesda, MD 20892-2560
Phone: 301-496-3583
Website: www.niddk.nih.gov

National Institute of Mental Health (NIMH)
6001 Executive Blvd.
Rm. 6200 MSC 9663
Bethesda, MD 20892-9663
Toll-Free: 866-615-6464
Phone: 301-443-4513
Toll-Free TTY: 866-415-8051
TTY: 301-443-8431
Fax: 301-443-4279
Website: www.nimh.nih.gov
E-mail: nimhinfo@nih.gov

National Institute of Neurological Disorders and Stroke (NINDS)
P.O. Box 5801
Bethesda, MD 20824
Toll-Free: 800-352-9424
Phone: 301-496-5751
TTY: 301-496-5981
Website: www.ninds.nih.gov

National Institute on Aging (NIA)
P.O. Box 8057
Gaithersburg, MD 20898
Toll-Free: 800-222-2225
Phone: 301-496-1752
Toll-Free TTY: 800-222-4225
Fax: 301-496-1072
Website: www.nia.nih.gov

National Institutes of Health (NIH)
9000 Rockville Pike
Bethesda, MD 20892
Phone: 301-496-4000
TTY: 301-402-9612
Website: www.nih.gov
E-mail: NIHinfo@od.nih.gov

National Women's Health Information Center (NWHIC)
200 Independence Ave. S.W.
Rm. 712E
Washington, DC 20201
Toll-Free: 800-994-9662
Phone: 202-690-7650
Fax: 202-205-2631
Website: www.womenshealth.gov

Office of Minority Health Resource Center (OMH-RC)
P.O. Box 37337
Washington, DC 20013-7337
Toll-Free: 800-444-6472
Phone: 800-444-6472
TDD: 301-251-1432
TTY: 301-230-7199
Fax: 301-251-2160
Website: www.minorityhealth.
hhs.gov
E-mail: info@minorityhealth.
hhs.gov

Substance Abuse and Mental Health Services Administration (SAMHSA)
5600 Fishers Ln.
Rockville, MD 20857
Toll-Free: 877-SAMHSA-7
(877-726-4727)
TDD: 800-487-4889
Website: www.samhsa.gov

U.S. Food and Drug Administration (FDA)
10903 New Hampshire Ave.
Silver Spring, MD 20993
Toll-Free: 888-INFO-FDA
(888-463-6332)
Phone: 301-796-8240
Fax: 301-847-8543
Website: www.fda.gov

U.S. National Library of Medicine (NLM)
8600 Rockville Pike
Bethesda, MD 20894
Toll-Free: 888-FIND-NLM
(888-346-3656)
Phone: 301-594-5983
Toll-Free TDD: 800-735-2258
Fax: 301-402-1384
Website: www.nlm.nih.gov
E-mail: custserv@nlm.nih.gov

Private Agencies That Provide Information about Disease Management

AbleData
103 W. Broad St.
Ste. 400
Falls Church, VA 22046
Phone: 800-227-0216
TTY: 703-992-8313
Fax: 703-356-8314
Website: www.abledata.com
E-mail: abledata@neweditions.net

Alzheimer's Association
225 N. Michigan Ave.
Fl. 17
Chicago, IL 60601
Toll-Free: 800-272-3900
Phone: 312-335-8700
TDD: 312-335-5886
Fax: 866-699-1246
Website: www.alz.org
E-mail: info@alz.org

American Academy of Family Physicians (AAFP)
11400 Tomahawk Creek Pkwy
Leawood, KS 66211-2680
Toll-Free: 800-274-2237
Phone: 913-906-6000
Fax: 913-906-6075
Website: www.aafp.org
E-mail: aafp@aafp.org

American Cancer Society (ACS)
250 Williams St. N.W.
Atlanta, GA 30303
Toll-Free: 800-227-2345
Website: www.cancer.org

American Health Information Management Association (AHIMA)
233 N. Michigan Ave.
21st Fl.
Chicago, IL 60601-5809
Toll-Free: 800-335-5535
Phone: 312-233-1100
Fax: 312-233-1090
Website: www.ahima.org

American Heart Association (AHA)
National Center
7272 Greenville Ave.
Dallas, TX 75231
Toll-Free: 800-242-8721
Website: www.heart.org

American Lung Association (ALA)
55 W. Wacker Dr.
Ste. 1150
Chicago, IL 60601
Toll-Free: 800-LUNGUSA
(800-548-8252)
Phone: 212-315-8700
Fax: 212-315-8800
Website: www.lung.org
E-mail: info@lung.org

American Medical Association (AMA)
330 N. Wabash Ave.
Ste. 39300
Chicago, IL 60611-5885
Toll-Free: 800-621-8335
Phone: 312-464-5000
Website: www.ama-assn.org

Cleveland Clinic
9500 Euclid Ave.
Cleveland, OH 44195
Toll-Free: 800-223-2273
Phone: 216-444-2200
TTY: 216-444-0261
Website: my.clevelandclinic.org

National Family Caregivers
Association (NFCA)
10400 Connecticut Ave.
Ste. 500
Kensington, MD 20895
Toll-Free: 800-896-3650
Phone: 301-942-6430
Fax: 301-942-2302
Website: www.caregiveraction.
com
E-mail: info@thefamilycaregiver.
org

National Healthcare Anti-
Fraud Association (NHCAA)
1220 L St. N.W.
Ste. 600
Washington, DC 20005
Phone: 202-659-5955
Fax: 202-785-6764
Website: www.nhcaa.org
E-mail: NHCAA@nhcaa.org

National Patient Advocate
Foundation (NPAF)
1100 H St. N.W.
Ste. 710
Washington, DC 20005
Phone: 202-347-8009
Fax: 202-347-5579
Website: www.npaf.org

National Patient Safety
Foundation (NPSF)
280 Summer St.
9th Fl.
Boston, MA 02210
Phone: 617-391-9900
Fax: 617-391-9999
Website: www.npsf.org
E-mail: info@npsf.org

National Rehabilitation
Information Center (NARIC)
8400 Corporate Dr.
Ste. 500
Landover, MD 20785
Toll-Free: 800-346-2742
Phone: 301-459-5900
TTY: 301-459-5984
Fax: 301-459-4263
Website: www.naric.com
E-mail: naricinfo@
heitechservices.com

The Nemours Foundation
1600 Rockland Rd.
Wilmington, DE 19803
Phone: 302-651-4046
Website: www.kidshealth.org
E-mail: info@kidshealth.org

Center for Children's Health
Media
300 Longwood Ave.
Boston, MA 02115
Phone: 617-355-5420
Website: cmch.tv
E-mail: cmch@childrens.
harvard.edu

Chapter 76

Directory of Health Insurance Information

Government Agencies That Provide Information about Health Insurance

Agency for Healthcare Research and Quality (AHRQ)
U.S. Department of Health and Human Services (HHS)
5600 Fishers Ln.
Rockville, MD 20857
Toll-Free: 800-358-9295
Phone: 301-427-1364
TDD: 888-586-6340
Website: www.ahrq.gov

Centers for Medicare and Medicaid Services (CMS)
7500 Security Blvd.
Baltimore, MD 21244
Toll-Free: 877-267-2323
Phone: 410-786-3000
Toll Free TTY: 866-226-1819
TTY: 410-786-0727
Website: www.cms.gov

Resources in this chapter were compiled from several sources deemed reliable; all contact information was verified and updated in January 2017.

Federal Trade Commission (FTC)
Consumer Response Center
600 Pennsylvania Ave. N.W.
Washington, DC 20580
Toll-Free: 877-FTC-HELP
(877-382-4357)
Phone: 202-326-2222
Website: www.ftc.gov

MedlinePlus Encyclopedia
Website: www.medlineplus.gov/
healthinsurance.html

U.S. Department of Labor (DOL)
Frances Perkins Bldg.
200 Constitution Ave. N.W.
Washington, DC 20210
Toll-Free: 866-4-USA-DOL
(866-487-2365)
Toll-Free TTY: 877-889-5627
Website: www.dol.gov

U.S. Department of the Treasury
Internal Revenue Service (IRS)
1500 Pennsylvania Ave. N.W.
Washington, DC 20220
Toll-Free: 800-829-1040
Phone: 202- 622-2000
Website: www.treasury.gov

Private Agencies That Provide Information about Health Insurance

AARP
601 E St. N.W.
Washington, DC 20049
Toll-Free: 888-OUR-AARP
(888-687-2277)
Phone: 202-434-2277
Website: www.aarp.org
E-mail: member@aarp.org

America's Health Insurance Plans (AHIP)
601 Pennsylvania Ave. N.W.
South Bldg.
Ste. 500
Washington, DC 20004
Phone: 202-778-3200
Website: www.ahip.org
E-mail: ahip@ahip.org

Coalition against Insurance Fraud (CAIF)
1012 14th St. N.W.
Ste. 200
Washington, DC 20005
Phone: 202-393-7330
Fax: 202-393-7329
Website: www.insurancefraud.
org
E-mail: info@insurancefraud.org

Families USA
1225 New York Ave. N.W.
Ste. 800
Washington, DC 20005
Phone: 202-628-3030
Fax: 202-347-2417
Website: www.familiesusa.org
E-mail: info@familiesusa.org

Insurance Information Institute (III)
110 William St.
24th Fl.
New York, NY 10038
Phone: 212-346-5500
Website: www.iii.org

Kaiser Family Foundation (KFF)
2400 Sand Hill Rd.
Menlo Park, CA 94025
Phone: 650-854-9400
Fax: 650-854-4800
Website: www.kff.org

National Association of Insurance Commissioners (NAIC)
1100 Walnut St., Ste. 1500
Kansas City, MO 64106-2197
Toll-Free: 866-470-NAIC
(866-470-6242)
Phone: 816-842-3600
Fax: 816-783-8175
Website: www.naic.org
E-mail: reslib@naic.org

Patient Advocate Foundation (PAF)
421 Butler Farm Rd., Ste. 200
Hampton, VA 23666
Phone: 800-532-5274
Fax: 757-873-8999
Website: www.patientadvocate.org
E-mail: help@patientadvocate.org

Chapter 77

Directory of Organizations That Provide Financial Assistance for Medical Treatments

Assistance with Paying for Medical Care and Procedures

Find A Health Center
5600 Fishers Ln.
Rockville, MD 20857
Website: findahealthcenter.hrsa.gov

Hill-Burton Facilities
Toll-Free:1-888-ASK-HRSA
(888-275-4772)
Phone: 900-638-0742
Website: www.hrsa.gov

Insure Kids Now
7500 Security Blvd.
Baltimore, MD 21244
Toll-Free: 1-877-KIDS-NOW
(1-877-543-7669)
Website: www.insurekidsnow.gov

This chapter includes text excerpted from "Financial Assistance Information," National Human Genome Research Institute (NHGRI), October 29, 2014; all contact information was verified and updated in January 2017.

Maternal and Child Health Bureau (MCHB)
Health Resources and Services
Administration (HRSA)
5600 Fishers Ln.
Rockville, MD 20857
Phone: 301-443-2170
Fax: 301-443-1797
Website: mchb.hrsa.gov
E-mail: ctibbs@hrsa.gov

U.S. Department of Health and Human Services (HHS)
200 Independence Ave. S.W.
Washington, DC 20201
Toll-Free: 1-877-696-6775
Website: www.hhs.gov

Financial Aid for Medical Treatments

Association of Maternal and Child Health Programs (AMCHP)
1825 K St.
Ste. 250
Washington, DC 20006
Phone: 202-775-0436
Fax: 202-478-5120
Website: www.amchp.org
E-mail: info@amchp.org

Families USA
1225 New York Ave. N.W.
Ste. 800
Washington, DC 20005
Phone: 202-628-3030
Fax: 202-347-2417
Website: www.familiesusa.org
E-mail: info@familiesusa.org

Family Voices
P.O. Box 37188
Albuquerque, NM 87176
Toll-Free: 888-835-5669
Phone: 505-872-4774
Fax: 505-872-4780
Website: www.familyvoices.org

National Patient Advocate Foundation (NPAF)
1100 H St. N.W.
Ste. 710
Washington, DC 20005
Phone: 202-347-8009
Website: www.npaf.org
E-mail: action@npaf.org

Patient Advocate Foundation (PAF)
421 Butler Farm Rd.
Hampton, VA 23666
Toll-Free: 800-532-5274
Fax: 757-873-8999
Website: www.patientadvocate.
org
E-mail: help@patientadvocate.
org

Social Security Administration (SSA)
Office of Earnings and
International Operations
P.O. Box 17775
Baltimore, MD 21235-7775
Phone: 410-965-2356
Fax: 877-385-0645
Website: www.ssa.gov

Assistance with Paying for Medications

National Organization for Rare Disorders (NORD)
55 Kenosia Ave.
Danbury, CT 06813-1968
Phone: 203-744-0100
Fax: 203-263-9938
Website: www.rarediseases.org
E-mail: orphan@rarediseases.org

The Partnership for Prescription Assistance (PPA)
Website: www.pparx.org

Assistance with Insurance Issues

Centers for Medicare and Medicaid Services (CMS)
7500 Security Blvd.
Baltimore, MD 21244
Toll-Free: 800-MEDICARE
(800-633-4227)
Phone: 410-786-3000
Toll-Free TTY: 866-226-1819
TTY: 410-786-0727
Website: www.cms.gov

Georgetown University Health Policy Institute (GUHPI)
3300 Whitehaven St.
Ste. 5000
Washington, DC 20057
Phone: 202-687-0880
Fax: 202-687-3110
Website: www.hpi.georgetown.edu

Health Care Choices (HCC)
6209 16th Ave.
Brooklyn, NY 11204
Phone: 718-234-0073
Website: www.Healthcarechoicesny.org

Kaiser Health News (KHN)
1330 G St. N.W.
Washington, DC 20005
Phone: 202-347-5270
Website: www.khn.org

Medicaid Waivers
Toll-Free: 888-444-3331
Phone: 727-841-8943
Website: www.medicaidwaiver.org

Index

Index

Page numbers followed by 'n' indicate a footnote. Page numbers in *italics* indicate a table or illustration